Medical Microbiology

Medical Microbiology

Editor: Erika Tanner

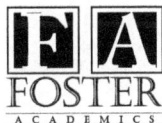

FA FOSTER
A C A D E M I C S

www.fosteracademics.com

www.fosteracademics.com

FA
FOSTER
ACADEMICS

Cataloging-in-Publication Data

Medical microbiology / edited by Erika Tanner.
    p. cm.
Includes bibliographical references and index.
ISBN 978-1-63242-703-8
1. Medical microbiology. 2. Microbiology. 3. Diagnostic microbiology. I. Tanner, Erika.
QR46 .M43 2019
616.904 1--dc23

Foster Academics,
118-35 Queens Blvd., Suite 400,
Forest Hills, NY 11375, USA

ISBN 978-1-63242-703-8 (Hardback)

Contents

Preface

Medical microbiology is the branch of medicine associated with the prevention, diagnosis and treatment of infectious diseases. It is a branch of microbiology and finds its applications in medical science. It is concerned with the treatment of infectious diseases caused by microbes such as bacteria, viruses, parasites and fungi. Epidemiology is considered to be a primary area of study under medical microbiology. It is concerned with identifying and analyzing the patterns of health and disease conditions in a given population. It also studies the causes and effects of such health related conditions. This book outlines the applications of medical microbiology in detail. It elucidates the concepts and innovative models around prospective developments with respect to this field. This book will prove to be immensely beneficial to students and researchers in this field.

This book is a comprehensive compilation of works of different researchers from varied parts of the world. It includes valuable experiences of the researchers with the sole objective of providing the readers (learners) with a proper knowledge of the concerned field. This book will be beneficial in evoking inspiration and enhancing the knowledge of the interested readers.

In the end, I would like to extend my heartiest thanks to the authors who worked with great determination on their chapters. I also appreciate the publisher's support in the course of the book. I would also like to deeply acknowledge my family who stood by me as a source of inspiration during the project.

Editor

Molecular characteristic of *mcr*-1 producing *Escherichia coli* in a Chinese university hospital

Qing-wen He[1,2†], Xiao-hong Xu[1†], Fang-jun Lan[1,2], Zhi-chang Zhao[3], Zhi-yun Wu[1,2], Ying-ping Cao[1] and Bin Li[1*]

Abstract

Background: Colistin has been considered as a last-line treatment option in severe infections caused by multidrug-resistant (MDR) gram-negative pathogens. However, the emergence of the mobile colistin resistance gene (*mcr*-1) has challenged this viewpoint. The aim of this study is to explore the prevalence of *mcr*-1 in *Escherichia coli* (*E. coli*) in a Chinese teaching hospital, and investigate their molecular characteristics.

Methods: A total of 700 *E. coli* isolates were used to screen *mcr*-1 by PCR and sequencing in a Chinese university hospital from August 2014 to August 2015. Susceptibility test of *mcr*-1-producing isolates was determined by Vitek -2 Compact system. 26 virulence factors (VFs), phylogenetic groups, Multi-locus sequence typing (MLST), and DNA Fingerprinting (ERIC-PCR) of strains were investigated by PCR.

Results: Four (0.6%) *mcr*-1 producing *E. coli* isolates were found in this study. The results of antibiotic susceptibility test showed that all four isolates were resistant to colistin, ciprofloxacin, levofloxacin, cefazolin, and trimethoprim/sulfamethoxazole, and were susceptible to amikacin, ertapenem and imipenem. In addition, all 4 isolates exhibited high-level resistance to aztreonam, cefotaxime and gentamicin. The numbers of VFs contained in *mcr*-1 positive isolates were no more than 4 in our study. MLST result demonstrated that these isolates were assigned to two sequence types: ST156 and ST167. The result of phylogenetic analysis showed that four *mcr*-1-positive isolates belong to two phylogenetic groups: A and B1 group. ERIC-PCR showed that four *mcr*-1 positive strains were categorized into three different genotypes.

Conclusions: Our study demonstrated a low prevalence of *mcr*-1 in *E. coli* clinical isolates in a Chinese teaching hospital, and we have gained insights into the molecular characteristics of these *mcr*-1-positive strains. Increasing the surveillance of these infections, as well as taking effective infection control measures are urgently needed to take to control the transmission of *mcr*-1 gene.

Keywords: *E. coli*, *mcr*-1, Colistin, Multidrug-resistant

Background

In recent years, colistin has been considered as an effective therapeutic option for the rapid increasing of multidrug-resistant (MDR) gram-negative pathogens [1, 2]. However, the prevalence of the mobile colistin resistance gene (*mcr*-1) in animals and human beings worldwide

has challenged this viewpoint [3, 4]. Resistance to polymyxins is mainly caused by the modification to bacterial outer membrane, which was usually considered as chromosomally mediated resistance [5, 6].

Since it was initially found, plasmid-mediated *mcr*-1 has been detected widely [3, 7]. Nowadays, *mcr*-1-producing bacteria have been reported in many regions in China [4, 8]. *Mcr*-1 was firstly found in *Escherichia coli* (*E. coli*), and now it has been spreading to other *Enterobacteriaceae* [9]. Several reports showed that the *mcr*-1 gene could coexist with other resistance genes (such as

*Correspondence: leonlee307@hotmail.com
†Qing-wen He and Xiao-hong Xu contributed equally to this work
[1] Department of Clinical Laboratory, Fujian Medical University Union Hospital, 29# Xinquan Road, Fuzhou 350001, Fujian, China
Full list of author information is available at the end of the article

CRE/ESBL) in *E. coli* and *Klebsiella pneumoniae*, which probably lead to the emergence pan-drug resistant and increase the difficulty of treatment [8, 10]. Therefore, the emergence and spread of *mcr-1* gene among human beings should be given close attention. The aim of this study was to evaluate the prevalence of *mcr-1* in *E. coli* clinical isolates in a Chinese teaching hospital, and to investigate the molecular characteristics of these strains.

Methods

Bacterial strains

A total of 700 *E. coli* clinical isolates were collected from the clinical laboratory of Fujian Medical University Union Hospital (Fuzhou, Fujian province, China) from August 2014 to August 2015. It is a 2200-bed tertiary care teaching hospital with approximately 95,000 hospital admissions per year, located in southeastern China. All isolates were identified by GNI card of the Vitek system (BioMèrieux, Missouri, France).

Antibiotic susceptibility testing

Antimicrobial susceptibility testing was performed using the AST-GN16 of Vitek-2 Compact system (Bio Mérieux, France). The antimicrobial agents tested included: tigecycline (glycycline); ertapenem and imipenem (carbapenems); cefazolin; cefoxitin; cefepime, and cefotaxime (cephalosporins); aztreonam (monobactam); amikacin and gentamicin (aminoglycosides); ciprofloxacin and levofloxacin (quinolone); piperacillin/tazobactam; trimethoprim/sulfamethoxazole. The results were interpreted by the Clinical and Laboratory Standards Institute (CLSI) [11]. The MIC of colistin was determined using agar dilution method, and the result was interpreted according to European Committee On Antimicrobial Susceptibility Testing (EUCAST) guidelines [12]. *E. coli* ATCC 25922 was used as a quality control.

DNA extraction

Several colonies were suspended in 50 µl of sterile distilled water for preparing genomic DNA of the isolates, and then the bacterial suspension was heated at 100 °C for 10 min as described previously [13].

MCR-1 detection

mcr-1 gene was screened in *E. coli* clinical isolates by PCR using primers as previously described [4]. All of the PCR products were sequenced and then compared with known sequences listed in the GenBank (http://www.ncbi.nlm.nih.gov/blast/).

Detection of virulence factor genes

Twenty six virulence factors (VFs) genes associated with extraintestinal virulence [14, 15] were detected using a multiplex PCR method as previously described [15]. These genes were as follows: adhesions (*pap*AH, *pap*EF, *pap*C, *pap*G allele I, *pap*G II/III, *pap*G allele II, *sfa/foc*DE, *afa/dra*BC, *fim*H, *gaf*D, *sfa*S, *foc*G and *nfa*E), toxins (*hly*A, *cnf*1 and *cdt*B), siderophores (*fyu*A and *iut*A), protections and invasions (*kps*MTII, *kps*MTIII, *tra*T, *cva*C, kpsMT and K1/K5), miscellaneous (*rfc* and PAI). The PCR products were sequenced and then compared with known sequences listed in the GenBank (http://www.ncbi.nlm.nih.gov/blast/).

Phylogenetic analysis

The phylogenetic groups (A, B1, B2, and D) of *mcr-1* producing *E. coli* isolates were identified by a triplex PCR as previously described [16].

Multi-locus sequence typing (MLST)

Mcr-1 positive strains were analyzed by multilocus sequence typing (MLST), which was based on 7 standard housekeeping genes (*adk*, *fumC*, *gyrB*, *icd*, *mdh*, *purA*, *recA*) (http://mlst.ucc.ie/mlst/mlst/dbs/Ecoli) [17].

DNA fingerprinting

Enterobacterial Repetitive Intergenic Consensus Sequences PCR (ERIC-PCR) was applied to typing *mcr-1* producing *E. coli* isolates with the primers ERIC-1 and ERIC-2 [18]. DNA fingerprints were compared by visual inspection, ERIC profiles were regarded as different if there were different bands on visual inspection [19].

Results and discussion

In this study, four isolates (0.6%) were confirmed to carry *mcr-1* gene, which is lower than previous study [4]. The age of the patients ranged between 38 and 80 years. These *mcr-1* producing strains were isolated from two different wards (Table 1). Two strains were isolated from the same patient. The clinical data of patients with *mcr-1* positive *E. coli* infection were shown in Table 2.

Mcr-1 was usually found to be co-localized with other resistance genes on plasmids, such as ESBL genes and carbapenemase genes [20], which might increase the emergence of pan-drug resistance. In our study, the results of antimicrobial susceptibility test showed a high drug resistance in the *mcr-1*-producing isolates. All of the *mcr-1* positive isolates were resistance to at least 3 different kinds of antibiotics (Table 1).

All four *mcr-1* positive strains detected in our study were resistant to colistin and the MICs ranged from 4 to 16 µg/ml. It will be worrisome once *mcr-1* coexists with other resistant genes, especially carbapenemase genes because of limited therapeutic options [20]. Previous studies revealed that *mcr-1* co-produced with carbapenem-resistant genes in *E. coli* [8, 21]. Fortunately, all of

Table 1 Main characteristics of the *mcr*-1 *E. coli*

Isolates	Data	Ward	Specimen	Phylogenetic groups	MLST	ERIC pattern	VFs	Antibiotic resistance
E321	2014.8	Colorectal surgery	Drainage-fluid	B1	ST156	1	*tra*T, *iut*A	COL, CFZ, FOX, CIP, LVX, SXT, TGC
E684	2015.1	Colorectal surgery	Secretion	B1	ST156	2	*fim*H, *tra*T, *iut*A	COL, CFZ, CTX, FEP, ATM, GEN, CIP, LVX, SXT
E921	2015.4	Hepatobiliary surgery	Secretion	A	ST167	3	*fyu*A, *tra*T, *iut*A	COL, CFZ, CTX, ATM, GEN, CIP, LVX, SXT
E1005	2015.5	Hepatobiliary surgery	Drainage-fluid	A	ST167	3	*fyu*A, *cva*C, *tra*T, *iut*A	COL, CFZ, CTX, ATM, GEN, CIP, LVX, SXT

CFZ cefazolin, *FOX* cefoxitin, *CTX* cefotaxime, *FEP* cefepime, *TZP* piperacillin/tazobactam, *ATM* aztreonam, *IPM* imipenem, *ETP* ertapenem, *AMK* amikacin, *GEN* gentamicin, *CIP* ciprofloxacin, *LVX* levofloxacin, *SXT* trimethoprim/sulfamethoxazole, *TIG* tigecycline, *COL* colistin, *MLST* multi-locus sequence typing, *ERIC* enterobacterial repetitive intergenic consensus, *VFs* virulence factor genes

Table 2 Clinical data of patients with mcr-1 positive *E. coli* infection

Isolates	Patients	Gender	Age (years)	Underlying diseases	Length of hospital stay (days)	Treatments used	Outcomes
E321	Patient 1	Female	80	Malignancy, hypertension, pulmonary tuberculosis	51	TZP	Survived
E684	Patient 2	Female	57	Perineal infection, hypertension	37	TZP	Survived
E921	Patient 3	Male	38	Hypertension, pancreatitis, diabetes	26	MEM	Survived
E1005	Patient 3	Male	38	Hypertension, pancreatitis, diabetes	26	MEM	Survived

TZP piperacillin/tazobactam, *MEM* meropenem

them were susceptible to carbapenems (IPM and ETP), which probably indicated that no carbapenem-resistant genes coexisted with *mcr*-1. Result of ERIC-PCR (Fig. 1) showed that four *mcr*-1 positive strains were categorized into three different genotypes, one of which contained 2 strains (from the same patient). These isolates which have different patterns suggest that they were non-clonal transmission. In a previous study, two *mcr*-1 positive *E. coli* isolates from a single fowl were belonging to phylogenetic B1 and D group [22]. The *mcr*-1-producing isolates in this study were belonged to phylogenetic groups A and B1, which were mainly distributed among human commensal *E. coli* isolates [23]. The *mcr*-1 producing isolates were assigned by MLST to two different sequence types: ST156 and ST167 (Table 1), which was similar to previous reports in other studies from China [8, 22]. *E. coli* ST156 has been found that it has connection with different ESBL genes [24, 25]. ST167 was belonged to ST10 complex and regarded as prevalent ST among ESBL-producing *E. coli* from human and animal sources [26]. In addition, *E. coli* ST167 was reported to be closely related to bla_{NDM}, which needed closely concern of spreading [27]. The similar molecular characterizations illustrated that *mcr*-1 positive isolates detected from the same department in our study were clonally related.

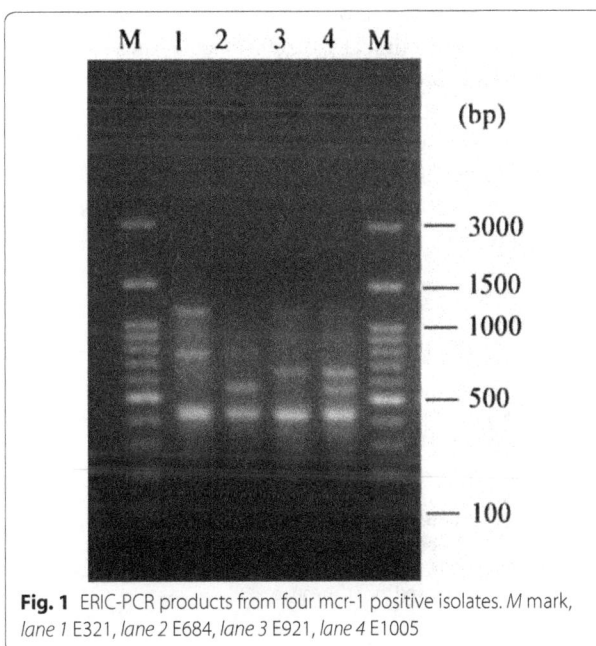

Fig. 1 ERIC-PCR products from four mcr-1 positive isolates. *M* mark, *lane 1* E321, *lane 2* E684, *lane 3* E921, *lane 4* E1005

VFs in *E. coli* were associated with colonization, bacterial fitness and virulence [28]. VFs include five main groups: (1) adhesions; (2) toxins; (3) siderophores; (4) capsule production and (5) protections and invasions.

Clinical *E. coli* strains often carry multiple VFs, and isolates belonging to groups A and B1 often have less VFs than those belonging to phylogroups B2 and D [28]. To the best of our knowledge, there is no study concerning about VFs in *mcr-1* producing *E. coli*. In our study, *mcr-1* producing isolates contained less than 4 different VFs (Table 1). Only five different kinds of VFs had been detected in our *mcr-1* positive isolates, which included *fim*H, *fyu*A, *tra*T, *iut*A and *cva*C. *fim*H is one of the most commonly VFs present in *E. coli*, which encodes the adhesion subunit of type 1 fimbriae and related to colonization [15]. Lee et al. reported that *fyu*A, *tra*T, and *iut*A were found to be independent predictors for pathogenicity. Meanwhile, *tra*T and *iut*A were thought to be closely related to ESBL genes [29]. Pitout et al. found that *cva*C was only present in non-CTX-M-producing isolates [30]. Previous reports suggested that antibiotic resistance has negative association with virulence factors [31], which could be interpreted by the loss of VFs associated with mutation to resistance [32].

It is noteworthy that two *mcr*-1 positive *E. coli* strains were isolated from the same patient but at different time (Table 1). Results of MLST and ERIC-PCR revealed that these isolates had identical genetic background. Result of antimicrobial susceptibility test showed that they had similar antibiograms. We speculate that the two isolates probably originated from a same source.

In conclusion, we have revealed a low prevalence of *mcr-1* in *E. coli* clinical isolates in a Chinese teaching hospital, and presented detailed molecular characteristics of these isolates. The presence of *mcr-1* in *E. coli* clinical isolates suggests that it will pose a threat to public healthcare. Effective infection control measures are urgently needed to take to control the transmission of *mcr*-1 gene.

Abbreviations

MCR-1: mobile colistin resistance gene; MDR: multi-drug resistant; PCR: polymerase chain reaction; CLSI: Clinical and Laboratory Standards Institute; MLST: multi-locus sequence typing; CRE: carbapenem-resistant *Enterobacteriaceae*; ESBL: extended-spectrum β-lactamase; ERIC-PCR: Enterobacterial Repetitive Intergenic Consensus Sequences PCR; VFs: virulence factors.

Authors' contributions

QH, XX, FL, ZZ and YC conducted laboratory assays. ZW collected clinical data. QH wrote the paper. BL designed the study and reviewed the manuscript. All authors read and approved the final manuscript.

Author details

[1] Department of Clinical Laboratory, Fujian Medical University Union Hospital, 29# Xinquan Road, Fuzhou 350001, Fujian, China. [2] The Union Clinical Medical College of Fujian Medical University, Fuzhou 350004, Fujian, China. [3] Department of Pharmacy, Fujian Medical University, Union Hospital, Fuzhou 350001, Fujian, China.

Acknowledgements

We thank Prof. Jianhua Liu and Yiyun Liu of South China Agricultural University, Guangzhou, China for kindly providing us the mcr-1 positive control. We also thank Prof. Min Chen and Department of Laboratory Medicine, Medical Technology and Engineering College, Fujian Medical University for their kindly help.

Competing interests

The authors declare that they have no competing interests.

Funding

This study was supported by the National Natural Science Foundation of China (Grant No. 81201328), the Fujian Provincial Funds for Distinguished Young Scientists in Colleges and Universities, China (Grant No. JA13134), and the Medical Elite Cultivation Program of Fujian, China (Grant No. 2015-ZQN-ZD-15).

References

1. Nation RL, Li J, Cars O, Couet W, Dudley MN, Kaye KS, Mouton JW, Paterson DL, Tam VH, Theuretzbacher U, et al. Framework for optimisation of the clinical use of colistin and polymyxin B: the Prato polymyxin consensus. Lancet Infect Dis. 2015;15(2):225–34.
2. Doi Y, Paterson DL. Carbapenemase-producing Enterobacteriaceae. Semin Respir Crit Care Med. 2015;36(1):74–84.
3. Skov RL, Monnet DL. Plasmid-mediated colistin resistance (mcr-1 gene): 3 months later, the story unfolds. Euro Surveill. 2016;21:9.
4. Liu YY, Wang Y, Walsh TR, Yi L, Zhang R, Spencer J, Doi Y, Tian G, Dong B, Huang X, et al. Emergence of plasmid-mediated colistin resistance mechanism MCR-1 in animals and human beings in China: a microbiological and molecular biological study. Lancet Infect Dis. 2016;16(2):161–8.
5. Giani T, Arena F, Vaggelli G, Conte V, Chiarelli A, Henrici De Angelis L, Fornaini R, Grazzini M, Niccolini F, Pecile P, et al. Large nosocomial outbreak of colistin-resistant, carbapenemase-producing *Klebsiella pneumoniae* traced to clonal expansion of an mgrB deletion mutant. J Clin Microbiol. 2015;53(10):3341–4.
6. Olaitan AO, Morand S, Rolain JM. Mechanisms of polymyxin resistance: acquired and intrinsic resistance in bacteria. Front Microbiol. 2014;5:643.
7. Du H, Chen L, Tang Y, Kreiswirth BN. Emergence of the mcr-1 colistin resistance gene in carbapenem-resistant Enterobacteriaceae. Lancet Infect Dis. 2016;16(3):287–8.
8. Yu H, Qu F, Shan B, Huang B, Jia W, Chen C, Li A, Miao M, Zhang X, Bao C, et al. Detection of mcr-1 colistin resistance gene in carbapenem-resistant Enterobacteriaceae from different hospitals in China. Antimicrob Agents Chemother. 2016;60(8):5033–5.
9. Schwarz S, Johnson AP. Transferable resistance to colistin: a new but old threat. J Antimicrob Chemother. 2016;71(8):2066–70.
10. Haenni M, Poirel L, Kieffer N, Chatre P, Saras E, Metayer V, Dumoulin R, Nordmann P, Madec JY. Co-occurrence of extended spectrum beta lactamase and MCR-1 encoding genes on plasmids. Lancet Infect Dis. 2016;16(3):281–2.
11. CLSI. Methods for dilution antimicrobial susceptibility tests for bacteria that grow aerobically; approved standard, 10th ed. CLSI document M07-A10. Wayne: Clinical and Laboratory Standards Institute; 2015.
12. EUCAST. Breakpoints tables for interpretation of MICs and zone diameters, version 6.0; 2016.
13. He Q, Chen W, Huang L, Lin Q, Zhang J, Liu R, Li B. Performance evaluation of three automated identification systems in detecting carbapenem-resistant Enterobacteriaceae. Ann Clin Microbiol Antimicrob. 2016;15(1):40.

14. Johnson JR, Russo TA. Molecular epidemiology of extraintestinal pathogenic (uropathogenic) *Escherichia coli*. Int J Med Microbiol. 2005;295(6–7):383–404.

15. Johnson JR, Stell AL. Extended virulence genotypes of *Escherichia coli* strains from patients with urosepsis in relation to phylogeny and host compromise. J Infect Dis. 2000;181(1):261–72.

16. Clermont O, Bonacorsi S, Bingen E. Rapid and simple determination of the *Escherichia coli* phylogenetic group. Appl Environ Microbiol. 2000;66(10):4555–8.

17. Johnson JR, Clermont O, Johnston B, Clabots C, Tchesnokova V, Sokurenko E, Junka AF, Maczynska B, Denamur E. Rapid and specific detection, molecular epidemiology, and experimental virulence of the O16 subgroup within *Escherichia coli* sequence type 131. J Clin Microbiol. 2014;52(5):1358–65.

18. Smith JL, Drum DJ, Dai Y, Kim JM, Sanchez S, Maurer JJ, Hofacre CL, Lee MD. Impact of antimicrobial usage on antimicrobial resistance in commensal *Escherichia coli* strains colonizing broiler chickens. Appl Environ Microbiol. 2007;73(5):1404–14.

19. Manges AR, Johnson JR, Foxman B, O'Bryan TT, Fullerton KE, Riley LW. Widespread distribution of urinary tract infections caused by a multidrug-resistant *Escherichia coli* clonal group. N Engl J Med. 2001;345(14):1007–13.

20. Schwarz S, Johnson AP. Transferable resistance to colistin: a new but old threat. J Antimicrob Chemother. 2016;71:2066–70.

21. Li A, Yang Y, Miao M, Chavda KD, Mediavilla JR, Xie X, Tang YW. Complete sequences of mcr-1-harboring plasmids from extended-spectrum-beta-lactamase- and carbapenemase-producing Enterobacteriaceae. Antimicrob Agents Chemother. 2016;60(7):4351–4.

22. Yang RS, Feng Y, Lv XY, Duan JH, Chen J, Fang LX, Xia J, Liao XP, Sun J, Liu YH. Emergence of NDM-5 and MCR-1-producing *Escherichia coli* clone ST648 and ST156 from a single muscovy duck (*Cairina moschata*). Antimicrob Agents Chemother. 2016;60:6899–902.

23. Pitout JD. Extraintestinal pathogenic *Escherichia coli*: an update on antimicrobial resistance, laboratory diagnosis and treatment. Exp Rev Anti Infect Ther. 2012;10(10):1165–76.

24. Cortes-Cortes G, Lozano-Zarain P, Torres C, Castaneda M, Moreno Sanchez G, Alonso CA, Lopez-Pliego L, Gutierrez Mayen MG, Martinez-Laguna Y, Rocha-Gracia RD. Detection and molecular characterization of *Escherichia coli* strains producers of extended-spectrum and CMY-2 type beta-lactamases, isolated from turtles in Mexico. Vector Borne Zoonotic Dis. 2016;16:595–603.

25. Pan YS, Liu JH, Hu H, Zhao JF, Yuan L, Wu H, Wang LF, Hu GZ. Novel arrangement of the blaCTX-M-55 gene in an *Escherichia coli* isolate coproducing 16S rRNA methylase. J Basic Microbiol. 2013;53(11):928–33.

26. Schink AK, Kadlec K, Kaspar H, Mankertz J, Schwarz S. Analysis of extended-spectrum-beta-lactamase-producing *Escherichia coli* isolates collected in the GERM-Vet monitoring programme. J Antimicrob Chemother. 2013;68(8):1741–9.

27. Huang Y, Yu X, Xie M, Wang X, Liao K, Xue W, Chan EW, Zhang R, Chen S. Widespread dissemination of carbapenem-resistant *Escherichia coli* sequence type 167 strains harboring blaNDM-5 in clinical settings in China. Antimicrob Agents Chemother. 2016;60(7):4364–8.

28. Smith JL, Fratamico PM, Gunther NW. Extraintestinal pathogenic *Escherichia coli*. Foodborne Pathog Dis. 2007;4(2):134–63.

29. Lee S, Yu JK, Park K, Oh EJ, Kim SY, Park YJ. Phylogenetic groups and virulence factors in pathogenic and commensal strains of *Escherichia coli* and their association with blaCTX-M. Ann Clin Lab Sci. 2010;40(4):361–7.

30. Pitout JD, Laupland KB, Church DL, Menard ML, Johnson JR. Virulence factors of *Escherichia coli* isolates that produce CTX-M-type extended-spectrum beta-lactamases. Antimicrob Agents Chemother. 2005;49(11):4667–70.

31. Skjot Rasmussen L, Ejrnaes K, Lundgren B, Hammerum AM, Frimodt Moller N. Virulence factors and phylogenetic grouping of *Escherichia coli* isolates from patients with bacteraemia of urinary tract origin relate to sex and hospital- vs. community-acquired origin. Int J Med Microbiol. 2012;302(3):129–34.

32. Vila J, Simon K, Ruiz J, Horcajada JP, Velasco M, Barranco M, et al. Are quinolone-resistant uropathogenic *Escherichia coli* less virulent? J Infect Dis. 2002;186(7):1039–42.

2

Detection of a CTX-M group 2 beta-lactamase gene in a *Klebsiella pneumoniae* isolate from a tertiary care hospital, Trinidad and Tobago

Paul Cheddie[1]* ⓘ, Francis Dziva[2]^ and Patrick Eberechi Akpaka[3]

Abstract

Background: Identification of the prevalence and spread of ESBL-mediated antibiotic resistance is essential especially in the hospital setting. It is for this reason, more and more studies are highlighting the importance of complementing phenotypic ESBL-detection techniques with molecular techniques in order to understand the basis and extent of this form of resistance among clinically evolved bacterial populations, especially those belonging to the *Enterobacteriaceae* family. However, in Trinidad and Tobago and other Caribbean countries, very little is known regarding ESBL detection rates and/or the prevalence of genes conferring ESBL resistance.

Methodology: Sixty-six *Klebsiella pneumoniae* isolates from clinical specimens phenotypically identified by the Microscan Walkaway-96 System as potential ESBL-producers were analysed in this study. Screening and confirmation of these isolates as ESBL producers was done by the Clinical and Laboratory Standards Institute (CLSI) approved methods. Polymerase chain reaction amplification of beta-lactamase genes bla_{TEM}, bla_{SHV}, bla_{CTX-M1}, bla_{CTX-M2} and bla_{AmpC} was performed to identify mechanisms of β-lactam resistance.

Results: ESBL-producing *K. pneumoniae* was confirmed in 78.8% (41/52) from isolates collected from a variety of sources during the period, April–July 2015. bla_{SHV} (84.8%) and bla_{CTX-M} (46.9%) were the predominant β-lactamase genes identified. A single *K. pneumoniae* isolate possessed a bla_{CTX-M} group 2 beta-lactamase gene. RAPD analysis identified a number of epidemiologically related isolates. However, current isolates were unrelated to isolates from previous years.

Conclusion: This study revealed that among *K. pneumoniae* isolates exhibiting extended spectrum β-lactam resistance, there was a high prevalence of bla_{SHV} and bla_{CTX-M} genes. This result highlights the need for a reliable epidemiological apparatus that involves the molecular characterisation of ESBL resistance.

Keywords: Extended-spectrum beta-lactamase, Polymerase chain reaction, Random amplification of polymorphic DNA, Trinidad and Tobago

Background

Organisms harbouring genes for extended spectrum β-lactamase (ESBL) production are a major public health concern especially given their association with

cephalosporin therapy failure, and the burden they place on infection control practices. Since the first reported case in *Klebsiella* isolates in Germany in the late twentieth century [1], they have increasingly been described worldwide, including in the Caribbean [2–4]. ESBLs are β-lactam hydrolysing enzymes capable of conferring bacterial resistance to the penicillins, 1st-, 2nd-, and 3rd-generation cephalosporins, and azetronam (but not the cephamycins or carbapenems), and which are inhibited

---

*Correspondence: paul.cheddie@gmail.com

^ Deceased

[1] Department of Medical Technology, University of Guyana, Georgetown, Guyana

Full list of author information is available at the end of the article

by β-lactamase inhibitors such as clavulanic acid [5, 6]. The clinical significance of these enzymes is underpinned by the fact that often times in vitro activity of antimicrobial drugs against ESBL-producing organisms does not always translate into clinical efficacy in patients [7].

Most *Klebsiella pneumoniae* ESBLs are plasmid-encoded enzymes derived classically from the TEM- and SHV- type β-lactamases [1] which belong to molecular class A, according to the classification scheme of Ambler, and Bush–Jacoby–Medeiros 2be group of β-lactamases [5]. TEM and SHV ESBLs are functionally similar to another group of rapidly proliferating β-lactamase enzymes, the CTX-M enzymes, that are related to chromosomally determined β-lactamases in species of *Kluyvera* [8, 9].

Due to the complex epidemiology of ESBL-producing *K. pneumoniae*, the frequency of isolation varies among institutions [10]. Exploring the population diversity of ESBL-harbouring *K. pneumoniae* in a single institution is essential to understanding the role of the genes, plasmids, and clones, involved in ESBL-production, and therapy failure with cephalosporins (and to some extent carbapenems) as well as providing useful information for infection prevention and control initiatives.

The presence and characterization of ESBL-producing genes in clinical isolates of *K. pneumoniae* and other *Enterobacteriaceae* have previously been described in Trinidad and Tobago [2, 3, 11]. However, this study sought to determine the evolving nature of these genes, specifically in the hospital setting, in order to provide data that could be useful in improving infection control measures and guide antimicrobial stewardship programmes.

Methods

Setting

The Eric Williams Medical Sciences Complex (EWMSC), a tertiary ambulatory regional hospital in Trinidad and Tobago that provides general healthcare for both paediatric and adult populations.

Clinical isolates

Seventy-two *K. pneumoniae* isolates were used in this study. This comprised 52 non-duplicate *K. pneumoniae* isolates recovered from the microbiology laboratory during the study period, April–July 2015, and identified as resistant to extended-spectrum β-lactam agents. Additionally, 20 isolates representing a subset recovered in 2008, 2009 and 2010—which were stored at −70 °C in BHI and 5% glycerol and were identified as β-lactamase producers—were also included in this study. Preliminary identification and susceptibility testing of the isolates

collected in the current study was determined using the Microscan WalkAway-96 (Beckman Coulter, Inc.). The procedures were performed in accordance with the manufacturer's recommendations. The breakpoints were interpreted in accordance with Clinical and Laboratory Standards Institute (CLSI) guidelines [12].

Antimicrobial susceptibility

Extended-spectrum β-lactamase production were confirmed according to the CLSI confirmatory testing guidelines [12]. Briefly, confirmatory testing was performed on Mueller–Hinton agar (BD) using cefotaxime 30 μg, ceftazidime 30 μg, cefotaxime/clavulanic acid 30/10 μg and ceftazidime 30/10 μg (Oxoid, Remel Inc, USA) (Additional file 1). Quality control of the test procedures was performed with *K. pneumoniae* ATCC 700603 and *Escherichia coli* ATCC 25922.

PCR amplification

From the sum total of isolates analysed (n = 72), 66 (consisting of 57 phenotypically confirmed ESBL producers and 9 non-ESBL producers randomly selected from the pool) were subjected to polymerase chain reaction (PCR) analysis. The non-ESBL producers were included to detect AmpC beta-lactamase production. The PCR amplification of *bla* genes, including bla_{TEM}, bla_{SHV}, $bla_{CTX-M-1}$, $bla_{CTX-M-2}$ and bla_{AmpC} were carried out with GoTaq® Green Master Mix (Promega, Madison, Wisconsin) using primers listed in Table 1. All PCR amplicons were separated by gel electrophoresis on a 1.5% (wt/vol) agarose gel. Staining of the gel was conducted with 0.5 μg/ml GelRed™ (Biotium, Hayward, CA).

Random amplification of polymorphic DNA (RAPD) typing

Bacteria were grown overnight on MacConkey agar (Hardy Diagnostics) at 37 °C. Genomic DNA was then extracted using the ChargeSwitch® gDNA Mini Bacteria Kit (Invirogen, Carlsbad, CA) following the specific manufacturer's instructions. Samples were initially screened for RAPD typing using five different primers:

Table 1 Primers used for PCR amplification of *bla* genes

Target	Primer name	Primer sequence (5'–3')
bla_{TEM}	TEM-F	GCGGAACCCCTATTTG
	TEM-R	ACCAATGCTTAATCAGTGAG
bla_{SHV}	SHV-F	TTATCTCCCTGTTAGCCACC
	SHV-R	GATTTGCTGATTTCGCTCGG
$bla_{CTX-M-1}$	CTX-M1-F	GGTTAAAAAATCACTGCGTC
	CTX-M1-R	TTGGTGACGATTTTAGCCGC
$bla_{CTX-M-2}$	CTX-M2-F	GATGAGACCTTCCGTCTGGA
	CTX-M2-R	CAGAAACCGTGGGTTACGAT
bla_{AmpC}	AmpC-F	ATGATGGGGGGGTCGTTATGC
	AmpC-R	TTGCAGCTTTTCAAGAATGCGC

All primers were obtained from Sigma-Aldrich (St. Louis, MO, USA)

RAPD1 (5′-CGTGGGCCT), RAPD2 (5′-TCGTCG-GCGT), RAPD3 (5′-GTGACGTAGG), RAPD4 (5′-CTTGAGTGGA), RAPD5 (5′-GAGATGACGA) (Sigma-Aldrich). RAPD–PCR was conducted under reaction conditions described by Ashayeri-panah et al. [13]. The amplified products were separated by electrophoresis in a 2.0% agarose gel containing GelRed™ run in 1 × TAE buffer at 65 V for 3 h 30 min until amplified fragments are separated. RAPD1 was chosen because it gave the best banding pattern. RAPD typing was then performed using selected isolates (Additional file 1). The resulting gel was photographed under UV light. RAPD fingerprints were analysed with PyElph version 1.4 gel analysis software [14], and a dendrogram generated using the unweighted pair group method with arithmetic averages (UPGMA).

Results

Description of isolates and CLSI confirmatory test results

Following initial testing, 52 *K. pneumoniae* isolates were identified during the study period, (April 2015–July 2015), by the Microscan Walkaway-96 as potential ESBL producers. Phenotypic AST confirmatory testing indicated that 41 (78.8%) of these isolates were indeed extended-spectrum β-lactamase producing. Additionally, of the subset of 20 *K. pneumoniae* isolates tested from previous years, 16 (80%) were identified as ESBL-producers after confirmatory testing. Four were *K. pneumoniae* isolated in 2008, nine were isolated in 2009, and three were isolated in 2010.

Detection and characterisation of *K. pneumoniae* isolates expressing extended-spectrum β-lactamase resistance

Of the 72 *K. pneumoniae* isolates, 66 were examined by PCR to detect the presence of bla_{TEM}, bla_{SHV}, bla_{CTX-M1}, bla_{CTX-M2} and bla_{AmpC}. This comprised the 41 ESBL-confirmed *K. pneumoniae* isolates collected during the study period along with the 16 ESBL-confirmed *K. pneumoniae* isolates collected between 2008 and 2010. Additionally, nine *K. pneumoniae* isolates identified as non-ESBL-producers were chosen randomly and added to the pool. 65 of the 66 isolates possessed a gene that may contribute to β-lactamase production (Table 2). bla_{TEM} was detected in 39 of the isolates tested, comprising n = 30 (2015), n = 2 (2008), n = 6 (2009) and n = 1 (2010) *K. pneumoniae* isolates respectively. bla_{SHV} was identified in n = 3 (2008), n = 9 (2009), n = 3 (2010), and n = 41(2015) of *K. pneumoniae* isolates respectively. bla_{CTX-M1} genes were detected in 30 of the isolates collected in 2015 as well as n = 2 (2008), n = 6 (2009) and n = 2 (2010). Interestingly, 88.9% (8/9) isolates, representing non-ESBL producing isolates that were tested with PCR, were positive for a

Table 2 Correlation between ESBL confirmatory results and PCR results

PCR result	Phenotypic confirmatory testing result (Not-confirmed isolates)		Phenotypic confirmatory testing result (Confirmed isolates)	
	Negative (9)	% Total	Positive (57)	% Total
Negative				
bla_{TEM}	8	88.8	18	31.6
bla_{SHV}	1	11.1	1	1.7
bla_{CTX-M1}	8	88.9	17	29.8
bla_{CTX-M2}	9	100	56	98.2
bla_{AmpC}	9	100	57	100
Positive				
bla_{TEM}	1	11.1	39	68.4
bla_{SHV}	8	88.9	56	98.2
bla_{CTX-M1}	1	11.1	40	70.2
bla_{CTX-M2}	0	0	1	1.7
bla_{AmpC}	0	100	0	100

bla_{SHV} gene. Only one *K. pneumoniae* isolate, recovered in 2015, tested positive for a bla_{CTX-M2} gene.

Twenty five isolates were positive for bla_{TEM}, bla_{SHV}, and bla_{CTX-M1} β-lactamase genes representing 21 of the *K. pneumoniae* isolates collected in 2015 in addition to 1 isolate from 2008 and 3 isolates from 2009. Notably, a single isolate collected in 2015 was positive for bla_{TEM}, bla_{SHV}, bla_{CTX-M1} and bla_{CTX-M2} genes.

The majority of the isolates, 80.5% (33/41), that were identified in 2015 as ESBL-producing were retrieved from urine specimens, whilst the remainder were recovered from blood, sputum, wound and genital sources. Records were not available for the 16 ESBL-positive isolates from previous years.

For the generation of DNA fingerprints using RAPD-PCR analysis, 18 isolates were used representing *K. pneumoniae* strains from 2008 to 2010 as well as isolates recovered during the duration of this study (Fig. 1). Banding patterns revealed DNA weights between 250 and 2000 bp (Fig. 1). RAPD analysis revealed that six *K. pneumoniae* isolates had the same banding patterns and these were placed into four genotypic groups. While there were similarities in some of the band positions of the remaining 12 *K. pneumoniae* isolates, their overall RAPD profiles were not similar. Therefore, the conclusion was that these isolates belonged to distinct genotypic groups.

The results from cluster analysis using UPGMA (Fig. 2) showed diversity between strains isolated from 2008 to 2010 and those isolated in 2015. However, relatedness was noted for one *K. pneumoniae* strain isolated in 2008 and another isolated in 2009. Also, two strains isolated in 2010 were also similar in their RAPD profiles. Finally, three separate pairs of *K. pneumoniae* strains isolated in

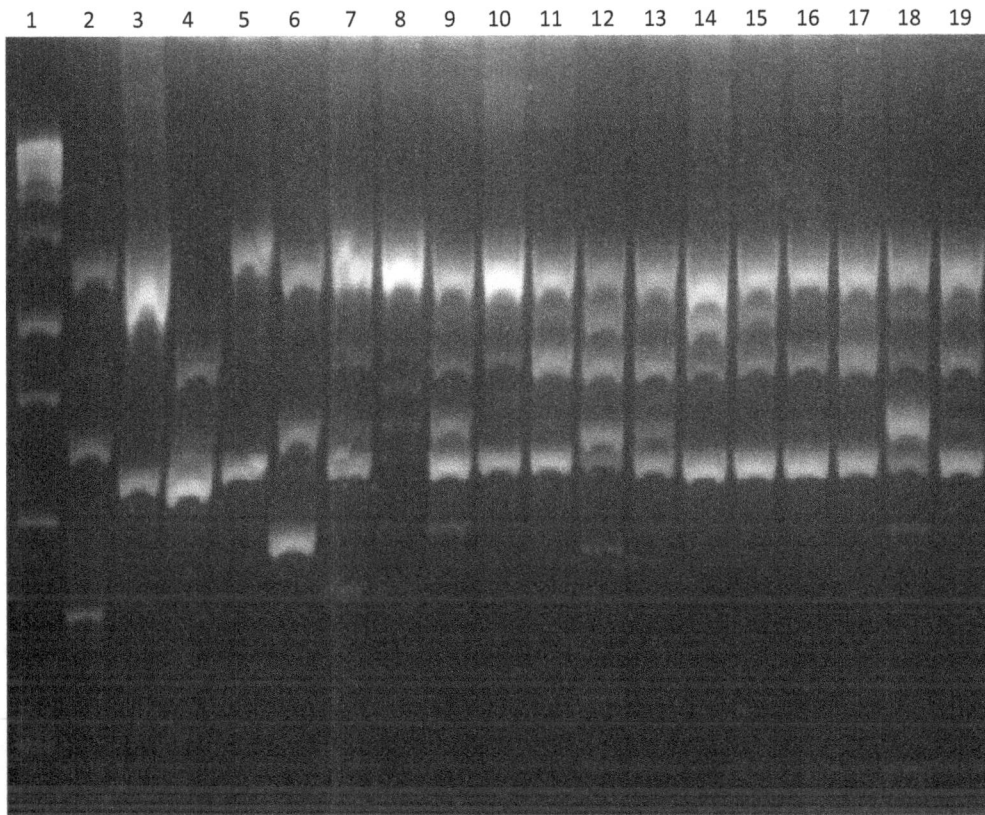

Fig. 1 RAPD profiles for a fraction of ESBL-producing *Klebsiella pneumoniae* isolates amplified by RAPD1 primers. From *left* to *right*: GeneRuler 1 kb ladder followed by isolates from 2008 (*lanes 2* and *3*), 2009 (*lanes 4* and *5*), 2010 (*lanes 6–8*) and 2015 (*lanes 9–19*)

2015 were found to be closely related based on their genotypic profiles.

Discussion

The CLSI disk diffusion ESBL confirmatory test proved suitable for the identification of *K. pneumoniae* isolates included in this study, correctly identifying 41 (78.85%) isolates as possessing β-lactamases capable of hydrolysing oximino-cephalosporins. Although it was not the intention of this study to evaluate the effectiveness of the Microscan WalkAway-96 System, the sensitivity being reported here is much less than that reported by Wiegand et al. [15] of 84 and 87% by Vespero et al. [16]. However, this 21.15% (11/52) "false positive" rate should be interpreted with caution as well as interest. In a SENTRY report authored by Bell et al. [17], they found that 20.3% of screen-positive isolates failed to show clavulanate synergy, and, subsequently, 75% of these nonconforming results were due to the presence of a plasmid-borne AmpC enzyme of the CIT or DHA type. Munier et al. [18] also found that 70% of ESBL screen-positive isolates (which were characterised by *E. coli*, *K. pneumoniae*, *K. oxytoca*, and *Proteus mirabilis*) were actually producing an AmpC β-lactamase, while

only 13% represented true ESBL producers. Although this study did assess whether isolates that produced negative confirmatory results possessed a gene that coded for an AmpC β-lactamase (data not shown), all of the isolates returned negative results. However, this finding does not rule out the possibility of these isolates harbouring other AmpC varieties, and further investigation is warranted.

Another possible reason that may be posited for the "high" number of false positives involves the influence of the inoculum effect. In their clinical update paper, Patterson and Bonomo highlight that in vitro, MICs of cephalosporins may rise as the inoculum of ESBL-producing organism increases [5]. This was further substantiated by Thauvin-Eliopoulos et al. [19] who showed that the cefotaxime MIC for a *K. pneumoniae* strain harbouring TEM-26 increased from 0.25 μg/ml at an inoculum of 10^5 CFU/ml to 64 μg/ml at an inoculum of 10^7 CFU/ml. Similarly, Bedenic et al. [20] found that SHV harbouring *klebsiellae* were more resistant to cephalosporin agents when the inoculum size was higher. This reason may certainly be applicable in the case of this study especially given that eight of nine negative confirmatory test isolates were

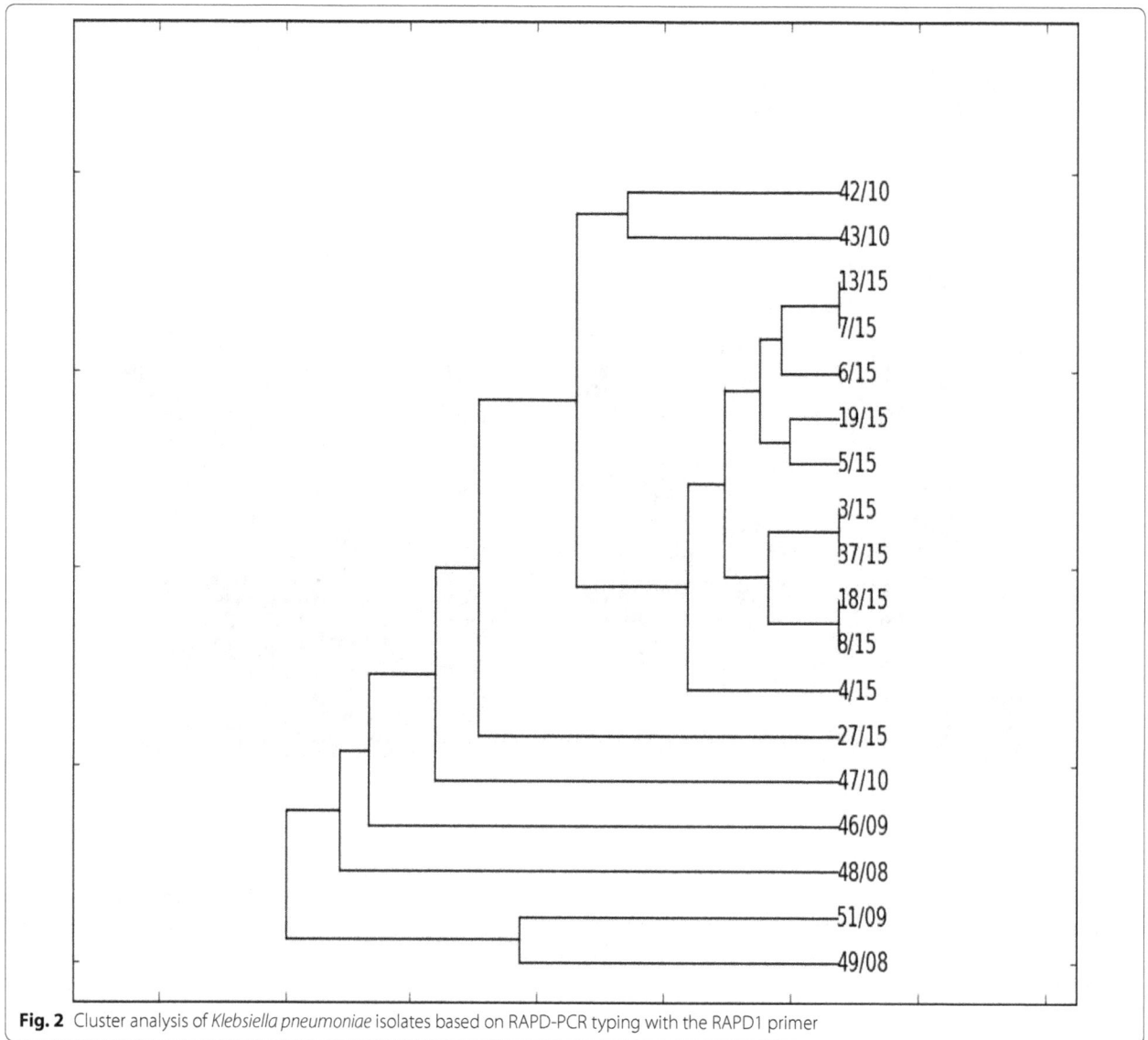

Fig. 2 Cluster analysis of *Klebsiella pneumoniae* isolates based on RAPD-PCR typing with the RAPD1 primer

identified as possessing a SHV-type β-lactamase gene when examined with a molecular assay.

It is also worth noting that even though there was PCR amplification of TEM and SHV genes in most of the isolates, without sequencing it cannot be determined whether these genes contributed to mediating extended spectrum beta-lactam resistance. Sequencing allows for the differentiation of the non-ESBL genes (e.g., TEM-1, -2, and SHV-1) from the ESBL variants (e.g., TEM-3 and SHV-2) [21].

The distribution of the three groups of ESBL-genes for *K. pneumoniae* identified in this study was different from what was reported at this institution by Akpaka et al. [2]. That study reported that there were 84.3% bla_{TEM}, 34.5% bla_{SHV} and 58.8% bla_{CTX-M} of the ESBL genes present in *K. pneumoniae* isolates recovered at the institution (EWMSC) over a 3-year period. In comparison, this study found lower rates for bla_{TEM} (59%; 39/66) and bla_{CTX-M} (46.9%; 31/66, bla_{CTX-M1} plus bla_{CTX-M2}), and a higher rate for bla_{SHV} (84.8%; 56/66). Most noteworthy is that 37.8% (25/66) of the *K. pneumoniae* isolates possessed all three β-lactamase genes. This suggests that one or more of these β-lactamase genes may have been acquired from transferrable plasmids, however, a conjugative assay was not performed at the time the study was conducted to confirm this. Moreover, this finding increases the likelihood that other genes such as plasmid-mediated fluoroquinolone and aminoglycoside resistance genes may also be co-transferred, thereby contributing to the dissemination of multidrug resistance mechanisms [22].

The emergence and spread of CTX-M continues to be well documented and reported across Latin America and the Caribbean [2, 9, 23, 24]. In this study there was widespread distribution of β-lactamases belonging to the CTX-M-1 group, and one instance of an isolate with a β-lactamase from the CTX-M-2 group- the first such account of this particular enzyme in *K. pneumoniae* from a Caribbean territory. This simultaneous production of both cefotaximase and ceftazidimase poses a serious problem to the characterization of resistance by clinical laboratories since these enzymes confer a higher level of resistance to oxyimino-cephalosporinases [25].

For RAPD typing, isolates that possessed two or more β-lactamase genes were chosen with the majority of isolates being those recovered in 2015. RAPD-PCR was chosen because it is a rapid and simple method which when optimized has proven competitive with the gold standard of pulse field gel electrophoresis [26, 27]. RAPD1, also referred to as Primer 640 by other authors [13, 26], proved to be optimal for DNA fingerprinting since it allowed the clear distinction of DNA banding patterns for all of the isolates tested. The resulting RAPD profiles for this select group of isolates showed that there was diversity among those isolated during 2008–2010 and those recovered in 2015. However, it was found that *K. pneumoniae* isolates with the same genotype possessed three or more extended-spectrum β-lactamase genes. This seems to suggest that these strains may have been epidemic in the hospital environment, but due to the lack of patient information this fact could not be proven with certainty.

This study was not without some limitations. The loss of transferrable genetic elements, i.e. plasmids, in stored *K. pneumoniae* isolates from 2008 to 2010 could not be accounted for, and, therefore, genes contributing to resistance might have been lost as has been highlighted by previous authors [5]. Secondly, RAPD-PCR was only conducted on a small subset of the isolates recovered due to inadequate resources for DNA extraction and purification.

Conclusion

This study serves as an important update on the ESBL genes conferring β-lactam antimicrobial resistance among clinical isolates of *K. pneumoniae* isolated from patients being treated at the EWMSC, Trinidad. Along with identifying the traditional bla_{TEM}, bla_{SHV}, and bla_{CTX-M1} genes, it also identified a previously uncharacterised gene belonging to the bla_{CTX-M2} group. These findings suggest that both phenotypic and genotypic methods are required to determine and describe the genes responsible for resistance in *K. pneumoniae*, and thus, better guide infection control and antimicrobial

stewardship measures directed at preventing the heterogeneous spread of plasmid-mediated resistance genes. Improving the results of studies, conducted at the EWMSC, similar to ours would require conducting plasmid conjugation transfer experiments and sequencing in order to determine: (1) the extent to which the resistance genes amplified by PCR are chromosomally-mediated or plasmid-mediated, and (2) what ESBL genotypes are prevalent among *K. pneumoniae* and other gram negative bacteria within the hospital setting.

Abbreviations

ATCC: American Type Culture; AST: antimicrobial sensitivity testing; *Bla*: used to designate "beta-lactamase" gene; CLSI: Clinical Laboratory Standards Institute; DNA: deoxyribonucleic acid; EWMSC: Eric Williams Medical Sciences Complex; ESBL: extended-spectrum beta (β)-lactamase; ID: identification; MIC: minimum inhibitory concentration; PCR: polymerase chain reaction; RAPD: random amplification of polymorphic DNA; UPGMA: unweighted pair group method with arithmetic averages.

Authors' contributions

PC was the principal investigator, participated in the planning and execution of the study, performed data entry and data analysis, laboratory work and was the main responsible author. FD and PEA coordinated the study, participated in planning, data analysis and writing. All authors read and approved the final manuscript.

Author details

[1] Department of Medical Technology, University of Guyana, Georgetown, Guyana. [2] Faculty of Medical Sciences, The University of the West Indies, St. Augustine, Trinidad and Tobago. [3] Department of Para-Clinical Sciences, Faculty of Medical Sciences, The University of the West Indies, St. Augustine, Trinidad and Tobago.

Acknowledgements

PC would like to acknowledge Ms. C. Dacron and others working in the Vet Laboratory, Eric Williams Medical Sciences Complex for use of the facilities during the different phases of laboratory testing as well as providing guidance about troubleshooting during the molecular-based testing phase of this research.

Competing interests

The authors declare that they have no competing interests

Funding

Funding was not provided for the completion of this research.

References

1. Philippon A, Arlet G, Lagrange PH. Origin and impact of plasmid-mediated extended spectrum beta-lactamases. Eur J Clin Microbiol Infect Dis. 1994;13(Suppl 1):S17–29.

2. Akpaka PE, Legall B, Padman J. Molecular detection and epidemiology of extended-spectrum beta-lactamase genes prevalent in clinical isolates of *Klebsiella pneumoniae* and *E. coli* from Trinidad and Tobago. West Indian Med J. 2010;59(6):591–6.

3. Nicholson AM, Gayle P, Roye-Green K. Extended spectrum beta-lactamase producing organisms at the University Hospital of the West Indies. West Indian Med J. 2004;53(2):104–8.

4. Akpaka PE, Swanston WH. Phenotypic detection and occurrence of extended-spectru beta-lactamases in clinical isolated of *Klebsiella pneumoniae* and *Escherichia coli* at a tertiary hospital in Trinidad and Tobago. Braz J Infect Dis. 2008;12(6):516–20.

5. Paterson DL, Bonomo RA. Extended-spectrum beta-lactamases: clinical update. Clin Microbiol Rev. 2005;18(4):657–86.

6. Lee JH, Bae IK, Lee SH. New definitions of extended-spectrum beta-lactamases conferring worldwide emerging antibiotic resistance. Med Res Rev. 2012;32(1):216–32.

7. Pitout JDD, Laupland KB. Extended-spectrum beta-lactamases-producing *Enterobacteriaceae*: an emerging public-health concern. Lancet. 2008;8:159–66.

8. Bush K, Jacoby GA. Updated functional classification of beta-lactamases. Antimicrob Agents Chemother. 2010;54(3):969–76.

9. Bonnet R. Growing group of extended-spectrum beta-lactamases: the CTX-M enzymes. Antimicrob Agents Chemother. 2004;48:1–14.

10. Coque TM, Oliver A, Perez-Diaz JC, Baquero F, Canton R. Genes encoding TEM-4, SHV-2, and CTX-M-10 extended-spectrum beta-lactamases are carried by multiple *Klebsiella pneumoniae* clones in a single hospital (Madrid 1989 to 2000). Antimicrob Agents Chemother. 2002;46(2):500–10.

11. Cherian BP, Singh N, Charles W, Prabhakar P. Extended spectrum beta-lactamase producing *Salmonella enteritidis* in Trinidad and Tobago. Emerg Infect Dis. 1999;5:181–2.

12. Clinical and Laboratory Standard Institute. M100-S24 Performance standards for antimicrobial susceptibility testing: twenty-fourth informational supplement. Performance standards for antimicrobial susceptibility testing. Pennsylvania: Clinical and Laboratory Institute; 2014. Report No.: M100-S24.

13. Ashayeri-panah M, Eftekhar F, Feizabadi M. Development of an optimized random amplified polymorphic DNA protocol for fingerprinting of *Klebsiella pneumoniae*. Lett Appl Microbiol. 2012;54(2):272–9.

14. Pavel AB, Vasile CL. PyElph- a software tool for gel images analysis and phylogenetics. BMC Bioinform. 2012;13(9):1–6.

15. Wiegand I, Geiss HK, Mack D, Sturenburg E, Seifert H. Detection of extended-spectrum beta-lactamases among *Enterobacteriaceae* by use of semiautomated microbiology systems and manual detection procedures. J Clin Microbiol. 2007;45(4):1167–74.

16. Vespero E, Perugini M, Saridakis H. Screening and confirmatory assays for detection of ESBLs (extended spectrum beta-lactamases) production by *Klebsiella pneumoniae* isolates. Semina Ciênc Biol e da Saúde Londrina. 2007;28(1):33–8.

17. Bell JM, Chitsaz M, Turnidge JD, Barton M, Walters LJ, Jones RN. Prevalence and significance of a negative extended-spectrum beta-lactamase (ESBL) confirmation test result after a positive ESBL screening test result for isolates of *Escherichia coli* and *Klebsiella pneumoniae*: results from the SENTRY Asia-Pacific surveillance program. J Clin Microbiol. 2007;45(5):1478–82.

18. Munier GK, Johnson CL, Snyder JW, Moland ES, Hanson ND, Thomson KS. Positive extended-spectrum-beta-lactamase (ESBL) screening results may be due to AmpC beta-lactamases more often than ESBLs. J Clin Microbiol. 2010;48(2):673–4.

19. Thauvin-Eliopoulos C, Tripodi MF, Moellering RC Jr, Eliopoulos GM. Efficacies of piperacillin–tazobactam and cefepime in rats with experimental intra-abdominal abscesses due to an extended-spectrum beta-lactamase-producing strain of *Klebsiella pneumoniae*. Antimicrob Agents Chemother. 1997;41:1053–7.

20. Bedenic B, Beader N, Zagar Z. Effect of inoculum size on the antibacterial activity of cefpirome and cefepime against *Klebsiella pneumoniae* producing SHV extended-spectrum beta-lactamases. Clin Microbiol Infect. 2001;7(11):626–35.

21. Shaikh S, Fatima J, Shakil S, Rizvi SM, Kamal MA. Antibiotic resistance and extended spectrum beta-lactamases: types, epidemiology and treatment. Saudi J Biol Sci. 2015;22(1):90–101.

22. Poulou A, Grivakou E, Vrioni G, et al. Modified CLSI extended-spectrum β-lactamase (ESBL) confirmatory test for phenotypic detection of ESBLs among *Enterobacteriaceae* producing various β-lactamases. Bourbeau P, ed. J Clin Microbiol. 2014;52(5):1483–9.

23. Espinal P, Garza-Ramos U, Reyna F, Rojas-Moreno T, Sanchez-Perez A, Carrillo B, et al. Identification of SHV-type and CTX-M-12 extended-spectrum beta-lactamases (ESBLs) in multiresistant *Enterobacteriaceae* from Colombian Caribbean hospitals. J Chemother. 2010;22(3):160–4.

24. Pallecchi L, Bartoloni A, Fiorelli C, Mantella A, Di Maggio T, Gamboa H, et al. Rapid dissemination and diversity of CTX-M extended-spectrum beta-lactamase genes in commensal *Escherichia coli* isolates from healthy children from low-resource settings in Latin America. Antimicrob Agents Chemother. 2007;51(8):2720–5.

25. Ryoo NH, Kim EC, Hong SG, Park YJ, Lee K, Bae IK, et al. Dissemination of SHV-12 and CTX-M-type extended-spectrum beta-lactamases among clinical isolates of *Escherichia coli* and *Klebsiella pneumoniae* and emergence of GES-3 in Korea. J Antimicrob Chemother. 2005;56(4):698–702.

26. Ashayeri-Panah MM, Eftekhar F, Ghamsari MM, Parvin M. Genetic profiling of *Klebsiella pneumoniae*: comparison of pulsed field gel electrophoresis and random amplified polymorphic DNA. Braz J Microbiol. 2013;7:823–8.

27. Eftekhar F, Nouri P. Correlation of RAPD-PCR profiles with ESBL production in clinical isolates of *Klebsiella pneumoniae* in Tehran. J Clin Diagn Res. 2015;9(1):DC01–3.

3

Assessment of antibiotic resistance in *Klebsiella pneumoniae* exposed to sequential in vitro antibiotic treatments

Jeongjin Kim[1], Ara Jo[1], Ekachai Chukeatirote[2] and Juhee Ahn[1,3*]

Abstract

Background: Bacteria treated with different classes of antibiotics exhibit changes in susceptibility to successive antibiotic treatments. This study was designed to evaluate the influence of sequential antibiotic treatments on the development of antibiotic resistance in *Klebsiella pneumoniae* associated with β-lactamase and efflux pump activities.

Methods: The antibiotic susceptibility, β-lactamase activity, and efflux activity were determined in *K. pneumoniae* grown at 37 °C by adding initial (0 h) and second antibiotics (8 or 12 h). Treatments include control (CON; no first and second antibiotic addition), no initial antibiotic addition followed by 1 MIC ciprofloxacin addition (CON-CIP), no initial antibiotic addition followed by 1 MIC meropenem addition (CON-MER), initial 1/4 MIC ciprofloxacin addition followed by no antibiotic addition (1/4CIP-CON), initial 1/4 MIC ciprofloxacin addition followed by 1 MIC ciprofloxacin addition (1/4CIP-CIP), and initial 1/4 MIC ciprofloxacin addition followed by 1 MIC meropenem addition (1/4CIP-MER).

Results: Compared to the CON, the initial addition of 1/4 MIC ciprofloxacin inhibited the growth of *K. pneumoniae* throughout the incubation period. The ciprofloxacin treatments (CON-CIP and 1/4CIP-CIP) showed significant reduction in the number of *K. pneumoniae* cells compared to meropenem (CON-MER and 1/4CIP-MER). The 1/4CIP-CIP achieved a further 1 log reduction of *K. pneumoniae*, when compared to the 1/4CIP-CON and 1/CIP-MER. The increase in sensitivity of *K. pneumoniae* to cefotaxime, kanamycin, levofloxacin, nalidixic acid was observed for CON-CIP. Noticeable cross-resistance pattern was observed at the 1/4CIP-CIP, showing the increased resistance of *K. pneumoniae* to chloramphenicol, ciprofloxacin, kanamycin, levofloxacin, nalidixic acid norfloxacin, sulphamethoxazole/trimethoprim, and tetracycline. The levels of β-lactamase activities were estimated to be 8.4 μmol/min/ml for CON, 7.7 μmol/min/ml for 1/4CIP-CON and as low as 2.9 μmol/min/ml for CON-CIP. Compared to the absence of phenylalanine-arginine-β-naphthylamide (PAβN), the fluorescence intensity of EtBr was increased in *K. pneumoniae* cells treated at the CON, CON-CIP, and CON-MER in the presence of PAβN. However, the efflux pump activity remained in *K. pneumoniae* cells treated at the 1/CIP, 1/CIP–CIP, and 1/CIP-MER in the presence of PAβN.

Conclusion: The results suggest that the pre-exposed antibiotic history, treatment order, and concentrations influenced the development of multiple antibiotic resistant associated with β-lactamase and efflux pump activities. This study highlights the importance of antibiotic treatment conditions, which would be taken into consideration when new antibiotic strategy is designed to prevent antibiotic resistance.

Keywords: β-Lactamase, Efflux pump system, Meropenem, Ciprofloxacin, Antibiotic resistance

*Correspondence: juheeahn@kangwon.ac.kr
[1] Department of Medical Biomaterials Engineering, Kangwon National University, Chuncheon, Gangwon 24341, South Korea
Full list of author information is available at the end of the article

Background

The overuse, underuse, and misuse of antibiotics have become major causes of the development of antibiotic resistance in bacteria [1]. The emergence and spread of antibiotic-resistant bacteria has been a growing concern over the last decade, which can lead to serious clinical and public health problems. *Klebsiella pneumoniae*, an opportunistic pathogen, is mainly responsible for nosocomial infections with high morbidity and mortality [2]. Recently, the rapid emergence of extended-spectrum β-lactamase (ESBL) producing *K. pneumoniae* has significantly increased the risk of developing serious nosocomial and community-acquired infections worldwide [3, 4]. Furthermore, multidrug-resistant *K. pneumoniae* strains can cause treatment failure with current antibiotic therapy [2].

The proposed resistance mechanisms of *K. pneumoniae* against different classes of antibiotics include release of antibiotic-inactivating enzymes, modification of antibiotic target sites, change in membrane permeability, activation of efflux pump systems, and alteration of metabolic pathways [2, 5]. Among these mechanisms, the enzymatic degradation and efflux pump systems play an important role in the development of multidrug resistance in *K. pneumoniae* [6]. *K. pneumoniae* strains produce enzymes, including extended-spectrum β-lactamases, metallo-β-lactamases, oxacillinases, and carbapenemases, that can degrade β-lactam antibiotics. The efflux pumps, belonging to the resistance-nodulation-division (RND) family, can extrude amphiphilic and charged antibiotics such as β-lactams, fluoroquinolones, and aminoglycosides [2].

The sequential and combination antibiotic therapies have currently been used to reduce not only the evolution of multidrug resistant bacteria but also the levels of antibiotics used in the treatment of bacterial infection [7–9]. The decreased selection pressure occurs when antibiotics are treated in appropriate order, which can prevent the emergence and spread of multidrug resistance [10]. From the practical viewpoint of antibiotic effectiveness, however, there is an important challenging question of whether the treatment history can cause potential carry-over effects on the additional antibiotic therapy. The pre-exposure to antibiotics influences the acquisition of resistance to second-line antibiotics [11]. The beneficial and adverse effects of current therapeutic approaches for treating bacterial infections are still under debate. Therefore, the objective of this study was to evaluate the impact of sequential antibiotic treatments on the antibiotic susceptibility and resistance mechanisms of *K. pneumoniae* in association with β-lactamase and efflux pump activities.

Methods

Bacterial strain and culture condition

Strain of *K. pneumoniae* ATCC 23357 was purchased from American Type Culture Collection (ATCC, Manassas, VA, USA). The strain was cultured in trypticase soy broth (TSB; BD, Becton, Dickinson and Co., Sparks, MD, USA) at 37 °C for 18 h. After cultivation, the culture was centrifuged at $3000{\times}g$ for 20 min at 4 °C. The harvested cells were washed twice with phosphate-buffered saline (PBS, pH 7.2) and diluted to 10^8 CFU/ml for assays.

Antibiotic susceptibility assay

The susceptibility of *K. pneumoniae* to ciprofloxacin and meropenem was evaluated according to the Clinical Laboratory Standards Institute (CLSI) procedure with slight modification [12]. All antibiotics used in this study were purchased from Sigma Chemicals (St. Louis, MO, USA). Antibiotic stock solutions were prepared by dissolving in glacial acetic acid for ciprofloxacin and distilled water for meropenem to obtain a final concentration of 10.24 mg/ml. The stock solutions of ciprofloxacin and meropenem (100 μl each) were serially (1:2) diluted to concentrations ranging from 2 to 0 μg/ml with TSB in 96-well flat-bottomed polystyrene microtiter plates (BD Falcon, San Jose, CA, USA). The test strain was inoculated at 10^5 CFU/ml and incubated at 37 °C for 18 h. Minimum inhibitory concentrations (MICs) of ciprofloxacin and meropenem were defined as the lowest concentration of each antibiotic at which no visible cell growth was observed.

Dynamic time-kill curve analysis

Time-kill curve assay was carried out to determine the antibiotic activities of ciprofloxacin and meropenem against *K. pneumoniae* using a sequential treatment scheme as described in Table 1. The initial population (10^5 CFU/ml) of *K. pneumoniae* was inoculated at 37 °C in TSB treated with (Treatments 1, 2, and 3) and without antibiotic (Treatments 4, 5, and 6). After being reached an optical density (OD) of 0.5, the non-adapted and ciprofloxacin-adapted *K. pneumoniae* cells were further treated with no (Treatments 1 and 4) and the increased concentrations of ciprofloxacin (Treatments 2 and 5) and meropenem (Treatments 3 and 6). The survival curves were measured at 600 nm at every 4 h interval throughout the incubation period. The cultured cells were collected for further analyses, including bacterial enumeration, disk diffusion, lactamase activity, and cartwheel tests.

Microbial analysis

The collected cells were serially diluted (1:10) with PBS and then plated on trypticase soy agar (TSA) using an Autoplate Spiral Plating System (Spiral Biotech Inc.,

Table 1 Sequential antibiotic treatments used in this study

Treatment	Antibiotic addition (h)		Abbreviation	Description
	0 h	8 or 12 h		
1	No (0)	No (8)	CON	No first and second antibiotic addition
2	No (0)	1 MIC CIP (8)	CON-CIP	No initial antibiotic addition followed by 1 MIC ciprofloxacin addition
3	No (0)	1 MIC MER (8)	CON-MER	No initial antibiotic addition followed by 1 MIC meropenem addition
4	1/4 MIC CIP (0)	No (12)	1/4CIP-CON	Initial 1/4 MIC ciprofloxacin followed by no antibiotic addition
5	1/4 MIC CIP (0)	1 MIC CIP (12)	1/4CIP-CIP	Initial 1/4 MIC ciprofloxacin followed by 1 MIC ciprofloxacin addition
6	1/4 MIC CIP (0)	1 MIC MER (12)	1/4CIP-MER	Initial 1/4 MIC ciprofloxacin followed by 1 MIC meropenem addition

CON, CIP, and MER denote no antibiotic addition, ciprofloxacin, and meropenem, respectively

Norwood, MA, USA). The plates were incubated at 37 °C for 24–48 h to enumerate viable cells using a QCount Colony Counter (Spiral Biotech Inc.). Log reduction (N_{TRT}/N_{CON}) was calculated for each treatment as compared to the control (CON). N_{CON} and N_{TRT} represent the numbers of control and treatments after incubation, respectively.

Disk-diffusion assay

The antibiotic susceptibility of cultured *K. pneumoniae* was determined by the disk-diffusion test. The cultured cells were evenly spread-plated on TSA and then allowed to dry for 5 min. Antibiotic disks (Becton, Dickinson and Company, NJ, USA), including cefotaxime (CTX; 30 μg), chloramphenicol (CHL; 30 μg), ciprofloxacin (CIP; 5 μg), kanamycin (KAN; 30 μg), levofloxacin (LEV; 5 μg), nalidixic acid (NAL; 30 μg), norfloxacin (NOR; 10 μg), sulphamethoxazole/trimethoprim (S/T; 25 μg), and tetracycline (TET; 30 μg), were placed on the surface of the agar using sterilized forceps. After incubation at 38 °C for 24 h, the diameters of inhibition zone were measured using a metric ruler.

β-Lactamase activity assay

The β-lactamase activity was evaluated using a nitrocefin hydrolysis assay [13]. The cultured cells were centrifuged at 3000×*g* for 20 min at 4 °C to collect cell-free supernatants. The cell-free supernatants were mixed with 20 μl of 1.5 mM nitrocefin (Biovision, Inc., CA, USA) and incubated at 37 °C. The absorbance was measured every 5 min up to 1 h at 515 nm [14].

Ethidium bromide (EtBr)-agar cartwheel assay

The cultured *K. pneumoniae* cells were centrifuged at 3000×*g* for 20 min at 4 °C, rinsed twice with PBS, and then suspended in PBS with and without efflux pump inhibitor (phenylalanine-arginine-β-naphthylamide; PAβN, 8 μg/ml) [15, 16]. The prepared cells were swabbed on EtBr-agar plates containing EtBr (1 μg/ml) and incubated at 37 °C for 18 h. After incubation, the swabbed

EtBr-agar plates exposed to UV light were photographed using a Gel-doc XR System (Bio-Rad, Hertfordshire, UK).

Statistical analysis

All analyses were conducted in duplicates for three replicates. Data were analyzed by the Statistical Analysis System (SAS) software. The General Linear Model (GLM) and least significant difference (LSD) procedures were used to compare treatments at $p < 0.05$.

Results

Effect of serial antibiotic treatments on the viability and antibiotic susceptibility

The MIC values of ciprofloxacin and meropenem were 0.03 and 0.06 μg/ml, respectively. The survival of *K. pneumoniae* was observed during the sequential antibiotic treatments (Fig. 1). The growth of *K. pneumoniae* was retarded by 1/4 MIC ciprofloxacin, showing that the non- and ciprofloxacin-treated *K. pneumoniae* cells reached OD of 0.5 after 8 and 12 h of incubation, respectively. The antibiotic effects of ciprofloxacin and meropenem on the growth of *K. pneumoniae* was noticeable in the non-adapted cells (CON-CIP and CON-MER) compared to the ciprofloxacin-adapted cells (1/4CIP-CIP and 1/4CIP-MER). The number of viable *K. pneumoniae* cells under 1/4CIP-CIP was significantly reduced by 1.8 log, followed by CON-CIP and 1/4CIP-MER (Fig. 2). The least reduction in *K. pneumoniae* cells was observed at the CON-MER. The reduction rate increased with increasing the concentration of CIP to 0.03 μg/ml (1/4CIP-CIP), while no significant reduction was observed for the 1/4CIP-MER switched from CIP to MER at the second treatment. The antibiotic resistance acquisition was evaluated in *K. pneumoniae* exposed to sequential antibiotic treatments (Fig. 3). The susceptibilities of *K. pneumoniae* to different classes of antibiotics varied in the treatments. The 1/4CIP-CIP treatment exhibited the decreased susceptibility to all antibiotics with exception of CTX, showing small clear zones (<10 cm). The enhanced susceptibility to all antibiotics tested was observed at the

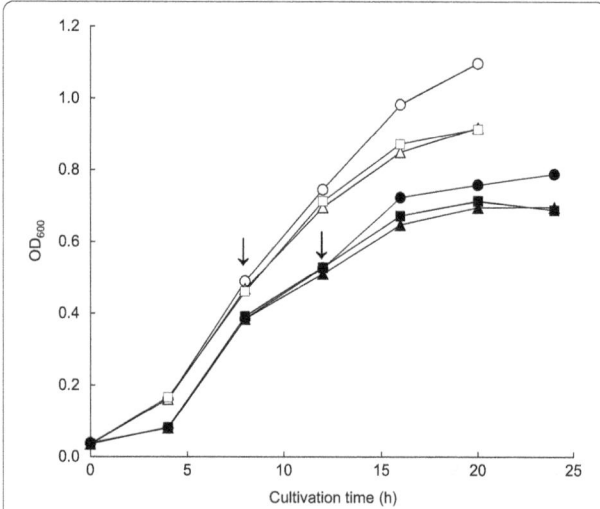

Fig. 1 Survival of *Klebsiella pneumonia* exposed to sequential antibiotics (CON, *open circle*; CON-CIP, *open triangle*; CON-MER, *open square*; 1/4CIP-CON, *closed circle*; 1/4CIP-CIP, *closed triangle*; 1/4CIP-MER, *closed square*). *Arrow* indicates the addition time

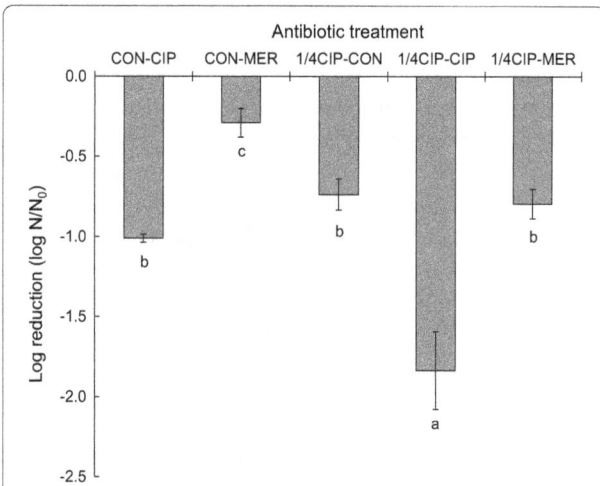

Fig. 2 Reduction of *Klebsiella pneumonia* exposed to sequential antibiotics. N_{CON} and N_{TRT} represent the numbers of control and treatments after incubation, respectively. Log reduction with different letters (*a–c*) are significantly different at $p < 0.05$

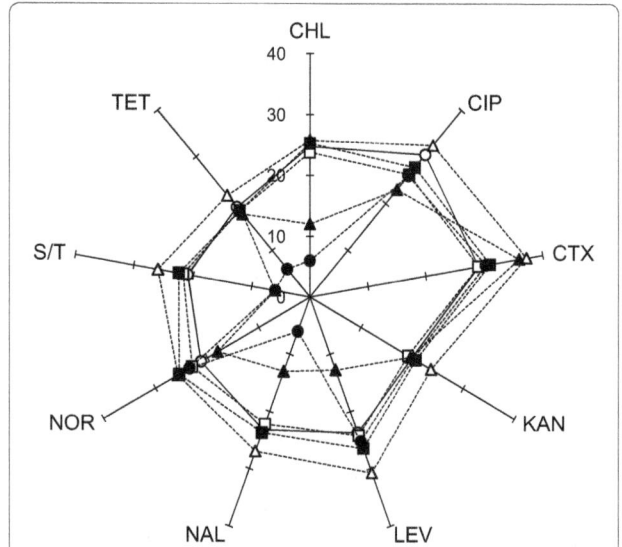

Fig. 3 Radar plot of antibiotic resistance profiles (disk diffusion in cm) of *Klebsiella pneumonia* exposed to sequential antibiotics (CON, *open circle*; CON-CIP, *open triangle*; CON-MER, *open square*; 1/4CIP-CON, *closed circle*; 1/4CIP-CIP, *closed triangle*; 1/4CIP-MER, *closed square*). Antibiotic discs include chloramphenicol (CHL; 30 μg), ciprofloxacin (CIP; 5 μg), cefotaxime (CTX; 30 μg), kanamycin (KAN; 30 μg), levofloxacin (LEV; 5 μg), nalidixic acid (NAL; 30 μg), norfloxacin (NOR; 10 μg), sulphamethoxazole/trimethoprim (S/T; 25 μg), and tetracycline (TET; 30 μg)

CON-CIP treatment, while the decreased susceptibilities to CIP and TET were observed at the treatments, CON-MER, 1/4CIP-CON, and 1/4CIP-MER. The treatments, CON-MER and 1/4CIP-MER, showed the similar resistance pattern as the CON.

Effect of sequential antibiotic treatments on β-lactamase and efflux pump activities

The β-lactamase activities were measured in *K. pneumoniae* cultured at sequential antibiotic treatments (Fig. 4). The highest β-lactamase activity was observed for the

CON (8.4 μmol/min/ml), followed by 1/4CIP-CON (7.7 μmol/min/ml) and CON-MER (6.0 μmol/min/ml).

The efflux activity of *K. pneumoniae* in the absence and presence of efflux pump inhibitor (EPI; PAβN) was evaluated on the EtBr-agar plates (Fig. 5). The efflux pump activity of *K. pneumoniae* was observed at all treatments in the absence of PAβN, showing the decreased fluorescence intensity (Fig. 5a). The increased EtBr accumulation was observed in the presence of PAβN at the CON, CON-CIP, and CON-MER, while relatively low EtBr accumulation was observed at the 1/4CIP-CON, 1/4CIP-CIP, and 1/4CIP-MER (Fig. 5b). The efflux pump activity in *K. pneumoniae* cells treated at the 1/4CIP-CIP, 1/4CIP-CIP, and 1/4CIP-MER was not reduced by the PAβN, suggesting that the EPI-insensitive efflux systems were activated in *K. pneumoniae* cells under sublethal concentration of ciprofloxacin.

Discussion

This study describes the effect of sequential antibiotic treatments on the development of antibiotic resistance in *K. pneumoniae*. Pathogenic bacteria exposed to different levels and various classes of antibiotics can exhibit various susceptibility to additional antibiotic treatments. However, few studies have been focused on the development of antibiotic resistance during the sequential

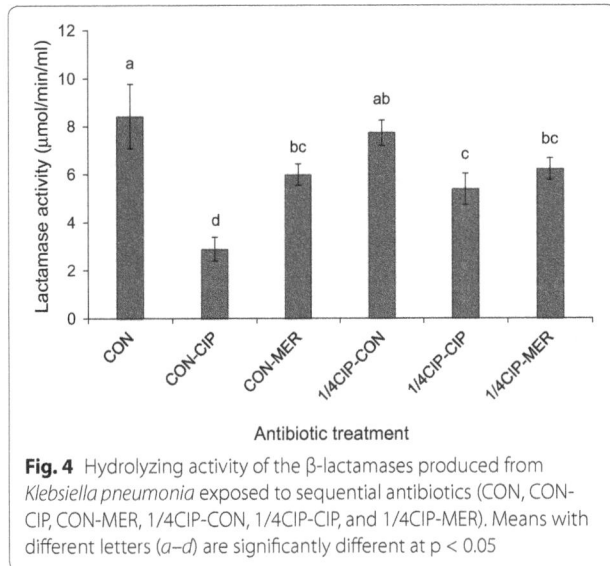

Fig. 4 Hydrolyzing activity of the β-lactamases produced from *Klebsiella pneumonia* exposed to sequential antibiotics (CON, CON-CIP, CON-MER, 1/4CIP-CON, 1/4CIP-CIP, and 1/4CIP-MER). Means with different letters (*a–d*) are significantly different at p < 0.05

antibiotic treatments [11]. Thus, this study highlights the pre-exposed antibiotic history as an important factor for the evolution of antibiotic resistance.

The CON-CIP was more effectively reduced the number of *K. pneumoniae* cells than the CON-MER, while no significant difference was observed between 1/4CIP-CON and 1/4CIP-MER (Fig. 2). The results indicate that meropenem was less effective against *K. pneumoniae* than ciprofloxacin. The lack of antibacterial activity of meropenem might be due to its short elimination half-life [17]. The successive ciprofloxacin treatment (1/4CIP-CIP) showed strong antibacterial activity against *K. pneumoniae* (Fig. 2). However, the cells exposed to 1/4CIP-CIP treatment induced were significantly resistant to different

classes of antibiotics such as CHL, CIP, LEV, NAL, and S/T, known as cross-resistance induction (Fig. 3). This suggests that the sequential single-antibiotic therapy at different levels can lead to the emergence of antibiotic resistant bacteria due to the phenotypic adaptation [18]. Previous studies have reported that antibiotic mono-therapy and combination therapy are the main causes of narrow- and broad-spectrum resistance, respectively [9]. The concentration of ciprofloxacin treated after the initial CIP exposure might be insufficient to suppress the development of antibiotic resistance [19]. The sequential antibiotic treatment, specifically 1/4CIP-CIP, can possibly cause a change in antibiotic resistance. This might be attributed to the mode of action of antibiotics, including time- and concentration-dependent activities. The time-dependent antibiotics include β-lactams and carbapenems, characterized by slow antibiotic activity according to exposure time above MIC [20, 21]. Ciprofloxacin is referred to as concentration-dependent antibiotic, showing antibiotic activity at high concentration [22]. Due to the bacterial adaptation, the sequential treatment of homogeneous antibiotic can reduce the susceptibility to same and different classes of antibiotics [19, 23]. Homogeneous treatment increases bacterial fitness and selection pressure, resulting in the development of antibiotic resistance [24, 25].

The strain of *K. pneumoniae* used in this study was intrinsically resistant to ampicillin (MIC > 256 µg/ml), piperazine (MIC > 16 µg/ml), cephalotin (MIC > 32 µg/ml), and cefoxitin (MIC > 16 µg/ml), resulted from the production of β-lactamases [26]. No significant change in β-lactamase activities was observed for 1/4CIP-CON when compared to the CON, while the β-lactamase

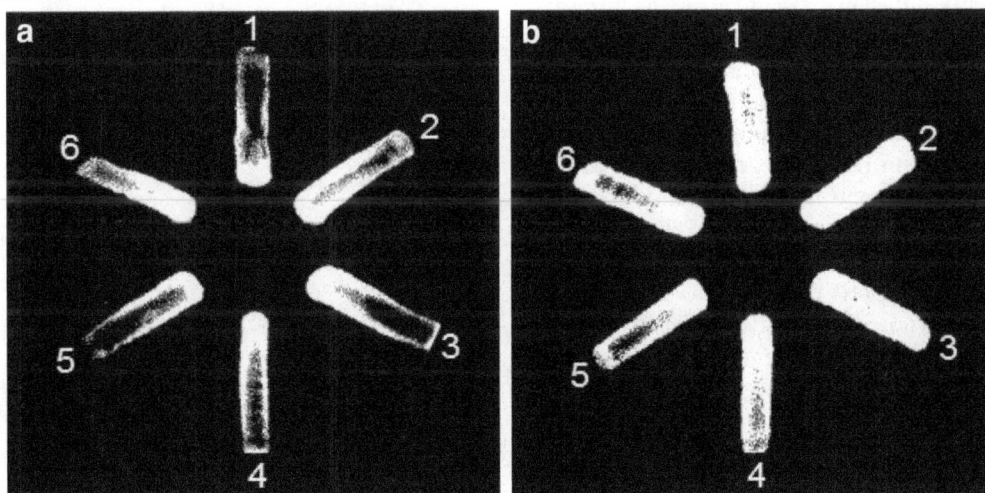

Fig. 5 Accumulation and efflux activity of *Klebsiella pneumonia* on EtBr agar plates containing without (**a**) and with (**b**) efflux pump inhibitor (PAβN). (*1* CON; *2* CON-CIP; *3* CON-MER; *4*, 1/4CIP-CON; *5* 1/4CIP-CIP; *6* 1/4CIP-MER)

activities were significantly decreased at the CON-CIP, CON-MER, 1/4CIP-CIP, and 1/4CIP-MER. The decrease in lactamase activity suggest that relatively fewer viable cells were observed at the treatments compared to the CON and the antibiotics used may act as a lactamase inhibitor [27]. *K. pneumoniae* cells exposed to CON-CIP showed the increased susceptibility to CTX (Fig. 3), which corresponds to the significant reduction in β-lactamase activity treated at CON-CIP (2.9 μmol/min/ml) (Fig. 4). The mechanisms of resistance to β-lactam antibiotics include not only the increase in β-lactamases-mediated hydrolysis but also the decrease in uptake through porin channels and the increase in efflux pump activity [6, 28]. The alteration in porin channel results in the decrease in membrane permeability to antibiotics such as β-lactams and quinolones, but not aminoglycosides that can enter the outer membrane through lipopolysaccharide (LPS) uptake system [19]. The results explain that the susceptibilities of *K. pneumoniae* cells grown at all treatments to KAN were constant regardless of the levels of β-lactamase activities (Fig. 3). Carbapenems such as imipenem and meropenem are stable to β-lactamases that can hydrolyze β-lactams [28–30]. The production of β-lactamases can contribute to the hydrolysis, resulting in the enhanced resistance to β-lactam antibiotics that cannot reach penicillin binding protein (PBP) [26]. This is in good agreement with the result of antibiotic susceptibility that *K. pneumoniae* possesses high intrinsic resistance to ampicillin (MIC > 256 μg/ml).

The efflux pump systems competitively expel substrates, which plays an important role in the development of multidrug resistance [2]. The specific substrates for efflux pumps in *K. pneumoniae* treated at 1/4CIP-CIP and 1/4CIP-CIP may include CHL, TET, NOR, NAL, and LEV, corresponding the enhanced multiple antibiotic resistance in disk-diffusion assay in Fig. 3. The intracellular concentrations of antibiotics substrates in bacteria are directly reduced by active efflux pump systems, leading to the decreased antibiotic susceptibility [31]. In other words, the inhibition of efflux pumps can restore antibiotic susceptibility in resistant bacteria, suggesting the EPI can be a possible control method against antibiotic-resistant bacteria [32–34]. The activation of efflux pumps is associated with the fast-acting antibiotic mechanism at the early stage of antibiotic resistance development [19]. The substrate-dependent efflux pump systems may contribute to cross-resistance to different classes of antibiotics [35].

Conclusions

This study highlights the influence of using sequential antibiotic treatment on the development of antibiotic resistance in *K. pneumoniae*. The difference in antibiotic activity against *K. pneumoniae* might be due to the time- and concentration-dependent modes of action of meropenem and ciprofloxacin, respectively. The antibiotic resistance mechanisms can occur within a short time in association with lactamase production, membrane permeability, and efflux pump activity. The efflux pump activities in *K. pneumoniae* cells treated at 1/4CIP-CON, 1/4CIP-CIP, and 1/4CIP-MER were still observed in the presence of PAβN, indicating that various types of substrate-dependent efflux pumps exist to reduce the intracellular concentrations of antibiotics. The induced efflux pump activity are responsible for the increased antibiotic resistance in *K. pneumoniae*. The most significant finding in this study was that *K. pneumoniae* treated with sequential antibiotics, specifically 1/4CIP-CIP, showed reduced susceptibility towards CHL, NOR, NAL, and LEV, leading to the multiple antibiotic resistance. Therefore, antibiotic therapies should take into account the history of pre-exposed antibiotics to prevent the development of antibiotic resistance. Further studies are needed to assess the risk of antibiotic resistance in sequential and combination antibiotic therapies, which is essential to design an effective strategy for controlling multiple antibiotic resistant bacteria.

Abbreviations

ESBL: extended-spectrum β-lactamase; MIC: minimum inhibitory concentration; CIP: ciprofloxacin; MER: meropenem; CTX: cefotaxime; CHL: chloramphenicol; KAN: kanamycin; LEV: levofloxacin; NAL: nalidixic acid; NOR: norfloxacin; S/T: sulphamethoxazole/trimethoprim; TET: tetracycline; CFU: colony forming unit; EtBr: ethidium bromide; EPI: efflux pump inhibitor; PAβN: phenylalanine-arginine-β-naphthylamide.

Authors' contributions

JK and AJ conducted all experiments and EC contributed to the writing and preparation of the manuscript. JA contributed to the experimental design, data interpretation, and manuscript writing. All authors read and approved the final manuscript.

Author details

[1] Department of Medical Biomaterials Engineering, Kangwon National University, Chuncheon, Gangwon 24341, South Korea. [2] School of Science, Mae Fah Luang University, Chiang Rai 57100, Thailand. [3] Institute of Bioscience and Biotechnology, Kangwon National University, Chuncheon, Gangwon 24341, South Korea.

Acknowledgements
Not applicable.

Competing interests
The authors declare that they have no competing interests.

Funding

This work supported by a grant of the Korea Health Technology R&D Project through the Korea Health Industry Development Institute (KHIDI), funded by the Ministry of Health & Welfare, Republic of Korea (Grant number: HI15C-1798-000016).

References

1. Odonkor ST, Addo KK. Bacterial resistance to antibiotics: recent trends and challenges. Int J Bio Med Res. 2011;2(4):1204–10.

2. HQ Zhong, Zhang S, Pan H, Cai T. Influence of induced ciprofloxacin resistance on efflux pump activity of *Klebsiella pneumoniae*. J Zhejiang Univ Sci B. 2013;14(9):837–43.

3. Brinkworth AJ, Hammer CH, Olano LR, Kobayashi SD, Chen L, Kreiswirth BN, et al. Identification of outer membrane and exoproteins of carbapenem-resistant multilocus sequence Type 258 *Klebsiella pneumoniae*. PLoS ONE. 2015;10(4):e0123219.

4. Latifpour M, Gholipour A, Damavandi MS. Prevalence of extended-spectrum beta-lactamase-producing *Klebsiella pneumoniae* isolates in nosocomial and community-acquired urinary tract infections. Jundishapur J Microbiol. 2016;9(3):e31179.

5. Tenover FC. Mechanisms of antimicrobial resistance in bacteria. Am J Med. 2006;119(6A):S3–10.

6. Pages J-M, Lavigne J-P, Leflon-Guibout V, Marcon E, Bert F, Noussair L, et al. Efflux pump, the masked side of β-lactam resistance in *Klebsiella pneumoniae* clinical isolates. PLoS ONE. 2009;4(3):e4817.

7. Nichol D, Jeavons P, Fletcher AG, Bonomo RA, Maini PK, Paul JL, et al. Steering evolution with sequential therapy to prevent the emergence of bacterial antibiotic resistance. PLoS Comput Biol. 2015;11(9):e1004493.

8. Perron GG, Kryazhimskiy S, Rice DP, Buckling A. Multidrug therapy and evolution of antibiotic resistance: when order matters. Appl Environ Microbiol. 2012;78(17):6137–42.

9. Vestergaard M, Paulander W, Marvig RL, Clasen J, Jochumsen N, Molin S, et al. Antibiotic combination therapy can select for broad-spectrum multidrug resistance in *Pseudomonas aeruginosa*. Int J Antimicrob Agent. 2016;47(1):48–55.

10. Warren DK, Hill HA, Merz LR, Kollef MH, Hayden MK, Fraser VJ, et al. Cycling empirical antimicrobial agents to prevent emergence of antimicrobial-resistant Gram-negative bacteria among intensive care unit patients. Crit Care Med. 2004;32(12):2450–6.

11. Gould IM, MacKenzie FM. Antibiotic exposure as a risk factor for emergence of resistance: the influence of concentration. J Appl Microbiol. 2002;92:78S–84S.

12. CLSI. Methods for dilution antimicrobial susceptibility tests for bacteria that grow aerobically. *Approved standard M07-A9*, 9th edn. Wayne, PA: Clinical and Laboratory Standards Institute; 2012.

13. Matsumoto Y, Hayama K, Sakakihara S, Nishino K, Noji H, Iino R, et al. Evaluation of multidrug efflux pump inhibitors by a new method using microfluidic channels. PLoS ONE. 2011;6(4):e18547.

14. Sharma S, Ramnani P, Virdi JS. Detection and assay of β-lactamases in clinical and non-clinical strains of *Yersinia enterocolitica* biovar 1A. J Antimicrob Chemother. 2004;54(2):401–5.

15. Costa SS, Falcão C, Viveiros M, Machado D, Martins M, Melo-Cristino J, et al. Exploring the contribution of efflux on the resistance to fluoroquinolones in clinical isolates of *Staphylococcus aureus*. BMC Microbiol. 2011;11(1):1–12.

16. Martins M, Viveiros M, Couto I, Costa SS, Pacheco T, Fanning S, et al. Identification of efflux pump-mediated multidrug-resistant bacteria by the ethidium bromide-agar cartwheel method. In Vivo. 2011;25(2):171–8.

17. Walsh F. Doripenem: a new carbapenem antibiotic a review of comparative antimicrobial and bactericidal activities. Ther Clin Risk Manag. 2007;3(5):789–94.

18. var der Horst MA, Schuurmans JM, Smid MC, Koenders BB, ter Kuile BH. De vovo acquisition of resistance to three antibiotics by *Escherichia coli*. Microb Drug Resist. 2011;17(2):141–7.

19. Wu BM, Sabarinath SN, Rand K, Johnson J, Derendorf H. Suppression of ciprofloxacin-induced resistant *Pseudomonas aeruginosa* in a dynamic kill curve system. Int J Antimicrob Agent. 2011;37(6):519–24.

20. Williamson R, Tomasz A. Inhibition of cell wall synthesis and acylation of the penicillin binding proteins during prolonged exposure of growing *Streptococcus pneumoniae* to benzylpenicillin. Eur J Biochem. 1985;151(3):475–83.

21. Jacobs MR. Optimisation of antimicrobial therapy using pharmacokinetic and pharmacodynamic parameters. Clin Microbiol Infect. 2001;7(11):589–96.

22. Levison ME, Levison JH. Pharmacokinetics and pharmacodynamics of antibacterial agents. Infect Dis Clin North Am. 2009;23(4):791–815.

23. Bergstrom CT, Lo M, Lipsitch M. Ecological theory suggests that antimicrobial cycling will not reduce antimicrobial resistance in hospitals. Proc Nat Acad Sci. 2004;101(36):13285–90.

24. Sandiumenge A, Diaz E, Rodriguez A, Vidaur L, Canadell L, Olona M, et al. Impact of diversity of antibiotic use on the development of antimicrobial resistance. J Antimicrob Chemother. 2006;57(6):1197–204.

25. Bonhoeffer S, Lipsitch M, Levin BR. Evaluating treatment protocols to prevent antibiotic resistance. Proc Nat Acad Sci. 1997;94(22):12106–11.

26. Zou L-K, Li L-W, Pan X, Tian G-B, Luo Y, Wu Q, et al. Molecular characterization of β-lactam-resistant *Escherichia coli* isolated from Fu River, China. World J Microbiol Biotechnol. 2012;28(5):1891–9.

27. Coleman K, Levasseur P, Girard A-M, Borgonovi M, Miossec C, Merdjan H, et al. Activities of ceftazidime and avibactam against β-lactamase-producing *Enterobacteriaceae* in a hollow-fiber pharmacodynamic model. Antimicrob Agent Chemother. 2014;58(6):3366–72.

28. Poole K. Resistance to β-lactam antibiotics. Cell Mol Life Sci. 2004;61(17):2200–23.

29. Franceschini N, Segatore B, Perilli M, Vessillier S, Franchino L, Amicosante G. Meropenem stability to β-lactamase hydrolysis and comparative in vitro activity against several β-lactamase-producing Gram-negative strains. J Antimicrob Chemother. 2002;49(2):395–8.

30. Nicoletti G, Russo G, Bonfiglio G. Recent developments in carbapenems. Expert Opin Investig Drug. 2002;11(4):529–44.

31. Aathithan S, French GL. Prevalence and role of efflux pump activity in ciprofloxacin resistance in clinical isolates of *Klebsiella pneumoniae*. Eur J Clin Microbiol Infect Dis. 2011;30(6):745–52.

32. Louw GE, Warren RM, Gey van Pittius NC, Leon R, Jimenez A, Hernandez-Pando R, et al. Rifampicin reduces susceptibility to ofloxacin in rifampicin-resistant *Mycobacterium tuberculosis* through efflux. Am J Respir Crit Care Med. 2011;184(2):269–76.

33. Askoura M, Mottawea W, Abujamel T, Taher I. Efflux pump inhibitors (EPIs) as new antimicrobial agents against *Pseudomonas aeruginosa*. Libyan J Med. 2011;6:5870.

34. Sun J, Deng Z, Yan A. Bacterial multidrug efflux pumps: mechanisms, physiology and pharmacological exploitations. Biochem Biophys Res Commun. 2014;453(2):254–67.

35. Blanco P, Hernando-Amado S, Reales-Calderon J, Corona F, Lira F, Alcalde-Rico M, et al. Bacterial multidrug efflux pumps: much more than antibiotic resistance determinants. Microorganisms. 2016;4(1):14.

4

The occurrence of ESBL-producing *Escherichia coli* carrying aminoglycoside resistance genes in urinary tract infections in Saudi Arabia

Essam J. Alyamani[1*], Anamil M. Khiyami[2], Rayan Y. Booq[1], Majed A. Majrashi[1], Fayez S. Bahwerth[3] and Elena Rechkina[4]

Abstract

Background: The infection and prevalence of extended-spectrum β-lactamases (ESBLs) is a worldwide problem, and the presence of ESBLs varies between countries. In this study, we investigated the occurrence of plasmid-mediated ESBL/AmpC/carbapenemase/aminoglycoside resistance gene expression in *Escherichia coli* using phenotypic and genotypic techniques.

Methods: A total of 58 *E. coli* isolates were collected from hospitals in the city of Makkah and screened for the production of ESBL/AmpC/carbapenemase/aminoglycoside resistance genes. All samples were subjected to phenotypic and genotypic analyses. The antibiotic susceptibility of the *E. coli* isolates was determined using the Vitek-2 system and the minimum inhibitory concentration (MIC) assay. Antimicrobial agents tested using the Vitek 2 system and MIC assay included the expanded-spectrum (or third-generation) cephalosporins (e.g., cefoxitin, cefepime, aztreonam, cefotaxime, ceftriaxone, and ceftazidime) and carbapenems (meropenem and imipenem). Reported positive isolates were investigated using genotyping technology (oligonucleotide microarray-based assay and PCR). The genotyping investigation was focused on ESBL variants and the AmpC, carbapenemase and aminoglycoside resistance genes. *E. coli* was phylogenetically grouped, and the clonality of the isolates was studied using multilocus sequence typing (MLST).

Results: Our *E. coli* isolates exhibited different levels of resistance to ESBL drugs, including ampicillin (96.61%), cefoxitin (15.25%), ciprofloxacin (79.66%), cefepime (75.58%), aztreonam (89.83%), cefotaxime (76.27%), ceftazidime (81.36%), meropenem (0%) and imipenem (0%). Furthermore, the distribution of ESBL-producing *E. coli* was consistent with the data obtained using an oligonucleotide microarray-based assay and PCR genotyping against genes associated with β-lactam resistance. ST131 was the dominant sequence type lineage of the isolates and was the most uropathogenic *E. coli* lineage. The *E. coli* isolates also carried aminoglycoside resistance genes.

Conclusions: The evolution and prevalence of ESBL-producing *E. coli* may be rapidly accelerating in Saudi Arabia due to the high visitation seasons (especially to the city of Makkah). The health authority in Saudi Arabia should monitor the level of drug resistance in all general hospitals to reduce the increasing trend of microbial drug resistance and the impact on patient therapy.

Keywords: ESBL, *E. coli*, *K. pneumonia*, Phenotyping, Genotyping, Saudi Arabia

*Correspondence: eyamani@kacst.edu.sa
[1] National Center for Biotechnology, King Abdulaziz City for Science and Technology, P.O. Box 6086, Riyadh 11442, Saudi Arabia
Full list of author information is available at the end of the article

The occurrence of ESBL-producing Escherichia coli carrying aminoglycoside resistance...

21

Background

Gram-negative bacteria that produce β-lactamases are a major concern in healthcare due to their ability to spread globally [1]. β-lactamases are produced by bacteria to hydrolyze the β-lactam ring in antibiotics, which results in ineffective drug treatment. Extended-spectrum β lactamases (ESBLs) are a major group of enzymes that confer resistance to several generations of β-lactam antibiotics, including third-generation cephalosporins [2, 3]. ESBL-producing Gram-negative bacteria are thought to be an important reason for cephalosporin therapy failure [4, 5]. Therefore, these bacteria should be monitored and reported by clinical laboratories to minimize their impact on patient therapy. ESBL resistance genes are primarily carried by plasmids. Plasmids may also carry genes encoding resistance to other antibiotic classes, such as ampA, ampC, aminoglycosides, chloramphenicol, macrolides, or quinolone. Therefore, treatment options are limited for bacteria that produce ESBLs due to the multiple resistance genes encoded in the plasmids. ESBL genes that are primarily encoded in plasmids include TEM, SHV, and CTX-M. Multiple variants of each gene are produced by altering the configuration of amino acids within the β-lactamase active site. Enterobacteriaceae, such as *Klebsiella pneumoniae* and *Escherichia coli*, are the major ESBL producers frequently isolated in clinical laboratories [6]. *Acinetobacter baumannii* is also an important ESBL-producing bacteria that has been reported globally [7]. Newer antibiotic classes, such as carbapenems, have been introduced by the pharmaceutical industry as treatment options for infections caused by ESBL-producing bacteria. Nevertheless, carbapenemase-producing bacteria have also been documented [8, 9]. Due to the increasing threat of multidrug-resistant bacteria, laboratory personnel, physicians, and clinical practitioners should implement a program to detect and report ESBLs as part of their infection control to limit the therapeutic failures caused by ESBL-producing bacteria. Molecular genotyping has been used concurrently with phenotyping techniques to detect and confirm antimicrobial drug resistance data and to detect Gram-negative ESBL producing bacteria [10]. PCR, multiplex PCR and oligonucleotide microarray-based assays have been developed and used to monitor the emergence of ESBLs and many other drug-resistant genes from *E. coli*, *K. pneumonia* and *A. baumannii* [11–15]. Strain characterization by multilocus sequence typing (MLST) is the method of choice in many clinical and research laboratories due to its high discriminatory power [16, 17]. The increased prevalence of ESBLs is being monitored and reported globally. Due to a lack of a solid data regarding the emergence of ESBLs from major Saudi general hospitals in the region of Makkah, this study reports the characterization of drug resistance genes for 58 *E. coli* isolates from an in-patient ward using phenotypic and genotypic approaches. Understanding the phenotypic and molecular nature of Enterobacteriaceae during the busy visitation Hajj season (pilgrimage season) in the city of Makkah, Saudi Arabia, is essential to reducing ESBL-strains prevalence.

Methods

Bacteriological culture

A total of 58 bacterial isolates were collected from two different general hospitals in the city of Makkah during the 2014–2015 Hajj (pilgrimage) season from patients with urinary tract infections. The bacterial isolates were phenotypically and genotypically investigated in microbiology laboratories at the King Abdulaziz City for Science and Technology (KACST). Single pure *E. coli* colonies were obtained from the all isolates. The bacteria were isolated from urine specimens using the clean-catch midstream urine sampling technique. Urine samples were inoculated using a calibrated 0.01 mL urine plastic loop on 5% sheep blood agar and MacConkey agar plates. The plates were incubated at 37 °C for 24 h. Urine samples were considered positive for UTIs if the number of colonies equaled or exceeded 10^5 CFU/mL. Gram staining was performed to identify urine specimens that contained more than 10^5 colony forming units (CFU)/mL of bacteria. A drop of well-mixed urine was fixed on a glass slide, stained, and examined under oil immersion (1000×) for the presence of at least one organism per oil immersion field.

Bacterial identification and antibiotic susceptibility testing

Bacterial identities were confirmed with a Vitek 2 GN ID card using the Vitek 2 system (bioMérieux, Marcy l'Etoile, France). Antibiotic susceptibility testing (AST) was completed using Vitek 2 cards (AST-N292) according to the manufacturer's recommendations (bioMérieux, Marcy l'Etoile, France). The Vitek ESBL susceptibility tests were interpreted according to the Clinical and Laboratory Standards Institute (CLSI) criteria using the Vitek system. *E. coli* ATCC 25922 was included in each Vitek testing step for quality control. The minimum inhibitory concentrations (MICs) were determined in Mueller–Hinton broth using microdilution plates [18]. The MICs of cefoxitin, ciprofloxacin, aztreonam, ceftazidime, meropenem, cefepime, cefotaxime, imipenem and ampicillin for all *E. coli* isolates were interpreted according to previous protocols (CLSI, 2014) [18]. Serial dilutions of the nine drugs were prepared (0.5, 1, 2, 4, 8, 16, 32, 64, 128, 256, 512 and 1024 µg/mL) in Mueller–Hinton broth and added to 96-well plates. Then, the bacterial suspensions were added to each well to achieve a final inoculum of

5×10^5 CFU/mL. The endpoint MIC was read visually and by spectrophotometer at 600 nm. The lowest concentration of antibiotic that inhibited visible bacterial growth after 24 h at 37 °C was defined as the MIC.

Amplification and sequencing of the 16S rRNA gene

The *E. coli* identity was confirmed using PCR and sequencing of the 16S rDNA gene [19–21]. Illustra PuRe-Taq Ready-To-Go PCR beads were used in the PCR reaction (GE Health Biosciences, USA). The 25-μL reaction was set up as follows: 2 μL of 10 pmol of each forward and reverse primer (IDT, Integrated DNA Technologies) were used with the 8-forward primer (AGA GTT TGA TCC TGG CTC AG) and 805-reverse primer (GAC TAC CAG GGT ATC TAA TC) [22]. Exactly 1 μL of DNA template was added to the beads, and the reaction was completed using 22 μL of nuclease-free ddH$_2$O (Promega). The amplification cycling conditions were 3 min for the initial incubation at 95 °C, followed by 35 cycles of 1 min at 95 °C, 1 min at 55 °C, and 2 min at 72 °C and a final extension at 72 °C for 7 min. All PCR amplicons were fractionated using 1% agarose gel electrophoresis prior to staining with ethidium bromide. Images were obtained with a gel documentation system under a UV transilluminator. The PCR amplicons were purified and sequenced in an ABI 3130 Genetic Analyzer (Life Technologies, Carlsbad, CA, USA) using the 16S rDNA forward primer with the ABI BigDye terminator cycle sequencing ready reaction kit according to the manufacturer's recommendations (Applied Biosystem, Foster City, CA, USA). The sequencing data were analyzed using the basic local alignment search tool BLAST-n (http://www.ncbi.nlm.nih.gov/BLAST) or the RDP database [23]. Unequivocal identification was obtained using 16S ribosomal DNA sequences.

Genetic background grouping of *E. coli* strains

The genetic background grouping of the *E. coli* isolates was explored. The grouping was performed based on Clermont phylo-typing method [24]. The majority of the pathogenic extra-intestinal *E. coli* strains belonged to groups B2. In contrast, the commensal *E. coli* strains belonged to groups A, B1, C, and F. The strains were subsequently phylogenetically inferred based on the presence or absence of the gene markers as follows: For group A, arpA+, chuA−, yjaA−, and TspE4.C2−, for group B1, arpA+, chuA−, yjaA−, and TspE4.C2+, for group F, arpA−, chuA+, yjaA−, and TspE4.C2−, for group B2, arpA−, chuA+, yjaA+, and TspE4.C2−, for group A or C, arpA+, chuA−, yjaA+, and TspE4.C2−, for group D or E, arpA+, chuA+, yjaA−, and TspE4.C2−. A standard 25-μL PCR reaction was used to investigate the genetic background of the *E. coli* strains used in our

study. Illustra PuReTaq Ready-To-Go PCR beads were used in the PCR reaction (GE Health Biosciences, USA) as described by Clermont to amplify the arpA (400 bp) ChuA (288 bp), YjaA (211 bp), TspE4C2 (152 bp), and an internal control trpA (489 bp). Primers and PCR cycling conditions were described in (Table 1).

Detection of ESBL, ampC and carbapenemase genes

Global genotyping utilizing an oligonucleotide micro-array-based assay and PCR genotyping were applied to identify and confirm the presence of drug resistance genes. For the microarray DNA analysis (Alere Technologies, Jena, Germany) [15], the ESBL/AmpC/carbapenemase genes were evaluated based on the manufacturer's protocols (bla_{ACC}, bla_{ACT}, bla_{CMY}, bla_{KHM}, $bla_{MOX-CMY9}$, $bla_{CTX-M-1}$, $bla_{CTX-M-15}$, $bla_{CTX-M 2}$, $bla_{CTX-M-8}$, $bla_{CTX-M-9}$, $bla_{CTX-M-26}$, bla_{DHA-1}, bla_{FOX}, bla_{GES-1}, bla_{G1M-1}, bla_{MI-3}, bla_{IMP}, bla_{KPC}, bla_{LAP-1}, bla_{LEN-1}, bla_{MOX}, bla_{OXA-1}, bla_{OXA-2}, bla_{OXA-7}, bla_{OXA-9}, bla_{OXA-23}, bla_{OXA-23}, bla_{OXA-40}, bla_{OXA-48}, bla_{OXA-51}, bla_{OXA-54}, bla_{OXA-55}, bla_{OXA-58}, bla_{OXA-60}, bla_{PER1}, bla_{PER2}, bla_{PSE-1}, bla_{SHF-1}, bla_{SHV}, bla_{SEM-1}, bla_{SPM-1}, bla_{TEM}, bla_{VEB-1}, and bla_{VIM}). For the PCR analysis, DNA templates were obtained by boiling 500 μL of bacterial cells (OD$_{600}$ = 1.0) in a sterile single 1.5 mL Eppendorf tube in a water bath at 100 °C. The DNA lysate was diluted 1:10 with ddH$_2$O and frozen at −20 °C before use for bacterial genotyping confirmation with gene-specific primers (Table 2) [10]. The primers detected the β-lactamase genes and their variants (TEM, SHV, and CTX-M groups 1, 15, 2, 8, 9, and 26). The PCRs were performed using a 9800 Thermal Cycler (Applied Biosystem, USA) in a total volume of 25 μL containing 10 pmol of primers, 25 μmol of dNTPs, 10 μL of gDNA/plasmid lysate, 2.5 μL of 10X *Taq* buffer, 2.5 mM MgCl$_2$ and 2.5 U of *Taq* polymerase. The cycling conditions used for the PCR were an initial denaturation at 94 °C for 10 min, 35 cycles of 94 °C for 40 s, 60 °C for 40 s and 72 °C for 1 min and a final extension step at 72 °C for 7 min [10]. All PCR amplicons were fractionated by 1% agarose gel electrophoresis prior to staining with ethidium bromide. Images were obtained with a gel documentation system under a UV transilluminator.

Bacterial genotyping by multilocus sequence typing

Fifty-eight *E. coli* isolates were subjected to multilocus sequence typing (MLST) as previously described [25]. The MLST schemes used to type *E. coli* were conducted using internal fragments of the following seven housekeeping genes: *Adk* (adenylate kinase), *fumC* (fumarate hydratase), *gyrB* (DNA gyrase), *mdh* (malate dehydrogenase), *purA* (adenylosuccinate dehydrogenase), *icd* (isocitrate/isopropylmalate dehydrogenase), *recA* (ATP/GTP binding motif) (ID Genomics Inc, Seattle, WA, USA). The primers

The occurrence of ESBL-producing Escherichia coli carrying aminoglycoside resistance...

23

Table 1 Primer sequences and PCR conditions for quadruplex phylo-grouping of *E. coli*

Target gene	Primer sequence	Size (bp)	PCR conditions	Reference
arpA (phylogenetic grouping)	F (5-AACGCTATTCGCCAGCTTGC-3) R (5-TCTCCCCATACCGTACGCTA-3)	400	PCR reactions were performed in a total volume of 25 μL by ready-to go PCR beads using 20 pmol of each primers for all targets except arpA (40 pmol) and trpA (12 pmol). The cycling conditions were as follow: denaturation 4 min at 94 °C, 30 cycles of 5 s at 94 °C and 20 s at 59 °C, 20 s at 72 °C and a final extension step of 5 min at 72 °C	[24]
chuA (phylogenetic grouping)	F (5-GACGAACCAACGGTCAGGAT-3) R (5-TGCCGCCAGTACCAAAGACA-3)	288		
yjaA (phylogenetic grouping)	F (5-TGAAGTGTCAGGAGACGCTG-3) R (5-ATGGAGAATGCGTTCCTCAAC-3)	211		
TspE4C2 (phylogenetic grouping)	F (5-GAGTAATGTCGGGGCATTCA-3) R (5-GCGCCAACAAAGTATTACG-3)	152		
Internal control trpA	F (5-CGGCGATAAAGACATCTTCAC-3) R (5-GCAACGCGGCCTGGCGGAAG-3)	489		

Table 2 Multiplex PCR-specific primers for ESBL gene detection in *Enterobacteriacaea*

Primer name	β-Lactamase target	Sequence (5′–3′)	Length (bases)	Amplicon size (bp)	Reference
Multiplex I TEM, SHV	TEM variants including TEM-1 and TEM-2	Multi- F CATTTCCGTGTCGCCCTTATTC Multi- R CGTTCATCCATAGTTGCCTGAC	22	800	[10]
	SHV variants including SHV-1	Multi-F AGCCGCTTGAGCAAATTAAAC Multi-R ATCCCGCAGATAAATCACCAC	21	713	
Multiplex II CTX-M group 1	Variants of CTX-M group 1 including CTX-M-1, CTX-M-3 and CTX-M-15	MultiCTX-M Gp1-F TTAGGAARTGTGCCGCTGYA MultiCTX-MGP1-R CGATATCGTTGGTGGTRCCAT	20 21	688	
Multiplex II CTX-M group 2	Variants of CTX-M group 2 including CTX-M-2	MultiCTX-MGp2-F CGTTAACGGCACGATGAC MultiCTXMGp2-R CGATATCGTTGGTGGTRCCA	18 21	404	
Multiplex II CTX-M group 9	Variants of CTX-M group 9 including CTX-M-9 and CTX-M-14	MultiCTX-MGp9-F TCAAGCCTGCCGATCTGGT MultiCTX-MGp9-R TGATTCTCGCCGCTGAAG	19 18	561	
Multiplex III CTX-M group 8/25	CTX-M-8, CTX-M-25, CTX-M-26 and CTX-M-39 to CTX-M-41	MultiCTX-MGg8/25-F AACRCRCAGACGCTCTAC MultiCTX-MGg8/25-R TCGAGCCGGAASGTGTYAT	18 19	326	

used for amplification and sequencing are illustrated in (Table 3) [25]. The PCR amplifications were performed using a 9800 Thermal Cycler (Applied Biosystem, USA) with the following conditions: initial denaturation at 94 °C for 7 min, followed by 35 cycles of denaturation at 94 °C for 30 s and an annealing temperature of 56 °C for 30 s, extension at 72 °C for 2 min and a final 7-min extension at 72 °C. The PCR amplicons were checked with 1% agarose gel electrophoresis prior to purification for sequencing. Forward and reverse sequencing reactions were performed for every isolate. Different allele sequences were assigned for each locus with an arbitrary allele number for identification. Each bacterial isolate was characterized by a pattern of numbers defining its sequence type (ST). The sequencing data of the MLST genes were analyzed using the *E. coli* MLST Database (Warwick Medical School, Coventry, UK database; http://mlst.warwick.ac.uk/mlst/dbs/Ecoli) [25]. The similarities of the allelic profiles were assessed using the Molecular Evolutionary Genetics Analysis (MEGA 6) software.

Phylogenetic analysis

Phylogenetic trees based on the concatenated alleles of seven MLST genes were constructed using the Molecular Evolutionary Genetics Analysis (Mega6) software for the *E. coli* dataset. The maximum likelihood trees were based on neighbor-joining (NJ) starting trees with Nearest-Neighbor Interchange branch swapping. The tree stability was assessed using the bootstrap method [26].

Results

Bacterial identification and antibiotic susceptibility testing

All obtained clinical *E. coli* isolates (n = 58) were phenotypically studied using the Vitek system and the microbroth dilution method to determine the MIC values against various antimicrobial drugs (cefoxitin, ciprofloxacin, aztreonam, ceftazidime, meropenem, cefepime, cefotaxime, imipenem and ampicillin), (Table 4). The greatest number of *E. coli* isolates was resistant to ampicillin (96.61%), followed by cefotaxime (76.27%), cefepime (74.58%), ceftazidime (81.36%), aztreonam (89.83%), and

Table 3 Primers used to amplify and sequence the seven housekeeping genes in the _E. coli_ isolates for the MLST analysis

Gene	Primer sequences	Usage
adk	F 5′-ATTCTGCTTGGCGCTCCGGG -3′ R 5′-CCGTCAACTTTCGCGTATTT-3′	Amp/seq
fumC	F 5′-TCACAGGTCGCCAGCGCTTC-3′ R 5′-GTACGCAGCGAAAAAGATTC-3′	Amp/seq
gyrB	F 5′-TCGGCGACACGGATGACGG-3′ R 5′-ATCAGGCCTTCACGCGCATC-3′	Amp/seq
icd	F 5′-ATGGAAAGTAAAGTAGTTGTTCCGGCACA-3′ R 5′-GGACGCAGCAGGATCTGTT-3′	Amp/seq
mdh	F 5′-ATGAAAGTCGCAGTCCTCGGCGCTGCTGGCGG-3′ R 5′-TTAACGAACTCCTGCCCCAGAGCGA- TATCTTTCTT-3′	Amp/seq
purA	F 5′-CGCGCTGATGAAAGAGATGA-3′ R 5′-CATACGGTAAGCCACGCAGA-3′	Amp/seq
recA	F 5′-CGCATTCGCTTTACCCTGACC-3′ R 5′-TCTCGATCAGCTTCTCTTTT-3′	Amp/seq

cefoxitin (15.25%). Meropenem and imipenem had rates of 0%, and the non-β-lactam ciprofloxacin had a rate of 79.66%. All _E. coli_ isolates were sensitive to meropenem and imipenem (Fig. 1).

ESBL-producing _E. coli_ genotyping

The genotyping of ESBL-producing _E. coli_ isolates by the global analysis of an oligonucleotide microarray-based assay and PCR identified a high proportion of β-lactamase genes among the _E. coli_ isolates. The _bla_CTX-M1, _bla_CTX-M15, blaOXA1 and _bla_TEM genotypes were more frequently identified and were more predominant among the _E. coli_ isolates than the _bla_CTX-M, _bla_OXA and _bla_SHV variants. The prevalence was 46.7% for _bla_CTX-M1 and _bla_CTX-M15, 48.3% for _bla_OXA1, and 38.7% for _bla_TEM. The genotypic prevalence of _bla_SHV was 3.2% among all isolates, which was considerably lower than the prevalence for _bla_CTX-M1, _bla_CTX-M15, _bla_OXA1 and _bla_TEM. No carbapenem-resistant _E. coli_ isolate was detected (Fig. 2).

Distribution of ESBL genes in _E. coli_

The β-lactam genes were studied to evaluate the distribution of the genes among our isolates. We found that 13.7% (8/58) of the _E. coli_ isolates harbored four major ESBL genes (bla$_{CTX-M1}$, bla$_{CTX-M15}$, bla$_{OXA1}$, and bla$_{TEM}$) and 17.2% (10/58) contained three ESBL genes (bla$_{CTX-M1}$, bla$_{CTX-M15}$, and bla$_{OXA1}$). Additionally, two positive ESBL genotypes (3.4%; 2/58) contained bla$_{OXA1}$ and bla$_{TEM}$ and two isolates contained only bla$_{SHV}$ (3.4%; 2/58). No carbapenemase genes were detected among the isolates according to the phenotypic and genotypic testing.

The phylogenetic grouping of _E. coli_ strains

The genetic background grouping of the _E. coli_ isolates was assigned based on the Clermont method which is very specific for _E. coli_ phylo-typing groups [24]. It has shown that 46.55% (27) of the ESBL-producing _E. coli_ isolate collection belonged to group B2, and 6.9% (4) belonged to group D or E, while 12% (7) belonged to group B1, 3.4% (2) belonged to group A, 24% (14) belonged to group A or C and 6.9% (4) belonged to group F. The majority of the pathogenic extra-intestinal _E. coli_ strains belonged to groups B2 (Fig. 3).

Prevalence of genes associated with aminoglycoside resistance in the _E. coli_ isolates

The prevalence of genes associated with aminoglycoside resistance among the 58 _E. coli_ isolates was investigated. A total of 44.8% of the _E. coli_ isolates carried the _aac6_ gene, 43% harbored _aac6Ib_, 42% contained _aadA4_, and 36% contained _strB_; these prevalences represented high proportions and were more common than the other aminoglycoside genes (15% for _aadA1_, 12% for _aadA2_, 4% for _aadB_, 4% for _ant2_, 12% for _aphA_ and 1% for _strA_) (Fig. 4).

Bacterial genotyping by MLST

In this study, 58 _E. coli_ isolates were assigned sequence types (ST) and ST complexes (STc) using a standard multi-locus sequence typing method (Fig. 5) [25]. Of the 58 _E. coli_ isolates, 7 isolates (12%) belonged to STc 10, 20 isolates (34.5%) to STc 131, and 4 isolates (7%) to STc 648 and STc 38. Other ST complexes (46, 448, 156, 155, 23, 12 and 73) were represented by 1–3 isolates (2–5%). The ST complex could not be determined for 14 isolates (24%). A new allele of the _rec_A gene was identified in isolate ID 4. This allele had one nucleotide substitution compared to allele 2 at position 40 from the beginning of the allele (C substituted by T). The allelic profile of one isolate (isolate ID 12) was not previously reported (Fig. 5).

Phylogenetic analysis

We conducted a phylogenetic analysis to examine the clonal diversity and phylogenetic relationships among the _E. coli_ isolates. The _E. coli_ isolates clustered in several monophyletic clades that corresponded to known phylogenetic groups. The majority of the _E. coli_ isolates fell into the phylogenetic groups B2: ST131 (20 isolates), ST1193 (3 isolates) [27], ST73 (1 isolate), ST12 (1 isolate) and ST127 (1 isolate). In this study, four _E. coli_ isolates appeared to belong to group E: ST38 (3 isolates) [27] ST315 (1 isolate), of which all isolates were from STc 38. Of the rest, one isolate belonged to phylogroup A, thirteen to phylogroup C, eight to phylogroup B1, two to phylogroup C, and four to phylogroup F. Most of the known virulent extraintestinal strains primarily belong to group

Table 4 Minimum inhibitory concentration (MIC) values of antimicrobial agents against ESBL-producing *E. coli*

Strains	Cefoxitin (µg/mL) R ≥ 32 MIC	Cefepime (µg/mL) R ≥ 16 MIC	Aztreonam (µg/mL) R ≥ 4 MIC	Ceftazidime (µg/mL) R ≥ 16 MIC	Cefotaxime (µg/mL) R ≥ 64 MIC	Ciprofloxacin (µg/mL) R ≥ 4 MIC	Meropenem (µg/mL) R ≥ 4 MIC	Imipenem (µg/mL) R ≥ 4 MIC	Ampecillin (µg/mL) R ≥ 32 MIC
1059	8	32	256	128	1024	1024	<0.5	<0.5	>1024
1129	8	<0.5	<0.5	<0.5	<0.5	16	<0.5	<0.5	1024
1060	4	64	64	64	>1024	>1024	<0.5	<0.5	>1024
1097	4	64	128	32	>1024	<0.5	<0.5	<0.5	>1024
4110	8	8	128	16	64	32	<0.5	<0.5	1024
7055	1	16	<0.5	32	1024	1	<0.5	<0.5	>1024
1015	16	16	32	8	64	1024	<0.5	<0.5	512
2001	4	<0.5	128	64	1024	64	<0.5	<0.5	>1024
1114	8	256	512	128	>1024	128	<0.5	<0.5	>1024
1007	8	16	128	32	128	128	<0.5	<0.5	>1024
1111	256	128	128	128	>1024	64	<0.5	<0.5	>1024
1128	16	16	64	16	256	1024	<0.5	<0.5	1024
1005	4	4	64	16	1024	16	<0.5	<0.5	>1024
1116	8	16	32	8	>1024	64	<0.5	<0.5	>1024
1010	2	<0.5	<0.5	<0.5	2	32	<0.5	<0.5	>1024
1041	512	1024	>1024	1024	>1024	1024	<0.5	1	>1024
1089	8	128	128	32	1024	64	<0.5	<0.5	>1024
1031	16	32	128	32	256	32	<0.5	<0.5	>1024
1055	16	256	256	256	>1024	1024	<0.5	<0.5	>1024
1057	16	64	512	128	1024	1024	<0.5	<0.5	>1024
1075	8	8	512	64	32	64	<0.5	<0.5	1024
1065	8	128	512	256	1024	<0.5	<0.5	<0.5	>1024
1085	32	64	64	16	512	64	<0.5	<0.5	>1024
1053	16	256	512	128	>1024	1024	<0.5	<0.5	>1024
1054	32	256	256	128	>1024	1024	<0.5	<0.5	>1024
1013	16	16	64	32	512	16	<0.5	<0.5	>1024
1011	16	64	256	64	1024	1024	<0.5	<0.5	>1024
1034	16	64	256	128	256	128	<0.5	<0.5	>1024
1028	8	32	256	64	512	<0.5	<0.5	<0.5	>1024
1045	16	4	128	8	32	1024	<0.5	<0.5	1024
1118	32	32	128	32	256	1024	<0.5	<0.5	1024
1096	1	<0.5	>1024	<0.5	<0.5	<0.5	<0.5	<0.5	<0.5
1110	8	128	256	64	512	1024	<0.5	<0.5	>1024
1025	8	16	>1024	32	256	32	<0.5	<0.5	>1024
1016	16	16	128	64	256	16	<0.5	<0.5	>1024
4003	8	16	256	64	512	1024	<0.5	<0.5	>1024
90003	32	128	>1024	512	>1024	64	<0.5	<0.5	>1024
1020	128	<0.5	4	32	8	<0.5	<0.5	<0.5	>1024
1094	16	32	256	64	512	64	<0.5	<0.5	>1024
1019	8	128	>1024	512	>1024	64	<0.5	<0.5	>1024
1012	16	<0.5	<0.5	4	<0.5	32	<0.5	<0.5	8
2002	8	16	1024	32	256	32	<0.5	<0.5	>1024
4045	8	8	128	32	256	64	<0.5	<0.5	>1024
1081	8	32	256	32	512	1024	<0.5	<0.5	>1024
1018	4	32	128	64	1024	<0.5	<0.5	<0.5	>1024
3043	4	<0.5	<0.5	<0.5	<0.5	16	<0.5	<0.5	1024
1091	16	128	512	256	>1024	1024	<0.5	<0.5	>1024

Table 4 continued

Strains	Cefoxitin (µg/mL) R ≥ 32 MIC	Cefepime (µg/mL) R ≥ 16 MIC	Aztreonam (µg/mL) R ≥ 4 MIC	Ceftazidime (µg/mL) R ≥ 16 MIC	Cefotaxime (µg/mL) R ≥ 64 MIC	Ciprofloxa-cin (µg/mL) R ≥ 4 MIC	Meropenem (µg/mL) R ≥ 4 MIC	Imipenem (µg/mL) R ≥ 4 MIC	Ampecillin (µg/mL) R ≥ 32 MIC
3067	32	<0.5	16	64	64	<0.5	<0.5	<0.5	>1024
2003	16	64	256	64	512	4	<0.5	<0.5	>1024
1103	32	32	16	2	64	1024	<0.5	<0.5	>1024
1120	16	32	64	32	256	32	<0.5	<0.5	>1024
1119	8	64	256	64	1024	1024	<0.5	<0.5	>1024
1098	8	8	128	32	128	64	<0.5	<0.5	1024
1124	8	64	512	256	1024	32	<0.5	<0.5	>1024
1104	16	16	16	1	64	<0.5	<0.5	<0.5	>1024
1125	8	32	128	64	512	<0.5	<0.5	<0.5	>1024
1102	8	64	256	64	512	128	<0.5	<0.5	>1024
1117	16	128	256	128	1024	<0.5	<0.5	<0.5	>1024
1105	8	<0.5	<0.5	<0.5	<0.5	<0.5	<0.5	<0.5	>1024

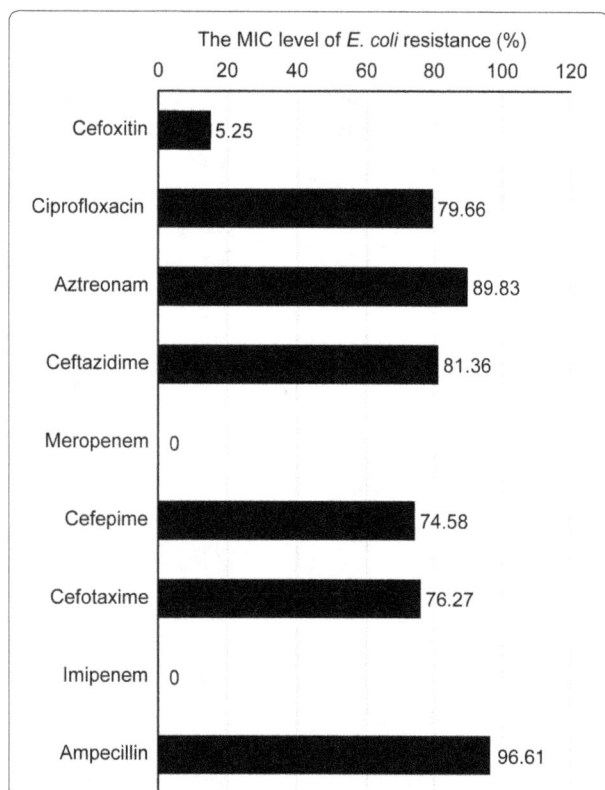

The MIC level of *E. coli* resistance (%)

Cefoxitin 5.25
Ciprofloxacin 79.66
Aztreonam 89.83
Ceftazidime 81.36
Meropenem 0
Cefepime 74.58
Cefotaxime 76.27
Imipenem 0
Ampicillin 96.61

Fig. 1 The level of *E. coli* resistance (in percentages) compared with the major ESBL drugs based on the MIC tests. No carbapenase phenotype was detected but Ciprofloxacin-resistance (fluoroquinolone resistance) was identified among the *E. coli* isolates

B2 and to a lesser extent to group D or E (4). Group A together with group B1, F, and C are considered predominant among commensal *E. coli* strains (5).

Discussion

During congested visitation seasons, especially during the religious pilgrimage (Hajj), the risk of spreading multidrug-resistant microbes increases substantially [28]. Therefore, this study investigated the prevalence of ESBL-producing *E. coli* in local general hospitals in Makkah during Hajj and the correlation between the ESBL phenotype and antimicrobial drug resistance using genotyping approaches. This study also explored multilocus sequence typing (MLST) to characterize these isolates and to enhance our understanding of the epidemiology of ESBL-producing *E. coli* in our region. Our data had demonstrated that our *E. coli* isolates exhibited varying levels of resistance to ESBL drugs and carried genes associated with aminoglycoside resistance. No carbapenem resistance genes were identified in any of the collected and investigated *E. coli* isolates (n = 58). All uropathogenic *E. coli* isolates in this study are classified as multidrug-resistant (MDR) according to the criteria by Magiorakos [29].

The distribution of ESBL-producing *E. coli* was consistent with the data obtained from an oligonucleotide microarray-based assay and PCR genotyping against genes associated with β-lactam resistance. The dominant sequence type lineage of the isolates was ST131, which is

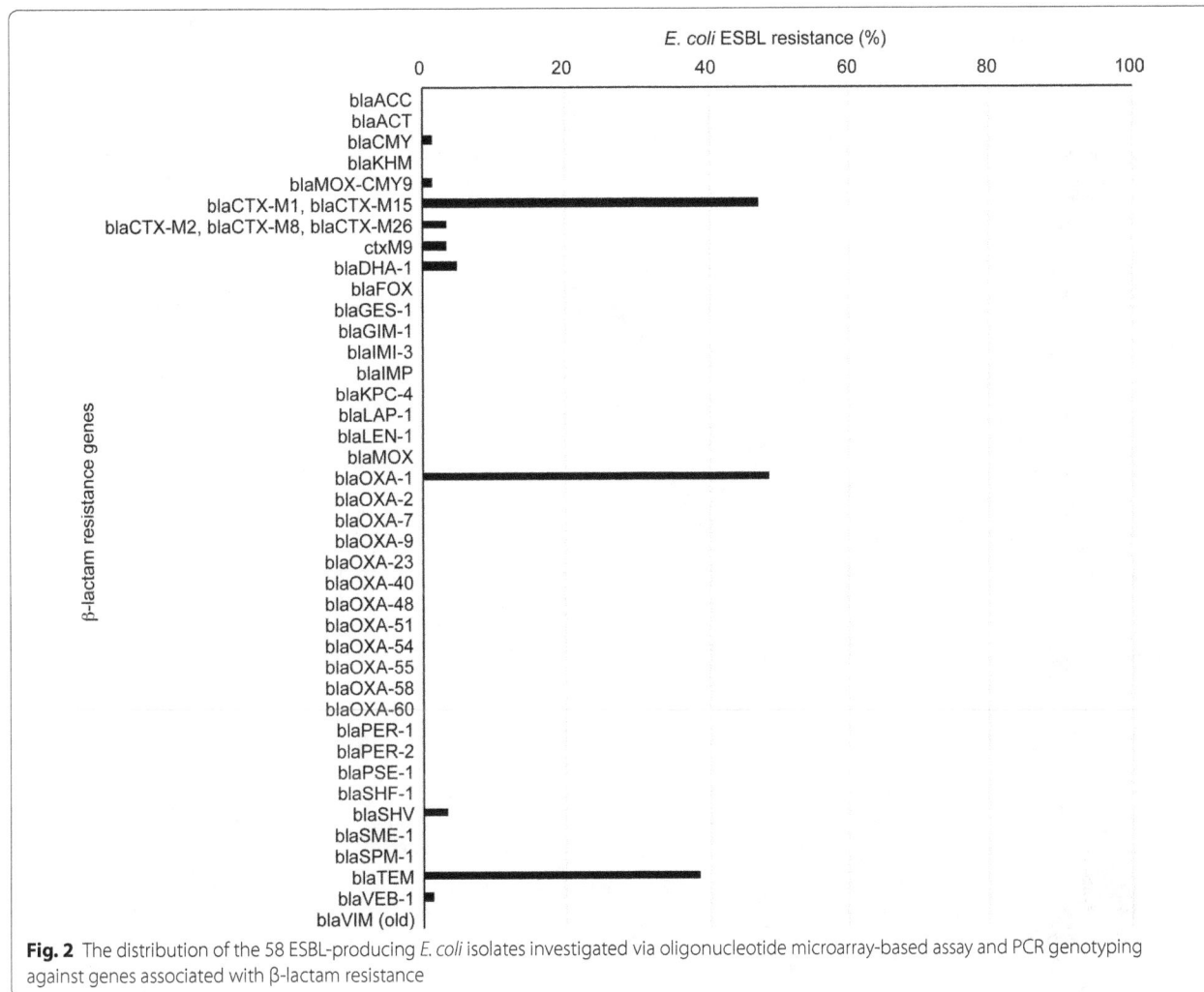

Fig. 2 The distribution of the 58 ESBL-producing *E. coli* isolates investigated via oligonucleotide microarray-based assay and PCR genotyping against genes associated with β-lactam resistance

the most uropathogenic *E. coli* lineage. The most commonly isolated bacterium from patients with urinary tract infections is *E. coli*. These isolates usually harbor different plasmids. Therefore, they have a tendency to acquire multidrug-resistant phenotypes and are difficult to treat.

Consistent with our study, studies have associated ST131/CTX-M15 human uropathogenic *E. coli* with ST410/CTX-M15, and ST648/CTX-M15. However, it was shown that ST410/CTX-M15, and ST648/CTX-M15 were also isolated from uropathogenic *E. coli* of cats and dogs (feline and canine) in Switzerland [30, 31]. These circulating STs may suggest that disease transmission between companion animals and humans may occur

by direct contact. Furthermore, three isolates of *E. coli* ST1193 were evident in this study. *E. coli* ST1193 is associated with urinary tract infection and fluoroquinolone-resistance, namely ciprofloxacin-resistance (Figs. 1, 5) [32, 33]. *E. coli* ST1193 may also be transmitted through household contact as suggested by a study from Japan [34].

It was demonstrated that multidrug-resistance (MDR) *E. coli* clone ST131 was globally disseminated in six different geographical countries. The rapid spread and emergence among countries may be due to high virulence factor gene-content, the presence of ESBL CTX-M-15, and fluoroquinolones resistance. Notably, the *E. coli* clone ST131 fluoroquinolone resistance phenotype was

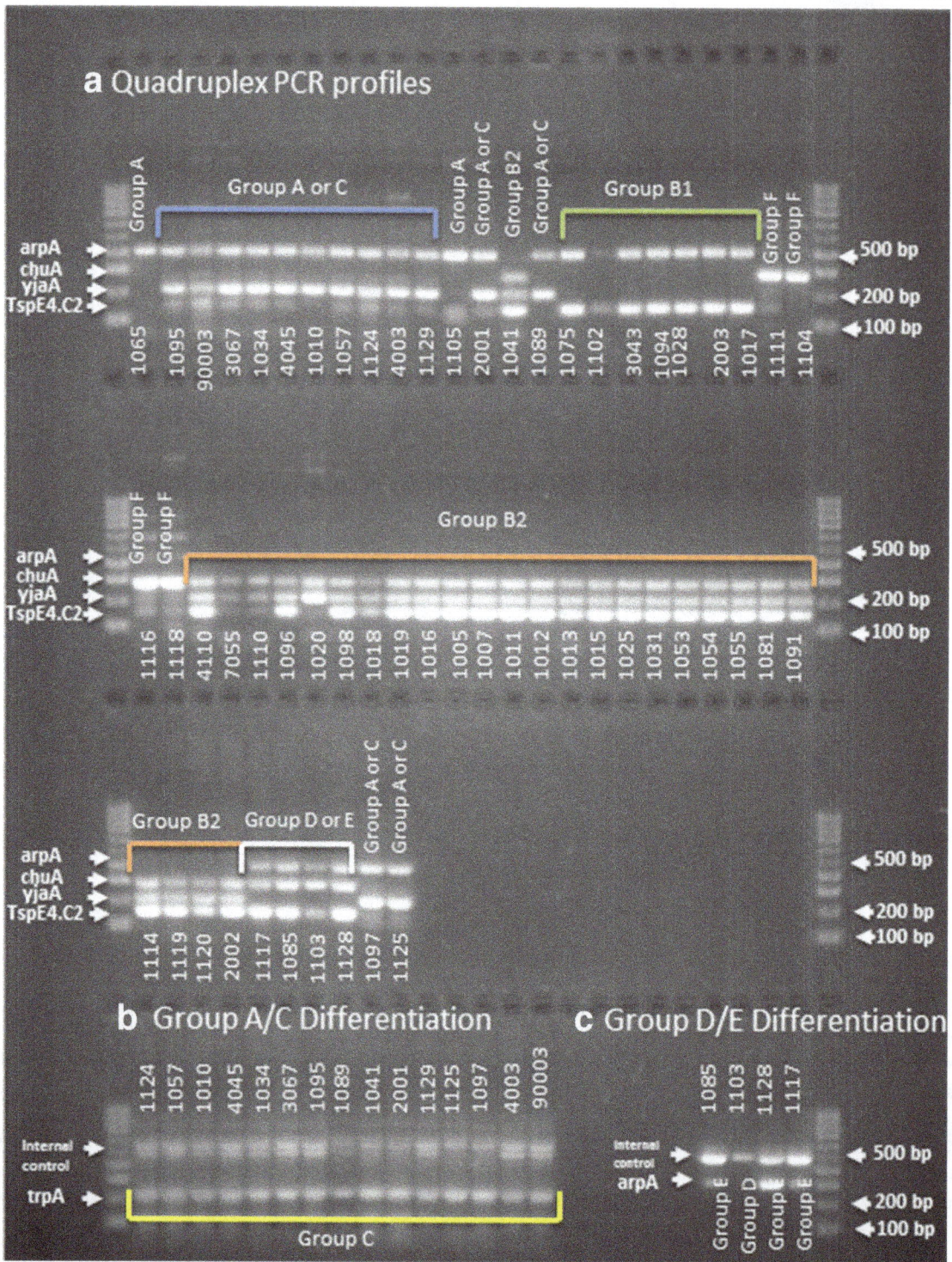

Fig. 3 **a** Quadruples PCR profiles of 58 *E. coli* MDR isolates. Isolate IDs shown under *each lane*. Data assignment were performed according to the presence or absence of signals of the following gene order arpA, chuA, yjaA, TspE4.C2. *Row 1, lanes 1, 12*—group A (+−−−); *lanes 2–11, 13, 15*—groups A or C (+−+−), lanes 16–22—group B1 (+−+), lane 14—group B2 (−+++), lanes 23–24—group F (−+−); Row 2, lanes 1–2—group F (−+−), lanes 3–24—group B2 (−+++) or (−++−) in lane 7; Row 3, lanes 1–4—group B2 (−+++), lanes 5–8—groups E or D (++−+), lanes 9–10—groups A or C (+−+−). **b** Groups A/C differentiation. In all *lanes*, both bands for internal control and Group C specific trpA fragment (219 bp) are present. **c** Groups D/E differentiation. *Lanes 1, 3* and *4*—both bands for internal control and Group E specific arpA fragment (301 bp) are present. *Lane 2*—only internal control present

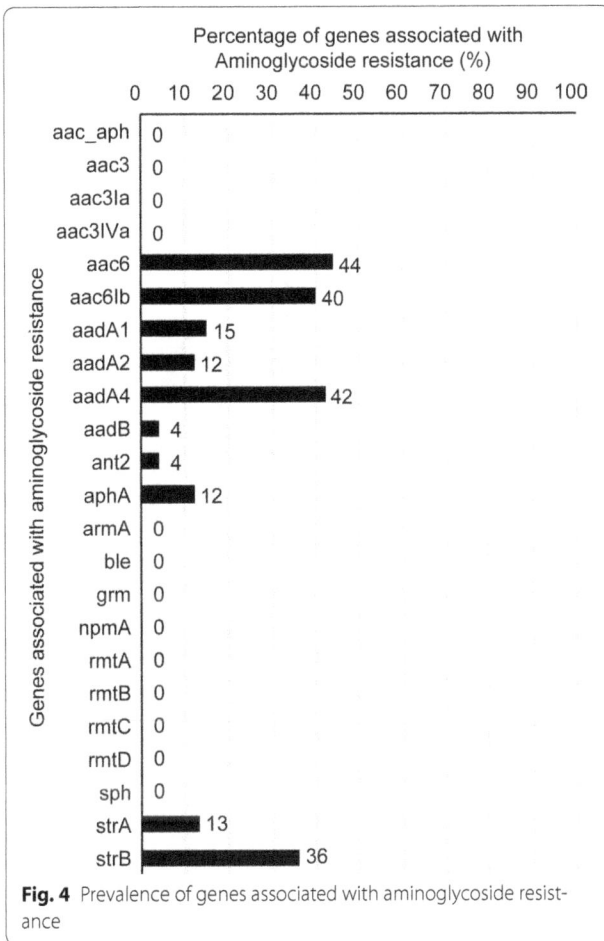

Fig. 4 Prevalence of genes associated with aminoglycoside resistance

the most prevalent geographically and was detected in this current study in Saudi Arabia (Figs. 1, 5) [35].

Studies have shown that pathogenicity island acquisition by uropathogenic *E. coli* may worsen urinary tract infections and aid in evasion of the host immune response, resulting in spreading in the bloodstream. Gene acquisition by intestinal pathogenic bacteria promotes their colonization in different intestinal regions; these genes may also alter the mechanism of bacterial-host interactions, causing distinct gastrointestinal pathology [27]. It was shown that a urinary sepsis niche for *E. coli* ST131 compared to bacteremia in non-ST131 *E. coli* clones [32, 36]. However, this niche could not be linked to the clinical manifestation of renal tract infections in

humans. No clinical focus to other sites of infection, such as intra-abdominal abscess, ascitic fluid, bones/joints, respiratory tract or bacteremia, has been established for the ST131 clone [37, 38]. There is evidence for a direct human-to-human route of transmission for ST131. For instance, an elderly father with pyelonephritis transmitted ST131 *E. coli* to his daughter, which initiated a similar illness in her. Similarly, an identical clone was identified from a young child with osteoarticular infection and a fecal sample from his mother [39, 40]. ST131 may contain genes for multiple antimicrobial resistance mechanisms, which may make therapy difficult. Carbapenems alone or in combination with amikacin were successfully used to treat infections caused by clones harboring CTX-M genes [32, 39]. A study demonstrated ESBL-producing *E. coli* acquisition among Makkah visitors after the Hajj (pilgrimage) season, especially CTX-M genes [28].

Molecular epidemiological studies have focused on the characterization and spread of the ST131 clone; however, global studies on the distribution and spread between humans and animals are limited, particularly in the developing world. There is a high frequency of infection by the drug-resistant ST131 clone in developing countries and a lack of timely countermeasures resulting in high morbidity and mortality rates [41–43].

Conclusion

In this study, 58 *E. coli* isolates were collected from patients with urinary tract infections from two local hospitals in the city of Makkah during the 2014–2015 Hajj (pilgrimage) season and screened for the production of ESBL/AmpC/carbapenemase/aminoglycoside resistance genes using phenotypic and genotypic analyses. Our data had demonstrated that our isolates primarily carried various ESBL and aminoglycoside resistance genes. The dominant sequence type lineage of the isolates was ST131, which was the most uropathogenic *E. coli* lineage. A genetic analysis of multiple isolates from the Middle Eastern regions may contribute to the development of rapid molecular detection methods and may lead to new therapies. Furthermore, controlling the endemicity of emerging MDR and decreasing the occurrence and prevalence of drug-resistant uropathogenic *E. coli* during heavy visitation seasons in the city of Makkah may involve the implementation of a stringent antidrug treatment policy.

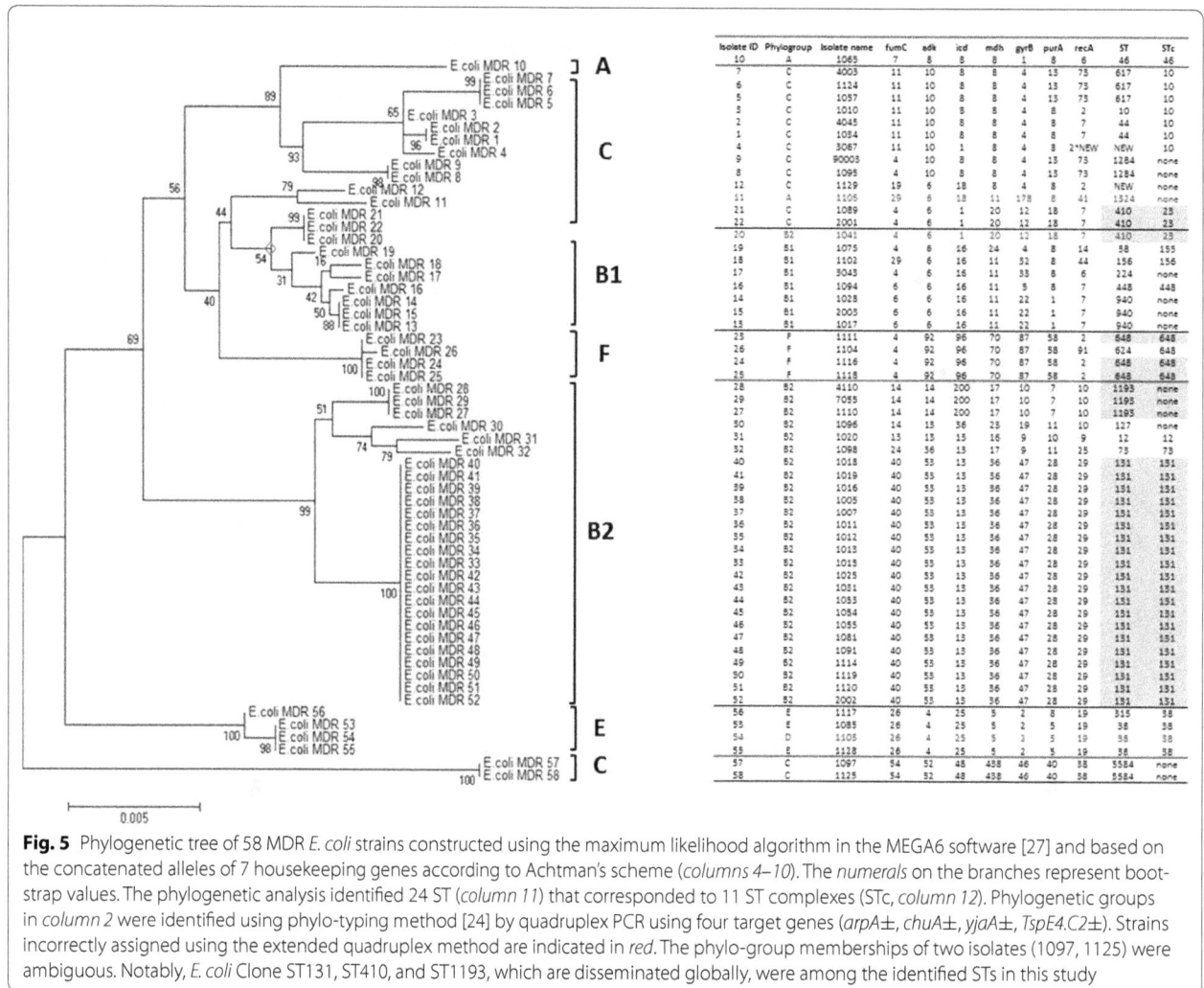

Fig. 5 Phylogenetic tree of 58 MDR *E. coli* strains constructed using the maximum likelihood algorithm in the MEGA6 software [27] and based on the concatenated alleles of 7 housekeeping genes according to Achtman's scheme (*columns 4–10*). The *numerals* on the branches represent bootstrap values. The phylogenetic analysis identified 24 ST (*column 11*) that corresponded to 11 ST complexes (STc, *column 12*). Phylogenetic groups in *column 2* were identified using phylo-typing method [24] by quadruplex PCR using four target genes (*arpA*±, *chuA*±, *yjaA*±, *TspE4.C2*±). Strains incorrectly assigned using the extended quadruplex method are indicated in *red*. The phylo-group memberships of two isolates (1097, 1125) were ambiguous. Notably, *E. coli* Clone ST131, ST410, and ST1193, which are disseminated globally, were among the identified STs in this study

Abbreviations

MDR: multi drug resistance; ESBL: extended-spectrum-β-lactamase; AmpC: AmpC beta-lactamases; MIC: minimum inhibitory concentration; MLST: multilocus sequence typing; ST: sequence typing; STc: sequence typing complex.

Authors' contributions

EA and AK contributed to the study design. RB, FB, MM, and ER collected the samples, and all authors contributed equally to the laboratory experiments. All authors contributed to the data interpretation. EA and AK drafted and revised the manuscript. All authors read and approved the final manuscript.

Author details

[1] National Center for Biotechnology, King Abdulaziz City for Science and Technology, P.O. Box 6086, Riyadh 11442, Saudi Arabia. [2] College of Medicine, Princess Nora Bint Abdul Rahman University, Riyadh 12484, Saudi Arabia. [3] Hera Hospital, Makkah, Saudi Arabia. [4] ID Genomics, Seattle, WA, USA.

Acknowledgements

All authors wish to acknowledge the Life Science & *Environment Research Institute and* the National Center for Biotechnology at KACST for supporting and facilitating this work.

Competing interests

All authors declare that they have no competing interests.

Consent for publication

All authors approve the publication of this work.

Funding

This work was funded by an internal grant from the Life Science & *Environment Research Institute and from* the National Center for Biotechnology at KACST.

References

1. Pitout JD, Laupland KB. Extended-spectrum beta-lactamase-producing Enterobacteriaceae: an emerging public-health concern. Lancet Infect Dis. 2008;8(3):159–66.

2. Knothe H, Shah P, Krcmery V, Antal M, Mitsuhashi S. Transferable resistance to cefotaxime, cefoxitin, cefamandole and cefuroxime in clinical isolates of *Klebsiella pneumoniae* and *Serratia marcescens*. Infection. 1983;11(6):315–7.

3. Philippon A, Labia R, Jacoby G. Extended-spectrum beta-lactamases. Antimicrob Agents Chemother. 1989;33(8):1131.

4. Drawz SM, Papp-Wallace KM, Bonomo RA. New beta-lactamase inhibitors: a therapeutic renaissance in an MDR world. Antimicrob Agents Chemother. 2014;58(4):1835–46.

5. Rawat D, Nair D. Extended-spectrum beta-lactamases in Gram Negative Bacteria. J Glob Infect Dis. 2010;2(3):263–74.

6. Livermore DM. Bacterial resistance: origins, epidemiology, and impact. Clin Infect Dis. 2003;36(Suppl 1):S11–23.

7. Antunes LC, Visca P, Towner KJ. *Acinetobacter baumannii*: evolution of a global pathogen. Pathog Dis. 2014;71(3):292–301.

8. Gupta N, Limbago BM, Patel JB, Kallen AJ. Carbapenem-resistant Enterobacteriaceae: epidemiology and prevention. Clin Infect Dis. 2011;53(1):60–7.

9. Kanj SS, Kanafani ZA. Current concepts in antimicrobial therapy against resistant gram-negative organisms: extended-spectrum β-lactamase—producing Enterobacteriaceae, carbapenem-resistant Enterobacteriaceae, and multidrug-resistant *Pseudomonas aeruginosa*. Mayo Clin Proc. 2011;86(3):250–9.

10. Dallenne C, Da Costa A, Decre D, Favier C, Arlet G. Development of a set of multiplex PCR assays for the detection of genes encoding important beta-lactamases in Enterobacteriaceae. J Antimicrob Chemother. 2010;65(3):490–5.

11. Trung NT, Hien TT, Huyen TT, Quyen DT, Binh MT, Hoan PQ, Meyer CG, Velavan TP, le Song H. Simple multiplex PCR assays to detect common pathogens and associated genes encoding for acquired extended spectrum betalactamases (ESBL) or carbapenemases from surgical site specimens in Vietnam. Ann Clin Microbiol Antimicrob. 2015;14(1):23.

12. Valverde A, Turrientes MC, Norman F, San Martín E, Moreno L, Pérez-Molina JA, López-Vélez R, Cantón R. CTX-M-15-non-ST131 *Escherichia coli* isolates are mainly responsible of faecal carriage with ESBL-producing Enterobacteriaceae in travellers, immigrants and those visiting friends and relatives. Clin Microbiol Infect. 2015;21(3):252.e251–4.

13. Tawfik AF, Alswailem AM, Shibl AM, Al-Agamy MH. Prevalence and genetic characteristics of TEM, SHV, and CTX-M in clinical *Klebsiella pneumoniae* isolates from Saudi Arabia. Microb Drug Resist. 2011;17(3):383–8.

14. Alyamani EJ, Khiyami MA, Booq RY, Alnafjan BM, Altammami MA, Bahwerth FS. Molecular characterization of extended-spectrum beta-lactamases (ESBLs) produced by clinical isolates of *Acinetobacter baumannii* in Saudi Arabia. Ann Clin Microbiol Antimicrob. 2015;14(1):38.

15. Braun SD, Monecke S, Thurmer A, Ruppelt A, Makarewicz O, Pletz M, Reibetaig A, Slickers P, Ehricht R. Rapid identification of carbapenemase genes in gram-negative bacteria with an oligonucleotide microarray-based assay. PLoS ONE. 2014;9(7):e102232.

16. Kitchel B, Rasheed JK, Patel JB, Srinivasan A, Navon-Venezia S, Carmeli Y, Brolund A, Giske CG. Molecular epidemiology of KPC-producing *Klebsiella pneumoniae* isolates in the United States: clonal expansion of multilocus sequence type 258. Antimicrob Agents Chemother. 2009;53(8):3365–70.

17. Salerno A, Deletoile A, Lefevre M, Ciznar I, Krovacek K, Grimont P, Brisse S. Recombining population structure of *Plesiomonas shigelloides* (Enterobacteriaceae) revealed by multilocus sequence typing. J Bacteriol. 2007;189(21):7808–18.

18. CLSI. Performance standards for antimicrobial susceptibility testing; twenty-fourth informational supplement (M100-S24). Wayne, PA: Clinical and Laboratory Standard Institute; 2014.

19. Weisburg WG, Barns SM, Pelletier DA, Lane DJ. 16S ribosomal DNA amplification for phylogenetic study. J Bacteriol. 1991;173(2):697–703.

20. Wilson KH, Blitchington RB, Greene RC. Amplification of bacterial 16S ribosomal DNA with polymerase chain reaction. J Clin Microbiol. 1990;28(9):1942–6.

21. James G. Universal bacterial identification by PCR and DNA sequencing of 16S rRNA gene. In: Schuller M, Sloots TP, James GS, Halliday CL, Carter IWJ, editors. PCR for clinical microbiology: an Australian and international perspective. New York: Springer; 2010. p. 209–14.

22. Srinivasan R, Karaoz U, Volegova M, MacKichan J, Kato-Maeda M, Miller S, Nadarajan R, Brodie EL, Lynch SV. Use of 16S rRNA gene for identification of a broad range of clinically relevant bacterial pathogens. PLoS ONE. 2015;10(2):e0117617.

23. Maidak BL, Olsen GJ, Larsen N, Overbeek R, McCaughey MJ, Woese CR. The ribosomal database project (RDP). Nucl Acids Res. 1996;24(1):82–5.

24. Clermont O, Christenson JK, Denamur E, Gordon DM. The Clermont *Escherichia coli* phylo-typing method revisited: improvement of specificity and detection of new phylo-groups. Environ Microbiol Rep. 2013;5(1):58–65.

25. Wirth T, Falush D, Lan R, Colles F, Mensa P, Wieler LH, Karch H, Reeves PR, Maiden MC, Ochman H. Sex and virulence in *Escherichia coli*: an evolutionary perspective. Mol Microbiol. 2006;60(5):1136–51.

26. Tamura K, Stecher G, Peterson D, Filipski A, Kumar S: MEGA6: molecular evolutionary genetics analysis version 6.0. Mol Biol Evol. 2013;30(12):2725–9.

27. Welch RA, Burland V, Plunkett G 3rd, Redford P, Roesch P, Rasko D, Buckles EL, Liou SR, Boutin A, Hackett J, et al. Extensive mosaic structure revealed by the complete genome sequence of uropathogenic *Escherichia coli*. Proc Natl Acad Sci USA. 2002;99(26):17020–4.

28. Leangapichart T, Dia NM, Olaitan AO, Gautret P, Brouqui P, Rolain JM. Acquisition of extended-spectrum beta-lactamases by *Escherichia coli* and *Klebsiella pneumoniae* in gut microbiota of pilgrims during the Hajj Pilgrimage of 2013. Antimicrob Agents Chemother. 2016;60(5):3222–6.

29. Magiorakos AP, Srinivasan A, Carey R, Carmeli Y, Falagas M, Giske C, Harbarth S, Hindler J, Kahlmeter G, Olsson-Liljequist B. Multidrug-resistant, extensively drug-resistant and pandrug-resistant bacteria: an international expert proposal for interim standard definitions for acquired resistance. Clin Microbiol Infect. 2012;18(3):268–81.

30. Huber H, Zweifel C, Wittenbrink MM, Stephan R. ESBL-producing uropathogenic *Escherichia coli* isolated from dogs and cats in Switzerland. Vet Microbiol. 2013;162(2–4):992–6.

31. Giufrè M, Graziani C, Accogli M, Luzzi I, Busani L, Cerquetti M: Escherichia coli of human and avian origin: detection of clonal groups associated with fluoroquinolone and multidrug resistance in Italy. J Antimicrob Chemother. 2012;67(4):860–7.

32. Johnson JR, Johnston B, Clabots C, Kuskowski MA, Pendyala S, DebRoy C, Nowicki B, Rice J. *Escherichia coli* sequence type ST131 as an emerging fluoroquinolone-resistant uropathogen among renal transplant recipients. Antimicrob Agents Chemother. 2010;54(1):546–50.

33. Rubin JE, Pitout JD. Extended-spectrum β-lactamase, carbapenemase and AmpC producing Enterobacteriaceae in companion animals. Vet Microbiol. 2014;170(1):10–8.

34. Kojima Y, Harada S, Aoki K, Ishii Y, Sawa T, Hasegawa K, Saji T, Yamaguchi K, Tateda K. Spread of CTX-M-15 extended-spectrum β-lactamase-producing *Escherichia coli* isolates through household contact and plasmid transfer. J Clin Microbiol. 2014;52(5):1783–5.

35. Petty NK, Zakour NLB, Stanton-Cook M, Skippington E, Totsika M, Forde BM, Phan M-D, Moriel DG, Peters KM, Davies M. Global dissemination of a multidrug resistant *Escherichia coli* clone. Proc Natl Acad Sci. 2014;111(15):5694–9.

36. Pitout JDD, Gregson DB, Campbell L, Laupland KB. Molecular characteristics of extended-spectrum-β-lactamase-producing *Escherichia coli* isolates causing bacteremia in the Calgary Health Region from 2000 to 2007: emergence of clone ST131 as a cause of community-acquired infections. Antimicrob Agents Chemother. 2009;53(7):2846–51.

37. Suzuki S, Shibata N, Yamane K, Wachino J, Ito K, Arakawa Y. Change in the prevalence of extended-spectrum-beta-lactamase-producing *Escherichia coli* in Japan by clonal spread. J Antimicrob Chemother. 2009;63(1):72–9.

38. Bert F, Johnson JR, Ouattara B, Leflon-Guibout V, Johnston B, Marcon E, Valla D, Moreau R, Nicolas-Chanoine MH. Genetic diversity and virulence profiles of *Escherichia coli* isolates causing spontaneous bacterial peritonitis and bacteremia in patients with cirrhosis. J Clin Microbiol. 2010;48(8):2709–14.

39. Lee MY, Choi HJ, Choi JY, Song M, Song Y, Kim SW, Chang HH, Jung SI, Kim YS, Ki HK, et al. Dissemination of ST131 and ST393 community-onset, ciprofloxacin-resistant *Escherichia coli* clones causing urinary tract infections in Korea. J Infect. 2010;60(2):146–53.

40. Ender PT, Gajanana D, Johnston B, Clabots C, Tamarkin FJ, Johnson JR. Transmission of an extended-spectrum-beta-lactamase-producing *Escherichia coli* (sequence type ST131) strain between a father and daughter resulting in septic shock and emphysematous pyelonephritis. J Clin Microbiol. 2009;47(11):3780–2.

41. Manges AR, Johnson JR, Foxman B, O'Bryan TT, Fullerton KE, Riley LW. Widespread distribution of urinary tract infections caused by

a multidrug-resistant *Escherichia coli* clonal group. N Engl J Med. 2001;345(14):1007–13.

42. Schaeffer AJ. Global molecular epidemiology of the O15:K52:H1 extraintestinal pathogenic *Escherichia coli* clonal group: evidence of distribution beyond Europe. J Urol. 2003;169(4):1612.

43. Oteo J, Pérez-Vázquez M, Campos J. Extended-spectrum β-lactamase producing *Escherichia coli*: changing epidemiology and clinical impact. Curr Opin Infect Dis. 2010;23(4):320–6.

5

Molecular characterization of penicillin non-susceptible *Streptococcus pneumoniae* isolated before and after pneumococcal conjugate vaccine implementation in Casablanca, Morocco

Idrissa Diawara[1,2]*, Abouddihaj Barguigua[3], Khalid Katfy[1,2], Kaotar Nayme[1,4], Houria Belabbes[1,2], Mohammed Timinouni[4], Khalid Zerouali[1,2] and Naima Elmdaghri[1,2]

Abstract

Background: *Streptococcus pneumoniae* is a major cause of morbidity and mortality worldwide, especially among children and the elderly. The ability to effectively treat pneumococcal infection has been compromised due to the acquisition of antibiotic resistance, particularly to β-lactam drugs. This study aimed to describe the prevalence and molecular evolution of penicillin non-susceptible *S. pneumoniae* (PNSP) isolated from invasive diseases before and after pneumococcal conjugate vaccine implementation in Casablanca, Morocco.

Methods: Isolates were obtained from the Microbiology Laboratory of Ibn Rochd University Hospital Centre of Casablanca. Serogrouping was done by Pneumotest Kit and serotyping by the Quellung capsular swelling. Antibiotic susceptibility pattern was determined by disk diffusion and E-test methods. The PNSP were analyzed by pulsed-field gel electrophoresis (PFGE) and by genotyping of *pbp1a*, *pbp2b*, and *pbp2x* genes.

Results: A total of 361 *S. pneumoniae* isolates were collected from 2007 to 2014. Of these isolates, 58.7% were obtained before vaccination (2007–2010) and 41.3% after vaccination (2011–2014). Of the 361 isolates, 80 were PNSP (22.2%). Generally, the proportion of PNSP between pre- and post-vaccination periods were 31 and 13% ($p = 0.009$), respectively. The proportion of PNSP isolated from pediatric and adult (age > 14 years) patients decreased from 34.5 to 22.9% ($p = 0.1$) and from 17.7 to 10.2% ($p = 0.1$) before and after vaccine implementation, respectively. The leading serotypes of PNSP were 14 (33 vs. 57%) and 19A (18 vs. 14%) before and after vaccination among children. For adults, serotypes 19A (53%) and 23F (24%) were the dominant serotypes in the pre-vaccination period, while serotype 14 (22%) was the most prevalent after vaccination. There were 21 *pbp* genotypes in the pre-vaccination period vs. 12 for post-vaccination period. PFGE clustering showed six clusters of PNSP grouped into three clusters specific to pre-vaccination period (clusters I, II and III), two clusters specific to post-period (clusters V and VI) and a cluster (IV) that contained clones belonging to the two periods of vaccination.

Conclusion: Our observations demonstrate a high degree of genetic diversity among PNSP. Genetic clustering among PNSP strains showed that they spread mainly by a restricted number of PNSP clones with vaccine serotypes. PFGE clustering combined with *pbp* genotyping revealed that vaccination can change the population structure of PNSP.

*Correspondence: diawaraidris@gmail.com
[1] Laboratoire de Microbiologie, Faculté de Médecine et de Pharmacie, Hassan II University of Casablanca, B.P 5696, Casablanca, Morocco
Full list of author information is available at the end of the article

Keywords: *Streptococcus pneumoniae,* Invasive pneumococcal disease, Penicillin-binding proteins, β-lactams, Serotypes, Antibiotic resistance, PFGE

Background

Streptococcus pneumoniae is a major cause of morbidity and mortality worldwide, especially among children and the elderly. Pneumococcal infections include serious diseases such as meningitis, bacteraemia, and pneumonia, as well as milder but more common illnesses, such as sinusitis and otitis media [1]. Disease rates and mortality are higher in developing than in industrialized settings, with the majority of deaths occurring in Africa and Asia. The ability to effectively treat pneumococcal infection has been compromised due to the acquisition of antibiotic resistance, particularly to β-lactam drugs [2].

Furthermore, antibiotic pressure, in combination with these horizontal recombination events, allows the acquisition of antibiotic-resistant genes or resistant strains which increases the resistance to a variety of antibiotics [3]. Pneumococcal resistance to β-lactams has been attributed to alterations of the penicillin-binding proteins (PBP) which reduce their affinity [4]. The first pneumococcal isolate resistant to penicillin was reported in 1967 from a patient in Australia [5], and resistant pneumococci have subsequently increased in prevalence worldwide. β-Lactam antibiotics exert their biological effects by interacting with the PBPs. PBPs are membrane enzymes that catalyze the polymerization and transpeptidation of glycan strands, during the assembly of the bacterial cell wall. β-Lactam resistance in clinical pneumococci is mediated by altered PBPs, specifically PBP1a, PBP2x and PBP2b [6, 7]. Penicillin resistance in *S. pneumoniae* is mediated by stepwise alterations of PBPs [8–10]. These three PBPs are considered to be the key targets for these agents and were therefore chosen for examination in this study.

In Morocco, the PCV-13 was introduced in the national immunization program in October 2010 in 2 + 1 schedule and replaced by the PCV-10 in July 2012. Before pneumococcal vaccine implementation in Morocco, the incidence rate of invasive pneumococcal diseases (IPD) in children aged to 2 years was 34.6/100,000 populations. The incidence rates of PCV-7, PCV-10 non-PCV-7 and PCV-13 non-PCV-10 serotypes were 18.0, 5.7 and 5.7/100,000 population in the same age, respectively [11]. In 2010, the use of the pneumococcal conjugate vaccine (PCV-13 and then PCV-10) dramatically reduced the prevalence of vaccine serotypes through active vaccination particularly among children less than 5 years of ages in Casablanca, Morocco. However, the introduction of vaccination was associated with a subsequent relative increase in non-vaccine serotypes [11]. This can be attributed to the phenomena of "serotype replacement", the expansion of preexisting NVT pneumococci, and/or serotype switching [12]. Vaccination has also reduced the incidence rate of antibiotic resistant serotypes, but we previously reported, a rebound due to the persistence of some vaccine serotypes like 6B and 14 [11]. Although several studies have described the genetic profile of the *pbp1a, pbp2b* and *pbp2x* genes in pneumococci from different countries [4, 13], actually, there are no studies on the characteristics of penicillin non- susceptible *S. pneumoniae* (PNSP) in Morocco.

This study aimed to describe the molecular evolution of penicillin non-susceptible *S. pneumoniae* isolated from invasive diseases before and after pneumococcal conjugate vaccine implementation in Morocco in 2010.

Methods

Bacterial strains, growth conditions and DNA extraction

Isolates, collected from 2007 to 2014, were obtained from the Microbiology Laboratory of Ibn Rochd University Hospital Centre of Casablanca (IR-UHC). All the non-duplicate invasive *S. pneumoniae* isolates recovered from patients, all ages included, during the study periods were included. Isolates obtained from normally sterile sites [cerebrospinal fluid (CSF), blood, pleural fluids, articular fluids or any other sterile site] were considered invasive.

The isolates were identified based on the typical colony morphology, Gram staining, optochin sensitivity test (Oxoid Company, Britain) on Mueller–Hinton agar plates supplemented with 5% sheep blood (BioMèrieux, Lyon, France) and bile solubility. The procedures employed for capsular typing and DNA extraction were previously described [14].

Antimicrobial susceptibility

Antibiotic susceptibility testing was done following Clinical Laboratory Standard Institute guidelines (CLSI, 2014). Erythromycin, tetracycline, chloramphenicol, and trimethoprim-sulfamethoxazole (cotrimoxazole), were tested by disk diffusion with antibiotic disks from Oxoid (Basingstoke, United Kingdom) on Mueller-Hinton Agar supplemented with 5% sheep blood (BioMèrieux, Lyon, France). A minimal inhibitory concentration (MIC) for penicillin G and ceftriaxone was determined on 5% sheep blood Mueller-Hinton agar with E-tests from Oxoid

(Oxoid, Basingstoke, UK). The breakpoints used for interpretation were those recommended by the CLSI in 2014. Quality control was conducted using *S. pneumoniae* ATCC 49619.

PCR- RFLP of *pbp* genes

Genetic polymorphism of the penicillin resistance genes *pbp1a*, *pbp2b*, and *pbp2x* of the penicillin-nonsusceptible isolates was investigated by restriction fragment length polymorphism (RFLP) analysis as described previously [15]. Briefly, we amplified a segment of 2.4, 1.5, and 2 kb of *pbp1a*, *pbp2b*, and *pbp2x* genes respectively by PCR. PCR amplifications were performed in simplex in a 25 µL reaction mixture containing 0.5 mM of dNTPs, 0.3 µM of each primer, 1× of PCR buffer, 2.5 mM of $MgCl_2$, 1U of Platinum *Taq* DNA polymerase (Invitrogen). The PCR cycle was 95 °C for 4 min followed by 30 amplification cycles of 94 °C for 1 min, 58 °C (*pbp1a*), 55 °C (*pbp2b*) and 60 °C (*pbp2x*) for 2 min, and 72 °C for 3 min; the final extension was 72 °C for 10 min. The amplification products were digested by restriction endonuclease *Hae*III and *Rsa*I and separated by agarose gel electrophoresis. Gels were scanned and analyzed by the Geldoc system (Bio-Rad). The different *pbp* genotypes received a three numbers code (e.g., x/y/z) referring to the RFLP patterns of the genes *pbp1a* (x), *pbp2b* (y), and *pbp2x* (z), respectively. As positive control for the three genes, we used 15 penicillin-susceptible *S. pneumoniae* (PSSP).

Pfge

PFGE was performed to determine the genetic relatedness among the same *pbp* genotypes of pneumococcus strains isolated before and after vaccination, following a standardized protocol developed by Bean et al. [16], Elliot et al. [17] and according to the recommendations of the pneumococcal molecular epidemiology network (PMEN). The gel images were processed and analyzed by BioNumerics Ver. 7.5 software (Applied Maths, Belgium). The images were normalized by use of standard molecular markers, and banding patterns were compared. Similarity analysis was performed using Dice coefficients and isolates were separated into similarity clusters by the unweighted pair group method using average linkages (UPGMA).

Statistical analysis

Data were analyzed with WHONET5.6, EpiInfo 7 (Centers for Disease Control, Atlanta, Georgia, USA) and Microsoft Excel. The Chi square test or Fisher's exact test was performed to compare proportion between collection periods. Differences were considered significant if the *p* value was <0.05.

Results

Prevalence of PNSP

A total of 361 *S. pneumoniae* isolates were collected from 2007 to 2014. Of these isolates, 58.7% were obtained before vaccination (2007–2010) and 41.3% after vaccination (2011–2014). Considering before and after vaccine introduction periods, isolates recovered from children (aged from 0 to 14 years) represented 54.7 and 41%, respectively. Of the 361 isolates, 80 were PNSP (22.2%). Consecutive PNSP, one per patient, were collected from blood cultures (43.5%), cerebrospinal fluid (40%), pleural fluid (4%) and other sterile body fluids (12.5%). Generally, the proportion of PNSP between pre- and post-vaccination periods were 31% and 13% ($p = 0.009$), respectively. The proportion of PNSP isolated from pediatric and adult (age $\leq$ 14 years) patients decreased from 34.5 to 22.9% ($p = 0.1$) and from 17.7% to 10.2% ($p = 0.1$) before and after vaccine implementation, respectively.

Of the 80 PNSP, according to CLSI breakpoints, we found co-resistance to other antibiotics: before vaccination, the proportion of PNSP resistant to cotrimoxazole was 66.7%, 40% to tetracycline, 21% to erythromycin and 5.1% to chloramphenicol and ceftriaxone. As for the post-vaccination period, among the 23 PNSP, 56.5% were resistant to cotrimoxazole, 47.8% to erythomycin and tetracycline, and 8.7% to ceftriaxone (intermediate susceptibility).

Serotype distribution among PNSP strains

Serotype distribution showed that vaccine serotypes and non-vaccine serotypes represented 90 and 10% among the PNSP isolated in children before vaccination; after, they represented 85.7 and 14.3%, respectively. In the adult population, vaccine and non-vaccine serotypes accounted for 82.4 and 17.6% before vaccination, while they represented 44.4 and 55.6% of PNSP after vaccination, respectively. The leading serotypes were 14 (33 vs. 57%) and 19A (18 vs. 14%) before and after vaccination among children. For adults, serotypes 19A (53%) and 23F (24%) were the dominant serotypes in the pre-vaccination period, while serotype 14 (22%) was the most prevalent after vaccination (Fig. 1).

pbp genotypes

A total of 10, 11 and 13 restriction profiles were found among the 80 PNSP strains after analysis of *pbp* gene by PCR–RFLP specific to *pbp1a*, *pbp2b*, and *pbp2x*, respectively (Fig. 2). For the 15 PSSP, control strains, we found only one profile for *pbp1a* while *pbp2b* and *pbp2x* presented different profiles with 4 and 3 profiles respectively (data none shown). *pbp* genotype of each strain was determined by combining the profiles of the three genes.

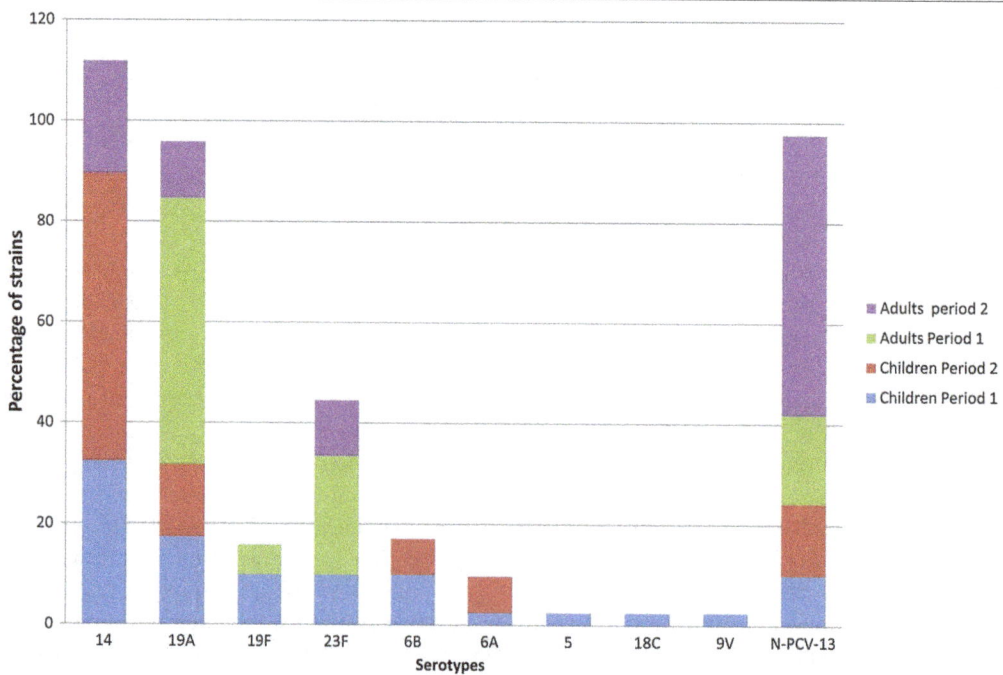

Fig. 1 Serotype distribution of the 80 penicillin non-susceptible *S. pneumoniae* isolated from IPD among children and adult, before and after vaccination in Casablanca, Morocco. Period 1 is the pre-vaccination period from 2007 to 2010 and Period 2 is the post-vaccination period from 2011 to 2014. The total number of PNSP was 40 and 14 strains for children, and 17 and 9 strains for adult, for period 1 and period 2, respectively

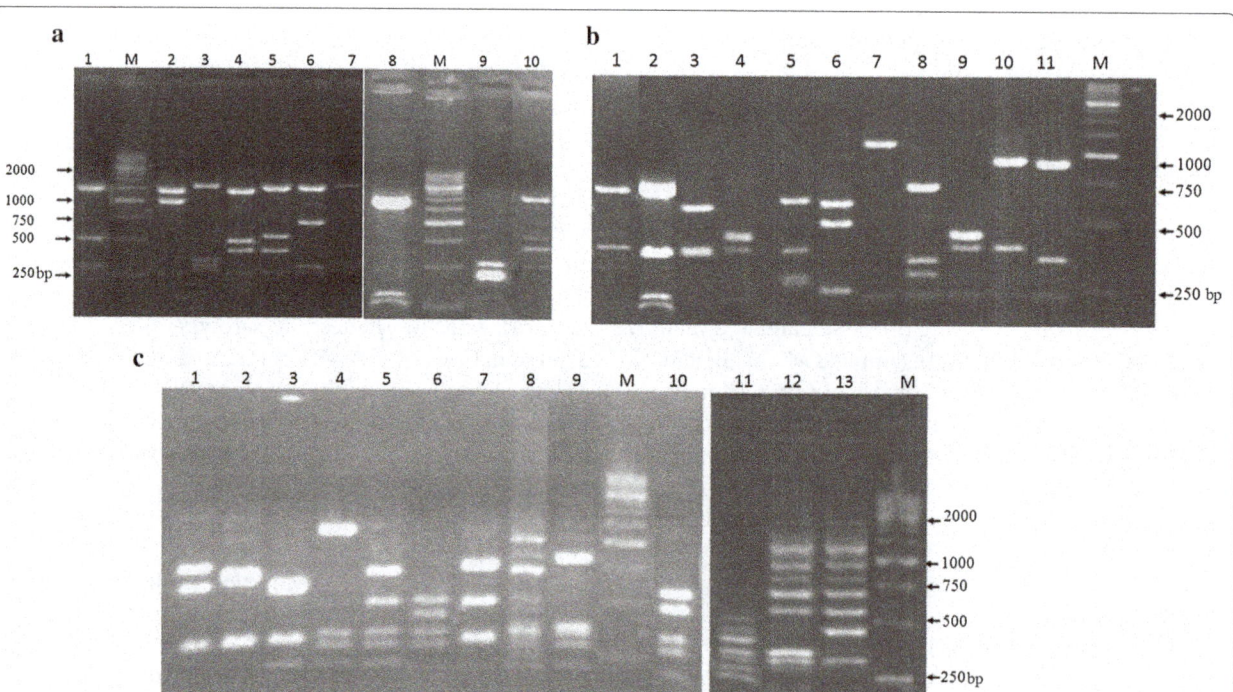

Fig. 2 PCR-RFLP profiles of the different *pbp* genes digested by *HaeIII* and *RsaI*. **a** Profile of *pbp1a* gene, *lanes* 1–10 correspond to RFLP profiles; **b** profile of *pbp2b* gene, *lanes* 1–11 correspond to RFLP profiles. **c** Profile of *pbp2x* gene, *lanes* 1–13 correspond to RFLP profiles. *Line M* corresponds to DNA size standards (250 base pairs)

This combination allowed to classify the strains collected in the pre-vaccination period into 21 different genotypes versus 12 for post-vaccination period. The different genotypes found during the two periods were illustrated in the Table 1. In general, the diversity of *pbp* genotype was associated to serotypes: serotype-dependent. This was highlighted for *pbp* genotype 1/5/1 associated to serotype 14 and for *pbp* genotype 4/2/5 associated to serotype 19A. However, several serotypes, grouped in a single genotype, were found in the two periods of vaccination.

A total of 58.3% (7/12) of *pbp* genotypes for the post-vaccination period were the same as those found in the pre-vaccination period. The dominant genotype in the pre-vaccination period was 4/2/5, carried by 16 strains of serotype 19A and one serotype19F. As for the post-vaccination period, the prevalent genotype was 4/2/2, carried

Table 1 PBP genotypes and serotypes distribution of the 80 penicillin non-susceptible *Streptococcus pneumoniae* isolated from invasive diseases in Casablanca, Morocco (2007–2014)

Genotype of pbp genes			Number of strains	MIC for PG (mg/L)	Serotype (number of strains)
pbp1a	*pbp2b*	*pbp2x*			
Pre-vaccination period					
1	3	7	1	1	23F (1)
1	*5*	*7*	*6*	*0.25–2*	*23F (2), 14 (2), 23A (1), 5 (1)*
1	*5*	*1*	*3*	*1–2*	*14 (3)*
1	7	7	1	2	9V (1)
1	9	6	1	2	14 (1)
2	4	6	1	2	14 (1)
2	5	7	4	0.5–2	14 (4)
2	*5*	*12*	*1*	*0.5*	*14 (1)*
2	5	8	1	2	19F (1)
2	5	1	1	2	14 (1)
2	7	8	2	0.5–2	6B (2)
2	*8*	*1*	*2*	*0.5–2*	*19F (2)*
3	6	9	1	0.25	23F (1)
4	2	5	17	0.125–0.5	19A (16), 19F (1)
4	2	2	4	0.5–1	24 (1) NT(2) 19F (1)
4	7	7	3	0.5	NT (3)
5	6	11	1	0.125–0.5	23F (1)
6	*3*	*3*	*2*	*0.125–0.25*	*6B (2)*
6	10	4	3	0.25	NT (3)
8	9	10	1	0.25	6A (1)
10	11	11	1	0.25	18C (1)
Post-vaccination period					
1	1	1	1	2	14 (1)
1	*5*	*1*	*1*	*2*	*14 (1)*
2	8	*1*	1	0.5	*19F (1)*
4	2	2	6	0.25–0.5	NT (3), 7F (1), 7A (2)
6	3	3	2	0.125–1	6B (1), 6A (1)
1	4	6	*1*	2	14 (1)
4	2	5	2	0.25	19A (2)
1	5	6	*1*	2	14 (1)
1	*5*	*7*	*5*	*0.5–1*	*14 (5)*
5	2	11	*1*	0.25	23F (1)
2	*5*	*12*	*1*	*2*	*14 (1)*
7	6	13	1	0.125	22F (1)

MIC minimal inhibitory concentration, *PG* penicillin G, *pbp* penicillin binding protein gene

Genotypes written in italics are those selected for PFGE typing

by 3 strains of non-vaccine serotypes, two strains of serotype 7A and one serotype 7F (Table 1).

PFGE pulsotypes

PFGE was performed to determine the genetic relatedness among the same *pbp* genotypes of pneumococcus strains isolated before (n = 12) and after (n = 8) vaccination. Isolates were assigned to the pulsed-field profiles designation as A1 to A12 for the 12 genotypes of the pre-vaccination period and B1 to B8 for the 8 genotypes of the post-vaccination period. The different pulsotypes as well as the associated genotypes are shown in the Table 2. Pulsotypes analysis of the pre-vaccination period, illustrated in Fig. 3a, showed a clonal and polyclonal dissemination of PNSP with 12 different pulsotypes. The pulsotypes A1 and A2 had a Dice similarity greater than 80% therefore belong to the same clone. These two clones belonged to the same serotype (serotype 14) and the same genotype (1/5/1). These clones were isolated only among children. Two other pulsotypes, A5 and A6, with the same serotype (19A) and the same *pbp* genotype (4/2/5), showed clonal dissemination among adults population.

A total of 8 pulsotypes were found among PNSP isolated during the post-vaccination period (Fig. 3b). Pulsotypes B3 and B4 constituted a single clone sharing the same *pbp* genotype and the both belonged to serotype 19A. This clone was present in both among adults and children. Pulsotype B5, B6 and B7 constituted a single clonal complex with the same *pbp* genotype and belonging to the serotype 14. This clonal complex diffused only among children.

The combined analysis of PNSP pulsotypes found during pre- and post-vaccination periods showed several clusters, as shown in the Fig. 3c. At the 60% level of Dice similarity, six clusters containing two or more isolates were found. The clusters I, II and III were specific to pre-vaccination period and clusters V and VI were specific to post-vaccination period. Interestingly, between these two cluster groups, there was the cluster IV that contained pulsotypes belonging to the pre- and post-vaccination periods. Analysis of this cluster showed that pulsotypes A6, B1 and A5, although present in the two periods, showed clonal dissemination before and after vaccination. However, while clones A5 and A6 are serotypes

Table 2 Pulsotype, PBP genotypes and serotypes distribution of penicillin non-susceptible *Streptococcus pneumoniae* isolated from invasive diseases in Casablanca, Morocco (2007–2014)

Pulsotypes	Genotypes of *pbp* genes			Number of strains	MIC of PG (mg/L)	Serotype (number of strains)
	plp1a	*plp2b*	*plp2x*			
Pre-vaccination period						
A1, A2	1	5	1	3	1−2	14 (3)
A12	1	5	7	3	0.25−2	23F (2), 23A (1)
ND	1	5	7	1	1	5 (1)
A3	1	5	7	2	1	14 (2)
A4	2	8	1	2	0.5−2	19F (2)
A2	2	5	12	1	0.5	14 (1)
A11	4	2	2	3	0.5−1	24 (1) NT (2)
A9	4	2	2	1	0.5	19F (1)
A6, A5	4	2	5	8	0.125−0.5	19A (8)
A5	4	2	5	3	0.125−0.5	19A (3)
A7	4	2	5	5	0.125−0.5	19A (5)
A8	4	2	5	1	0.125	19F (1)
A10	6	3	3	2	0.125−0.25	6B (2)
Post-vaccination period						
B8	1	5	1	2	2	14 (1)
B5, B6, B7	1	5	7	5	0.5−1	14 (5)
B1	2	8	1	1	0.5	19F (1)
B6	2	5	12	1	2	14 (1)
ND	4	2	2	3	0.25−0.5	NT (3)
B8	4	2	2	3	0.25−0.5	7F (1), 7A (2)
B3, B4	4	2	5	2	0.25	19A (2)
B2	6	3	3	2	0.125−1	6B (1), 6A (1)

MIC minimal inhibitory concentration, *PG* penicillin G, *pbp* penicillin-binding protein gene, *ND* not determined

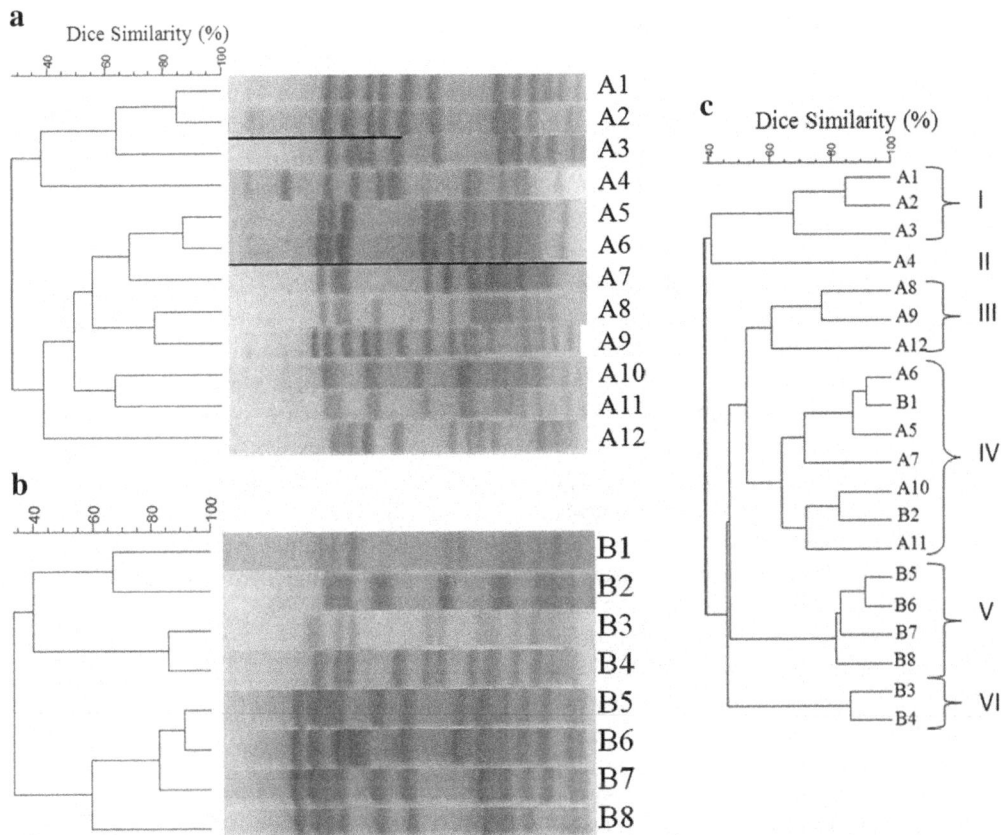

Fig. 3 PFGE dendrogram analysis generated by BioNumerics for Molecular typing of penicillin non-susceptible *S. pneumoniae* (PNSP).isolates. **a** PFGE dendrogram for PNSP isolated before vaccination (2007–2010). **b** PFGE dendrogram for PNSP isolated after vaccination (2011–2014). **c** PFGE dendrogram obtained by combined analysis of PNSP pulsotypes found during pre- and post-vaccination periods, the clusters at 60% of dice coefficient are from I to VI

19A, pulsotype B1 is a 19F. The Pulsotypes A10 and B2 also showed clonal dissemination between the two periods. These two clones belonged to serogroup 6 and had the same *pbp* genotypes.

Discussion

Antibiotic resistance in *S. pneumoniae* is a serious concern globally [18]. One of the added benefits of the PCVs in Casablanca has been the decline in *S. pneumoniae* antibiotic resistance, most notably for the PNSP and cotrimoxazole non-susceptible strains in children under 2 years of age, as reported elsewhere [11]. This is not surprising since the majority of serotypes associated with penicillin resistance in Casablanca are serotypes found in the PCV-10 and PCV-13. Although vaccination has reduced the incidence rate of antibiotic resistant serotypes, but the persistence of some vaccine serotypes constitutes a serious concern and needed to be analyzed.

This study describes the prevalence, serotype distribution, genetic diversity of *pbp* genes and molecular evolution of PNSP isolated in Casablanca before and after PCV-13 and PCV-10 introduction in Moroccan NIP. Vaccine coverage of PCVs vaccines in children aged to 2 years of age was estimated to 88% at the Grand Casablanca in 2014 as declared by the observatory regional of epidemiology service of health of Casablanca. The overall prevalence of PNSP was 22.2% from 2007 to 2014. This rate of resistance decreased from 34.5 to 22.9% and from 17.7 to 10.2% before and after vaccine implementation, among children and adults respectively. Significant reduction of PNSP occurred in several countries after the use of PCV [19–23]. The maximal level of resistance of PNSP responsible of IPD is relatively low with MICs = 2 mg/L compared to MICs of PNSP in many countries where MICs $\geq$ 8 mg/L were reported [4, 24]. Serotypes among PNSP were mainly 6B, 14, 19A, 19F and 23F in children and adults. These serotypes are included in the currently vaccine program (PCV-10) in Morocco except 19A. As previously published, resistance, particularly high-level penicillin resistance, is mainly associated with seven serotypes commonly carried in children: 6A, 6B, 9V, 14, 19A, 19F, and 23F [25].

Analysis of genetic diversity of *pbp* genes of these serotypes showed a high similarity between pre- and post-vaccine periods. Analyzes of genetic diversity have already been published [15, 26] but this is the first time that a study has analyzed this diversity before and after the introduction of PCV. The genetic profile of the *plp1a*, *plp2b* and *plp2x* genes shows that *plp1a* exhibited high genetic stability followed by *plp2x* and finally *plp2b* as shown by analysis of PSSP strains. However, genetic diversity of *pbp* genes showed that 58.33% of the *pbp* genotypes of post-vaccine period were the same as those found before vaccination. Furthermore, we found that *pbp* genotypes were closely related to serotypes "serotype-dependent". This close linkage is probably due to the position of the *cps* loci between *pbp1a* gene in upstream and *plp2x* gene in downstream [12, 27]. This configuration could promote co-transfer and a genetic harmony between serotype and *pbp* genotypes.

To study the same *pbp* genotypes found before and after vaccination, we used PFGE. The molecular epidemiology profile, as obtained by PFGE, showed that despite the genotypic diversity of the *pbp* genes in PNSP before vaccination, there was a clonal dissemination. The same situation was observed after vaccination. Thus, prior to vaccination, we found clonal dissemination of serotypes 19A and 14, where serotypes 19A had the same *pbp* genotypes. Depending to the level of penicillin resistance and to the type of *pbp* genotype, the clonal dissemination of serotype 14 was different to serotype 19A. These data suggest that the same PNSP clone can harbor different genotypes of *pbp* genes as previously suggested by Gherardi et al. [15] in the USA. The genotyping of *pbp* genes showed that several serotypes can belong to the same *pbp* genotype. One of the benefits of PFGE method was to differentiate these serotypes in different pulsotypes (clone), which showed a higher degree of resolution of PFGE compared to the genotyping of the *pbp* genes. The prevalence and distribution of serotypes among a population of pneumococci are an important consideration, especially in the context of post-vaccine period to evaluate vaccine efficacy.

In this study, PFGE clustering combined with *pbp* genotyping revealed that vaccination can change the population structure of PNSP. These findings suggest that probably, the clones specific to pre-vaccine periods was eliminated by large scale vaccination in Casablanca. For the clones specific to the post-period, they could be an emerging of new clones that escaped to the vaccination. As for the clones belonging to the clusters IV, they probably escaped to the vaccination and they remained before and persistent after vaccination. Molecular epidemiology study by whole genome sequencing will be the next step of the current study to corroborate our results.

Conclusions

This study investigated the prevalence of the molecular characteristics of PNSP causing IPD in Casablanca. Our observations demonstrated a high degree of genetic diversity among PNSP. Genetic clustering among PNSP strains showed that they spread mainly by a restricted number of PNSP clones with vaccine serotypes. PFGE clustering combined with *pbp* genotyping revealed that vaccination can change the population structure of PNSP. In Casablanca, as previously published, IPD are reduced by PCVs, this should normally result in a reduction of antibiotic prescription rate in children and adults. Limiting antibiotic prescription and large-scale vaccination using pneumococcal conjugate vaccines containing all vaccine serotypes would probably contribute to control this problem. Surveillance of antibiotic-resistant pneumococci in Casablanca should be continued in the era of multivalent pneumococcal conjugate vaccines, with due attention to the mechanisms of antibiotics resistance.

Authors' contributions

ID and NE conceived and designed the study. ID, KZ, KK and HB conducted the case surveillance and collected clinical data. ID and KN conducted the laboratory assays. ID, KZ, AB, and NE analyzed the data. ID, AB and KZ drafted the manuscript. All authors read and approved the final manuscript.

Author details

[1] Laboratoire de Microbiologie, Faculté de Médecine et de Pharmacie, Hassan II University of Casablanca, B.P 5696, Casablanca, Morocco. [2] Service de Microbiologie, CHU Ibn Rochd, B.P 2698, Casablanca, Morocco. [3] Laboratoire Polyvalent en Recherche et Développement, département de Biologie-Géologie, Faculté polydisciplinaire, Université Sultan Moulay Slimane, Beni Mellal, Morocco. [4] Molecular Bacteriology Laboratory, Institut Pasteur du Maroc, Casablanca, Morocco.

Acknowledgements

We thank all members of Bacteriology of Virology and Hospital Hygiene Laboratory, University Hospital Centre Ibn Rochd, Morocco for their collaboration. We would like to acknowledge Pr. Mohamed Benbachir for his generous scientific advisories.

Competing interests

The authors declare that they have no competing interests.

Consent for publication

All authors, participants (The patients/legal guardians) and partners agreed the publication of data presented in this manuscript.

Funding

This work was supported by an unrestricted, investigator-initiated grant from Pfizer (No. W1172148). The authors conceived the study and the study design was developed and agreed to by the authors without any input from the funding body. The study concept and design was peer reviewed prior to award of the grant from the funding body. The funding body was not involved in and, had no influence over, study design, data collection, data analyses, interpretation of results, report writing or in the decision to submit the paper for publication. All study data are held solely by the authors.

References

1. Organisation Mondiale de la Santé. Pneumococcal vaccines WHO position paper-2012-recommendations. Vaccine. 2012;30(32):4717–8.
2. Appelbaum PC. Resistance among *Streptococcus pneumoniae*: implications for drug selection. Clin Infect Dis. 2002;34(12):1613–20.
3. Song JH, Dagan R, Klugman KP, Fritzell B. The relationship between pneumococcal serotypes and antibiotic resistance. Vaccine. 2012;30(17):2728–37.
4. Zhou X, Liu J, Zhang Z, Liu Y, Wang Y, Liu Y. Molecular characteristics of penicillin-binding protein 2b, 2x and 1a sequences in *Streptococcus pneumoniae* isolates causing invasive diseases among children in Northeast China. Eur J Clin Microbiol Infect Dis. 2016;35(4):633–45.
5. Hansman DB. M. M. : a resistant pneumococcus. Lancet. 1967;2:245–245.
6. Ghuysen JM. Serine beta-lactamases and penicillin-binding proteins. Annu Rev Microbiol. 1991;45:37–67.
7. Hakenbeck R, Ellerbrok H, Briese T, Handwerger S, Tomasz A. Penicillin-binding proteins of penicillin-susceptible and -resistant pneumococci: immunological relatedness of altered proteins and changes in peptides carrying the beta-lactam binding site. Antimicrob Agents Chemother. 1986;30(4):553–8.
8. Nagai K, Davies TA, Jacobs MR, Appelbaum PC. Effects of amino acid alterations in penicillin-binding proteins (PBPs) 1a, 2b, and 2x on PBP affinities of penicillin, ampicillin, amoxicillin, cefditoren, cefuroxime, cefprozil, and cefaclor in 18 clinical isolates of penicillin-susceptible, -intermediate, and -resistant Pneumococci. Antimicrob Agents Chemother. 2002;46(5):1273–80.
9. Barcus VA, Ghanekar K, Yeo M, Coffey TJ, Dowson CG. Genetics of high level penicillin resistance in clinical isolates of *Streptococcus pneumoniae*. FEMS Microbiol Lett. 1995;126(3):299–303.
10. Cafini F, del Campo R, Alou L, Sevillano D, Morosini MI, Baquero F, Prieto J. Alterations of the penicillin-binding proteins and *murM* alleles of clinical *Streptococcus pneumoniae* isolates with high-level resistance to amoxicillin in Spain. J Antimicrob Chemother. 2006;57(2):224–9.
11. Diawara I, Zerouali K, Katfy K, Zaki B, Belabbes H, Najib J, Elmdaghri N. Invasive pneumococcal disease among children younger than 5 years of age before and after introduction of pneumococcal conjugate vaccine in Casablanca. Morocco. Int J Infect Dis. 2015;40:95–101.
12. Wyres KL, Lambertsen LM, Croucher NJ, McGee L, von Gottberg A, Linares J, Jacobs MR, Kristinsson KG, Beall BW, Klugman KP, et al. Pneumococcal capsular switching: a historical perspective. J Infect Dis. 2013;207(3):439–49.
13. Bogaert D, Syrogiannopoulos GA, Grivea IN, de Groot R, Beratis NG, Hermans PW. Molecular epidemiology of penicillin-nonsusceptible *Streptococcus pneumoniae* among children in Greece. J Clin Microbiol. 2000;38(12):4361–6.
14. Diawara I, Zerouali K, Katfy K, Barguigua A, Belabbes H, Timinouni M, Elmdaghri N. Phenotypic and genotypic characterization of *Streptococcus pneumoniae* resistant to macrolide in Casablanca, Morocco. Infect Genet Evol. 2016;40:200–4.

15. Gherardi G, Whitney CG, Facklam RR, Beall B. Major related sets of antibiotic-resistant Pneumococci in the United States as determined by pulsed-field gel electrophoresis and *pbp1a-pbp2b-pbp2x-dhf* restriction profiles. J Infect Dis. 2000;181(1):216–29.
16. Bean DC, Ikram RB, Klena JD. Molecular characterization of penicillin non-susceptible *Streptococcus pneumoniae* in Christchurch. New Zealand. J Antimicrob Chemother. 2004;54(1):122–9.
17. Elliott JA, Farmer KD, Facklam RR. Sudden increase in isolation of group B streptococci, serotype V, is not due to emergence of a new pulsed-field gel electrophoresis type. J Clin Microbiol. 1998;36(7):2115–6.
18. Linares J, Ardanuy C, Pallares R, Fenoll A. Changes in antimicrobial resistance, serotypes and genotypes in *Streptococcus pneumoniae* over a 30-year period. Clin Microbiol Infect. 2010;16(5):402–10.
19. Tan TQ. Pediatric invasive pneumococcal disease in the United States in the era of pneumococcal conjugate vaccines. Clin Microbiol Rev. 2012;25(3):409–19.
20. Demczuk WH, Martin I, Griffith A, Lefebvre B, McGeer A, Lovgren M, Tyrrell GJ, Desai S, Sherrard L, Adam H, et al. Serotype distribution of invasive *Streptococcus pneumoniae* in Canada after the introduction of the 13-valent pneumococcal conjugate vaccine, 2010–2012. Can J Microbiol. 2013;59(12):778–88.
21. von Gottberg A, de Gouveia L, Tempia S, Quan V, Meiring S, von Mollendorf C, Madhi SA, Zell ER, Verani JR, O'Brien KL, et al. Effects of vaccination on invasive pneumococcal disease in South Africa. N Engl J Med. 2014;371(20):1889–99.
22. Richter SS, Heilmann KP, Dohrn CL, Riahi F, Diekema DJ, Doern GV. Pneumococcal serotypes before and after introduction of conjugate vaccines, United States, 1999-2011(1.). Emerg Infect Dis. 2013;19(7):1074–83.
23. dos Santos SR, Passadore LF, Takagi EH, Fujii CM, Yoshioka CR, Gilio AE, Martinez MB. Serotype distribution of *Streptococcus pneumoniae* isolated from patients with invasive pneumococcal disease in Brazil before and after ten-pneumococcal conjugate vaccine implementation. Vaccine. 2013;31(51):6150–4.
24. Liu EY, Chang JC, Lin JC, Chang FY, Fung CP. Important Mutations contributing to high-level penicillin resistance in Taiwan19F-14, Taiwan23F-15, and Spain23F-1 of *Streptococcus pneumoniae* Isolated from Taiwan. Microb Drug Resist. 2016;22(8):646–54.
25. Dagan R, Klugman KP. Impact of conjugate pneumococcal vaccines on antibiotic resistance. Lancet Infect Dis. 2008;8(12):785–95.
26. Yee EK, Melkerson-Watson LJ, Bloch CA, Pierson CL, Blackwood RA. Genomic analysis of penicillin-resistant *Streptococcus pneumoniae* in Southeastern Michigan. J Infect. 2004;49(2):126–35.
27. Hakenbeck R, Kaminski K, Konig A, van der Linden M, Paik J, Reichmann P, Zahner D. Penicillin-binding proteins in beta-lactam-resistant *Streptococcus pneumoniae*. Microb Drug Resist. 1999;5(2):91–9.

6

Comparison of methods for the identification of microorganisms isolated from blood cultures

Aydir Cecília Marinho Monteiro[1], Carlos Magno Castelo Branco Fortaleza[2], Adriano Martison Ferreira[3], Ricardo de Souza Cavalcante[4], Alessandro Lia Mondelli[5], Eduardo Bagagli[1] and Maria de Lourdes Ribeiro de Souza da Cunha[1,2]*

Abstract

Background: Bloodstream infections are responsible for thousands of deaths each year. The rapid identification of the microorganisms causing these infections permits correct therapeutic management that will improve the prognosis of the patient. In an attempt to reduce the time spent on this step, microorganism identification devices have been developed, including the VITEK® 2 system, which is currently used in routine clinical microbiology laboratories.

Methods: This study evaluated the accuracy of the VITEK® 2 system in the identification of 400 microorganisms isolated from blood cultures and compared the results to those obtained with conventional phenotypic and genotypic methods. In parallel to the phenotypic identification methods, the DNA of these microorganisms was extracted directly from the blood culture bottles for genotypic identification by the polymerase chain reaction (PCR) and DNA sequencing.

Results: The automated VITEK® 2 system correctly identified 94.7 % (379/400) of the isolates. The YST and GN cards resulted in 100 % correct identifications of yeasts (15/15) and Gram-negative bacilli (165/165), respectively. The GP card correctly identified 92.6 % (199/215) of Gram-positive cocci, while the ANC card was unable to correctly identify any Gram-positive bacilli (0/5).

Conclusions: The performance of the VITEK® 2 system was considered acceptable and statistical analysis showed that the system is a suitable option for routine clinical microbiology laboratories to identify different microorganisms.

Keywords: Blood culture, Phenotypic identification, Genotypic identification, Automated VITEK® 2 system

Background

Sepsis is a global health problem and an estimated 17 million cases of sepsis occur each year in the world [1]. The early initiation of appropriate antibiotic therapy is determinant for the prognosis and survival of patients with bloodstream infections [2]. Patients receiving antibiotic therapy that is adapted based on the susceptibility profile of the infectious agent isolated from blood cultures exhibit lower mortality than those treated initially with inadequate antibiotic therapy [3]. In addition, technological advances that permit the rapid and reliable identification of most pathogens involved in infectious diseases have long been recognized to have clinical benefits, including shorter hospital stays and lower mortality, as well as financial benefits by reducing healthcare costs [4].

The objective of this study was to evaluate the sensitivity of the VITEK® 2 system, a system that automatically performs the processes required for microorganism identification and for the determination of antimicrobial susceptibility using a standard primary inoculum isolated from subcultures of positive

*Correspondence: cunhamlr@ibb.unresp.br
[1] Departamento de Microbiologia e Imunologia, Instituto de Biociências de Botucatu, UNESP–Univ. Estadual Paulista, Distrito de Rubião Junior, s/n, Botucatu, SP CEP: 18618-970, Brazil
Full list of author information is available at the end of the article

blood cultures. Although classical identification methods are still considered the gold standard, these methods are slow, time consuming and prone to subjective interpretations. On the other hand, the VITEK® 2 system reduces the time necessary for identification and permits the standardization of inter- and intra-laboratory results, the storage of results, issuing rapid epidemiological reports, and simultaneous identification and antimicrobial susceptibility testing; however, the system is poorly efficient in identifying certain species of Gram-positive cocci [42].

Studies using direct inoculation of VITEK® 2 cards from blood culture bottles have been conducted in an attempt to further reduce the time of identification of microorganisms that cause bloodstream infections, but the results were acceptable only for Gram-negative bacilli and were inaccurate for Gram-positive cocci [5, 6]. For this reason, the present study used inocula of microorganisms cultured previously on solid media for 24 h.

The difference of this study was the prospective evaluation of the VITEK® 2 system during the routine work of a clinical microbiology laboratory in a university hospital using 400 microorganisms isolated from blood cultures collected during the hospitalization period of patients rather than to conduct a retrospective study of samples stored for years.

Methods
Isolates studied
Four hundred microorganisms isolated from positive blood cultures of patients hospitalized in intensive care units of the Botucatu University Hospital between August 2012 and February 2014 were identified. The blood samples were inoculated into blood culture bottles and incubated in the BACTEC™ 9050 apparatus.

Identification of microorganisms in positive blood cultures
Automated phenotypic identification
Samples exhibiting microbial growth were submitted to Gram staining and cultured on solid media directly from the blood culture bottles. After subculture on blood and MacConkey agar, the isolates were inoculated into the following specific identification cards of the automated VITEK® 2 system using the standard protocol: Gram-positive cocci (GP), Gram-positive bacilli (GN), Gram-negative bacilli (ANC), and yeasts (YST). Gram-positive cocci, Gram-positive bacilli and yeast were inoculated into the cards from colonies grown on blood agar and Gram-negative bacilli from colonies grown on Mac-Conkey agar, all diluted in saline (0.9 % NaCl) to a 0.5 McFarland standard.

Phenotypic identification by conventional methods
Phenotypic identification consisted of Gram staining for the observation of morphology and specific staining, followed by a series of biochemical tests specific for each group of microorganisms. Gram-positive cocci were submitted to the catalase test for differentiation between *Staphylococcus* and *Enterococcus*. The following biochemical test battery was used for the identification of species of the genus *Staphylococcus*: coagulase, sugar fermentation (sucrose, maltose, trehalose, xylose, and mannitol), anaerobic growth on semi-solid sodium thioglycolate medium and, if necessary, ornithine and urease production and novobiocin susceptibility [7]. Isolates previously identified as Gram-positive, catalase-negative, bile esculin-positive, NaCl-positive (growth in brain heart infusion broth with 6.5 % NaCl) and pyrrolidonyl-aminopeptidase test-positive cocci were submitted to biochemical tests of fermentation of mannitol, arabinose, arginine and sorbitol, motility, and presence or absence of a pigment on sheep blood agar. Gram-negative bacilli were first tested for glucose fermentation. Glucose-fermenting bacilli were submitted to manual biochemical tests known as EPM/MILi/Citrate, an identification system based on the following tests: production of H_2S, urease and L-tryptophan desaminase; motility; indol production; lysine decarboxylase production, and the ability to use citrate as a single carbon source. Non-glucose-fermenting Gram-negative bacilli were identified based on motility, growth at a temperature of 42 °C, and production of DNAse. Yeasts were isolated on Sabouraud agar, replated on CHROMagar, and identified based on the color, texture and shape of their colonies [8].

DNA extraction from the isolates
Extraction of bacterial DNA Bacterial DNA was extracted directly from the blood sample of the blood culture bottle using the Illustra Kit (GE Healthcare) according to the protocol of the manufacturer, with modifications in the first centrifugation [9] and the addition of 800 μL benzyl alcohol [10]. For sample collection, the lid of the blood culture bottle was first disinfected with cotton soaked in 70 % alcohol. Next, 1.5 mL of the culture was aspirated with a sterile needle and syringe and transferred to sterile microtubes. The microtubes were centrifuged at 850g for 2 min and the supernatant was removed by aspiration with a micropipette and sterile tips and the supernatant stored (directly in a DNA-free microtube) at −20 °C until the time of extraction.

For DNA extraction, the sample was centrifuged at 10,000g for 1 min, the supernatant was discarded, and 500 μL lysozyme was added to the sediment. The mixture was vortexed, 800 μL benzyl alcohol was added, and the mixture was again shaken and centrifuged at 7000g for 5 min. Next, 300 μL of the supernatant was carefully removed and transferred to a new sterile microtube (which was used for extraction). Ten microliter lysozyme (10 mg/mL) was added and the microtube was left to stand at room temperature for 15 min, with vortexing every 5 min. After this period, 10 μL proteinase K (20 mg/mL) was added and the mixture was vortexed. The microtube was incubated for 15 min at 56 °C, with vortexing every 5 min. This mixture was then transferred to an extraction microcolumn and centrifuged at 11,000g for 1 min. The filtrate was discarded and 500 μL washing solution was added to the microcolumn. The column was again centrifuged at 11,000g for 3 min. The supernatant was discarded, the microcolumn was transferred to a new sterile microtube, and 200 μL Milli-Q water previously heated to 70 °C was added. The microcolumn was kept at room temperature for 1 min and centrifuged at 11,000g for 1 min. The columns were discarded and the filtered material was frozen until analysis by the polymerase chain reaction (PCR).

Extraction of yeast DNA   Yeast DNA was extracted according to the protocol proposed by McCullough et al. [11]. The isolates were seeded onto inclined Sabouraud agar and incubated for 36 h at 37 °C. A loopful of this culture was resuspended in a 2-mL tube containing 1 mL 1 M sorbitol, 125 mM EDTA, and 500 mg glass beads. The tube was shaken twice in a Precellys® homogenizer for 45 s and centrifuged at 13,000g for 10 min. The supernatant was discarded and the sediment together with the glass beads was resuspended in 500 μL of a buffer solution containing 50 mM Tris–HCl, 50 mM EDTA and 2 % SDS and incubated for 1 h at 65 °C. After incubation, 500 μL 3 M sodium acetate was added. The mixture was homogenized by inverting the tube and kept on ice for 2 h, followed by centrifugation for 10 min at 25 °C. The supernatant was transferred to a 1.5-mL centrifugation microtube containing 1 mL ice-cold absolute ethanol, homogenized by inversion, and centrifuged for 10 min at 4 °C. The supernatant was discarded and the DNA retained on the tube wall was resuspended in 50 μL autoclaved Milli-Q water and frozen until the time of PCR.

Genotypic identification of the isolates

Polymerase chain reaction of bacteria   Gram-positive bacteria of the genus *Staphylococcus* that belonged to the group of coagulase-negative staphylococci (CoNS) were identified by internal transcribed spacer PCR (ITS-PCR) using primers targeting conserved sequences adjacent to the 16S and 23S genes: G1 (5′-GAAGTCGT AACAAGG-3′) and L1 (5′-CAAGGCATCCACCGT-3′) [12, 13].

The remaining isolates of Gram-positive cocci and Gram-negative bacilli were submitted to PCR carried out in 0.2-mL microtubes containing 15.8 μL Milli-Q water, 10 pM of the forward primer and 10 pM of the reverse primer, 100 μM triphosphate desoxyribonucleotides (GE Healthcare), 10 U Taq DNA polymerase (Biotools), 20 mM MgCl$_2$-free buffer (Biotools), 0.75 mM MgCl$_2$ (Biotools), and 3 μL DNA. Primers targeting conserved sequences of each species were used for DNA amplification. The temperature and time parameters and number of amplification cycles reported in the literature and described in Table 1 were used.

The efficiency of the amplifications was monitored by electrophoresis on 2 % agarose gel prepared in 1× TBE buffer (89 mM Tris (pH 7.6), 89 mM boric acid, and 2 mM EDTA) and stained with SYBR® Safe at 90 V for 60 min (Figs. 1, 2). The following international reference strains were used as controls: *Acinetobacter baumannii* (ATCC 19606), *Enterobacter cloacae* (ATCC 23355), *Enterococcus faecalis* (ATCC 29212), *Enterococcus faecium* (ATCC 6569), *Escherichia coli* (ATCC 10536), *Klebsiella pneumoniae* (ATCC 4352), *Morganella morganii* (ATCC 8019), *Proteus mirabilis* (ATCC 15290), *Pseudomonas aeruginosa* (ATCC 15442), *Serratia marcescens* (ATCC 14756), *Staphylococcus aureus* (ATCC 25923), and *Stenotrophomonas maltophilia* (ATCC 13637).

Figures 1 and 2 illustrate the genotypic identification of *Enterobacter cloacae* and *Escherichia coli*, respectively.

DNA sequencing of bacteria   The yeast and Gram-positive bacillus isolates were sequenced for identification to species level. Gram-negative bacilli identified as *Enterobacter aerogenes* by the conventional phenotypic methods and by the automated test were sequenced for species confirmation.

Amplification and purification of bacterial DNA for sequencing   The bacterial isolates identified as Gram-positive bacilli by Gram staining and the Gram-negative bacilli identified as *Enterobacter aerogenes* by the conventional phenotypic methods and automated test were submitted to simple PCR. The efficiency of the reactions was monitored as described in item 2.4.1. For PCR, protocols described in the literature were followed using universal primers for Gram-positive bacilli [14] and primers of enterobacteria for *Enterobacter aerogenes* isolates [15]. The temperature and time parameters and number of amplification cycles are shown in Table 1. The amplified DNA fragments were purified using the HiYield Gel/PCR DNA Fragments Extraction Kit (RBC).

Amplification and purification of yeast DNA   The yeast isolates were submitted to ITS-PCR as described by

Table 1 Primers used for the identification of some bacterial species by PCR

Microorganism	Gene	Annealing temperature (°C)	Amplicon size (bp)	Reference
Acinetobacter baumannii	*bla*OXA_51-like	52	353	[44]
Acinetobacter lwoffii	*bla*OXA_154-like	52	223	[45]
Enterobacter cloacae	Hsp60 (housekeeping)	52	343	[46]
Enterococcus faecalis	16S chromosomal region	60	143	[47]
Enterococcus faecium	sodA (superoxide dismutase)	45	216	[21]
Escherichia coli	gadA (alpha-glutamate decarboxylase)	65	373	[48]
Klebsiella pneumoniae	rpoB (β subunit of RNA polymerase)	52	364	[49]
Morganella morganii	16S chromosomal region	62	809	[50]
Proteus mirabilis	rsbA (quorum sensing)	55	236	[51]
Pseudomonas aeruginosa	Genome fragment	55	724	[52]
Serratia marcescens	16S chromosomal region	52	1058	[53]
Staphylococcus aureus	16S chromosomal region	52	442	[54]
Stenotrophomonas maltophilia	atpD (housekeeping)	52	854	[55]
Bacillus spp.	rpoB (β subunit of RNA polymerase)	72	400	[14]
Enterobacter aerogenes	16SrDNA	55	280	[15]

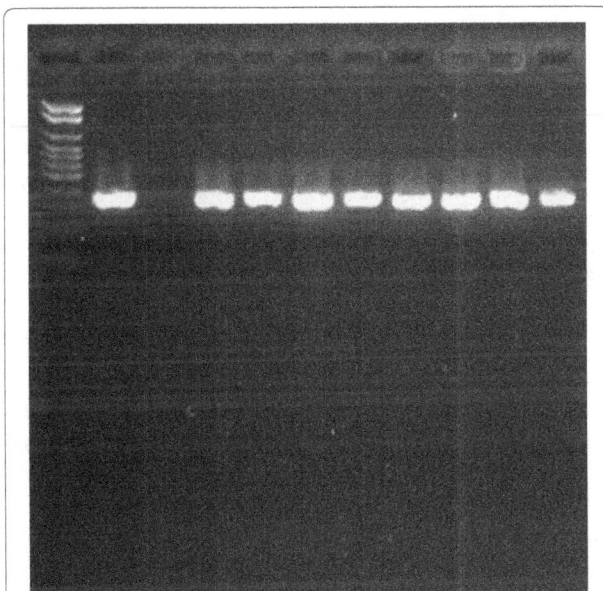

Fig. 1 Agarose gel electrophoresis for detection of Hsp60 (343 bp) in *Enterobacter cloacae* (stained with SYBR® Safe) showing the amplified products positive control, negative control and some samples studied. A 100-bp ladder was used as molecular size marker

Kurtzman et al. [16]. These reactions were carried out in 0.2-mL microtubes containing a mixture of 6.7 μL Milli-Q water, 10 μM forward primer and 10 μM reverse primer, 12.5 μL GoTaq®Green Master Mix, and 3 μL DNA. The efficiency of the amplifications was monitored by electrophoresis (60 min, 80 V) on 1.5 % agarose gel prepared in 1× TBE buffer and stained with SYBR® Safe. Strains previously identified at the Laboratory of Fungal Biology,

Department of Microbiology and Immunology, IBB, were used as controls. The amplified fragments were purified using the Illustra™ ExoProStar™ Kit (GE Healthcare Life Sciences).

DNA sequencing reaction of yeast and bacteria The sequencing reactions were carried out in a mixture containing 3.25 μL water, 1.75 μL 5× BigDye buffer (Applied Biosystems), 1 μL of each primer (5 pmol/μL), 2 μL of the PCR product, and 2 μL BigDye (Applied Biosystems). The cycle sequencing reaction was initiated at 96 °C for 1 min, followed by 40 cycles of denaturation at 96 °C for 30 s, annealing at 60 °C for 30 s and extension at 72 °C for 4 min. The sequencing reaction product was precipitated with 1 μL 125 mM EDTA, 1 μL 3 M sodium acetate, and 25 μL 100 % ethanol. After homogenization, the solution was left to stand for 15 min and then centrifuged at 3000g for 15 min at 4 °C. The supernatant was removed by inverting the tube and 35 μL 70 % ethanol was added. The solution was centrifuged at 1650g for 15 min at 4 °C. After removal of the supernatant by inversion, 10 μL HiDi formamide (Applied Biosystems) was added and the mixture was left to stand for 5 min at 95 °C and for 2 min on ice. The product was run on an 8-capillary ABI 3500 sequencer (50 cm) using POP7 polymer (Applied Biosystems).

Analysis of the DNA sequences of yeast and bacteria The MEGA 5.0 (Molecular Evolutionary Genetics Analysis) and Lasergene programs were used for visualization and alignment of the DNA sequences obtained, which were compared to sequences published and stored in the GenBank database.

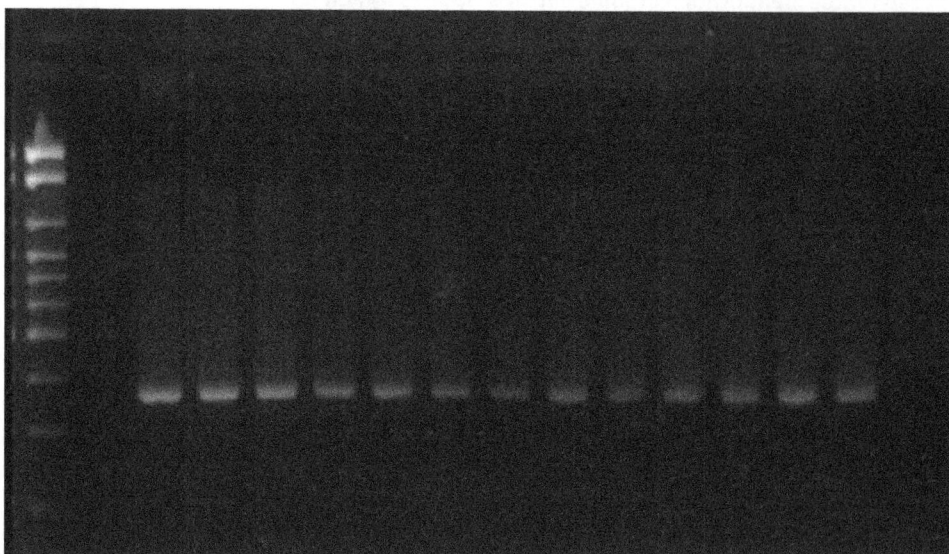

Fig. 2 Agarose gel electrophoresis for detection of *gad*A (373 bp) in *Escherichia coli* (stained with SYBR® Safe) showing the amplified products positive control, negative control and some samples studied. A 100-bp ladder was used as molecular size marker

Statistical analysis

Agreement between the results obtained with the different identification methods was analyzed statistically by the kappa test using the SPSS 20 program (IBM, Armonk, NY, USA). Genotypic identification was used as the gold standard. The accuracy of the conventional phenotypic identification methods and identification by the VITEK® 2 system was evaluated by calculating sensitivity and specificity according to Fletcher et al. [17].

Results

The results of identification with the automated VITEK® 2 system showed overall agreement of 94.7 % with the results of the genotypic methods (Tables 2, 3). Overall agreement of 98.7 % was observed between the results obtained by phenotypic identification using conventional methods and the results of the genotypic methods.

All yeast isolates (15/15) were correctly identified by the VITEK® 2 system using the YST card. The same result was obtained with the GN card for the identification of Gram-negative bacilli, with 100 % correct identifications of the 165 strains isolated.

The rate of correct identification obtained with the GP card used for the identification of Gram-positive cocci was 92.6 % for the microorganisms isolated (199/215). The agreement between the results of automated identification and those obtained with the other identification methods for *Enterococcus* spp. was 91.7 % due to the incorrect identification of one *Enterococcus faecalis* strain by the VITEK® 2 system. The agreement between species of the genus *Staphylococcus* was 97.5 % (198/203). The

VITEK® 2 system correctly identified all *Staphylococcus aureus* isolates (17/17) and incorrectly identified 15 of the 186 (9.19 %) isolates belonging to the group of CoNS. The highest rate of incorrect identification was observed for *Enterococcus faecalis* with 12.5 % (7/8), followed by *Staphylococcus epidermidis* with 12.3 % (10/81), *Staphylococcus hominis* with 8.6 % (3/35), *Staphylococcus capitis* with 5.5 % (1/18), and *Staphylococcus haemolyticus* with 2 % (1/50).

The VITEK® 2 system incorrectly identified the isolates because some biochemical tests failed during the identification process performed by the device, exhibiting divergent characteristics of the species isolated. These errors are shown in Table 4.

Fewer errors occurred when the conventional phenotypic methods were used for identification compared to the automated VITEK® 2 system. Among Gram-positive cocci, the conventional phenotypic methods correctly identified 211/215 (98.1 %) isolates and the few errors observed mainly occurred in the identification of CoNS species, showing divergent results for a given species. The conventional phenotypic methods correctly identified all yeasts (15/15) and 164/165 (99.4 %) Gram-negative bacilli, with the errors described in Table 4.

One hundred percent discrepant results were obtained for the identification of five isolates of Gram-positive bacilli by the VITEK® 2 system (ANC card) and the genotypic identification methods.

Statistical analysis of the identification results revealed a kappa value of 0.945 (p < 0.001), indicating almost perfect agreement according to the criteria of Landis and Koch [18] (Table 5).

Table 2 Comparison of the results of identification of blood culture isolates obtained with the automated VITEK® 2 system, conventional phenotypic methods, and genotypic methods

Microorganism isolated (number)	Automated identification	Conventional methods	Genotypic identification
Bacillus licheniformis (N = 2)	0	NP	2
Corynebacterium amycolatum (N = 3)	0	NP	3
Enterococcus faecalis (N = 8)	7	8	8
Staphylococcus epidermidis (N = 81)	71	81	81
Staphylococcus hominis (N = 35)	32	33	35
Staphylococcus capitis (N = 18)	17	18	18
Staphylococcus haemolyticus (N = 50)	49	48	50
Staphylococcus aureus (N = 17)	17	17	17
Enterobacter cloacae (N = 13)	13	13	13
Proteus mirabilis (N = 5)	5	5	5
Escherichia coli (N = 13)	13	13	13
Serratia marcescens (N = 22)	22	22	22
Acinetobacter baumannii (N = 39)	39	39	39
Acinetobacter lwoffii (N = 3)	3	3	3
Candida albicans (N = 5)	5	5	5
Candida glabrata (N = 5)	5	5	5
Candida krusei (N = 2)	2	2	2
Candida tropicalis (N = 3)	3	3	3
Enterobacter aerogenes (N = 8)	8	8	8
Enterococcus faecium (N = 4)	4	4	4
Klebsiella pneumoniae (N = 43)	43	42	43
Morganella morganii (N = 3)	3	3	3
Pseudomonas aeruginosa (N = 15)	15	15	15
Staphylococcus cohnii (N = 1)	1	1	1
Staphylococcus warneri (N = 1)	1	1	1
Stenotrophomonas maltophilia (N = 1)	1	1	1

NP identification not performed

Table 3 Discrepant results between the automated VITEK® 2 system and the other identification methods of blood culture isolates

No.	Automated identification	Conventional methods	Genotypic identification
4	*Staphylococcus hominis*	*Staphylococcus epidermidis*	*Staphylococcus epidermidis*
3	*Corynebacterium urealyticum*	NP	*Corynebacterium amycolatum*
2	*Corynebacterium urealyticum*	NP	*Bacillus licheniformis*
2	*Staphylococcus lentus*	*Staphylococcus epidermidis*	*Staphylococcus epidermidis*
2	*Staphylococcus haemolyticus*	*Staphylococcus hominis*	*Staphylococcus hominis*
1	*Enterococcus gallinarum*	*Enterococcus faecalis*	*Enterococcus faecalis*
1	*Staphylococcus cohnii*	*Staphylococcus capitis*	*Staphylococcus capitis*
1	*Staphylococcus haemolyticus*	*Staphylococcus haemolyticus*	*Staphylococcus epidermidis*
1	*Staphylococcus lugdunensis*	*Staphylococcus epidermidis*	*Staphylococcus epidermidis*
1	*Staphylococcus scuri*	*Staphylococcus epidermidis*	*Staphylococcus epidermidis*
1	*Staphylococcus capitis*	*Staphylococcus epidermidis*	*Staphylococcus epidermidis*
1	*Staphylococcus warneri*	*Staphylococcus haemolyticus*	*Staphylococcus haemolyticus*
1	*Staphylococcus haemolyticus*	*Staphylococcus haemolyticus*	*Staphylococcus hominis*

NP identification not performed

Table 4 Biochemical tests that failed during the identification process by the VITEK® 2 system and by the conventional phenotypic methods

No.	Genotypic identification	Conventional phenotypic method	VITEK® 2 system		
	Identification	Identification	Incorrect test	Identification	Incorrect test
3	*Staphylococcus epidermidis*	*Staphylococcus epidermidis*	0	*Staphylococcus hominis*	dMNE−; TRE +
2	*Staphylococcus epidermidis*	*Staphylococcus epidermidis*	0	*Staphylococcus lentus*	PolyB−
1	*Staphylococcus epidermidis*	*Staphylococcus epidermidis*	0	*Staphylococcus cohnii*	SUC−; dTRE +
3	*Staphylococcus hominis*	*Staphylococcus hominis*	0	*Staphylococcus haemolyticus*	PyrA+; dMAN+
2	*Staphylococcus hominis*	*Staphylococcus epidermidis*	THIO+	*Staphylococcus hominis*	0
2	*Staphylococcus haemolyticus*	*Staphylococcus warneri*	URE+	*Staphylococcus haemolyticus*	0
1	*Enterococcus faecalis*	*Enterococcus faecalis*	0	*Enterococcus gallinarum*	dSOR−; dRAF+
1	*Staphylococcus capitis*	*Staphylococcus capitis*	0	*Staphylococcus cohnii*	βGAL+; βGUR+; SUC−; dTRE+
1	*Staphylococcus epidermidis*	*Staphylococcus haemolyticus*	URE−	*Staphylococcus haemolyticus*	PyrA+; URE−, PolyB−; TRE+; dMNE−
1	*Staphylococcus epidermidis*	*Staphylococcus epidermidis*	0	*Staphylococcus lugdunensis*	PyrA+; dTRE+
1	*Staphylococcus epidermidis*	*Staphylococcus epidermidis*	0	*Staphylococcus scuri*	PolyB−; βGUR+; NAG (+); dMAN+; dTRE+
1	*Staphylococcus epidermidis*	*Staphylococcus epidermidis*	0	*Staphylococcus capitis*	SUC−; dMAL−; PolyB−; URE−
1	*Staphylococcus haemolyticus*	*Staphylococcus haemolyticus*	0	*Staphylococcus warneri*	0
1	*Klebsiella pneumoniae*	*Klebsiella oxytoca*	Indol+	*Klebsiella pneumoniae*	0

dMNE D-mannose, *dTRE* D-trehalose, *PolyB* polymyxin B, *SUC* sucrose, *PyrA* L-pyrrolidonylarylamidase, *dMAN* D-mannitol, *dSOR* D-sorbitol, *dRAF* D-raffinose, *URE* urea, *βGAL* beta-galactosidase, *THIO* thioglycolatebroth, *βGUR* beta-glucuronidase, *NAG* N-acetylglucosamine, 0 no errors in the tests

Table 5 Kappa value according to Landis and Koch

Kappa value	Level of agreement
<0.00	No agreement
0.00–0.20	Slight
0.21–0.40	Fair
0.41–0.60	Moderate
0.61–0.80	Substantial
0.81–1.00	Almost perfect

Agreement between the conventional phenotypic methods and genotypic identification was higher than that between the genotypic method and automated identification by the VITEK® 2 system (Table 6).

Comparison of the sensitivity of the conventional phenotypic methods and the VITEK® 2 system showed a better performance of the former (Table 7).

Discussion

The need for the rapid and efficient identification of microorganisms isolated from blood cultures has encouraged studies that investigated automated identification systems to reduce the time of identification. Several of these studies have used direct inoculation from blood culture bottles, but the results were not as efficient as those obtained in studies using standard inocula from subcultures of microorganisms grown for 24 h

on solid media. The poor performance of the VITEK® 2 system for the identification of microorganisms using direct inoculation from blood culture bottles is probably due to the small number of cells or to contamination with other microorganisms that impair the correct identification of the causative agent of infection [19–22]. The VITEK system has been investigated for more than two decades and improvement of the ID-GPC (Gram-positive cocci) and ID-GNB (Gram-negative bacilli) identification cards to the GP (Gram-positive cocci) and GN (Gram-negative bacilli) cards has made the system more efficient. Wallet et al. [23] compared the old and new identification cards and found that the GP and GN cards correctly identified 235/249 (94.4 %) Gram-positive cocci and 321/331 (97 %) Gram-negative bacilli, while the ID-GPC and ID-GNB correctly identified 218/249 (87.5 %) and 295/331 (89.1 %) isolates, respectively.

The present study was conducted over a period of 18 months and evaluated the accuracy of the VITEK® 2 system in identifying 400 microorganisms (Gram-positive cocci, Gram-positive bacilli, Gram-negative bacilli, and yeasts) isolated from blood cultures and inoculated by the standard method onto GP, GN, YST (yeast) and ANC (Gram-positive bacilli) cards. The results were compared to genotypic identification (gold standard) and 94.7 % agreement was observed. Similar rates have been reported by De Cueto et al. [24] (95.0 %, 95/100)

Table 6 Kappa values of agreement between automated identification by the VITEK®2 system, the conventional phenotypic methods, and genotypic identification

Group	Number of isolates	Kappa	
		Conventional method × genotypic method	Automated method × genotypic method
Gram-positive cocci	255	0.969	0.904
CoNS	186	0.969	0.886
Gram-negative bacilli	165	0.993	1.000
Gram-positive bacilli	5	NP	0
Yeasts	15	1.000	1.000
Total	400	0.958	0.945

CoNS coagulase-negative staphylococci, NP not performed

and by Nakasone et al. [25] (95.8 %, 454/474) who also used standard inocula. Studies using direct inoculation from blood cultures bottles obtained lower agreement of 91.4 % [5] and 81.0 % [6].

All 15 yeasts isolated during the study period were correctly identified by the VITEK® 2 system. Correct identification of all yeast isolates (56/56) has also been observed by Nakasone et al. [25]. Studies involving a larger number of strains and species found lower agreement, 92.1 % (222/241) reported by Graf et al. [26] and 78.9 % (277/351) by Won et al. [27].

The VITEK® 2 system has shown satisfactory identification rates of Gram-negative bacilli for decades, as also observed in this study in which 100 % correct identifications of the isolates were obtained. Funke et al. [28] and Ling et al. [29] analyzed 845 and 281 isolates, with correct identification rates of 84.7 % (716/845) and 95 % (267/281), respectively. Nakasone et al. [25], Gherardi et al. [5] and Prod'hom et al. [6] analyzed 181, 91 and 95 Gram-negative bacilli and obtained correct identifications of 96.7 % (175/181), 100 % (91/91) and 98.8 % (92/95), respectively, with the VITEK® 2 system.

Studies using direct inoculation from blood culture bottles reported lower rates of correct identification of 82 [30] and 93 % [31]. De Cueto et al. [24] compared direct inoculation from blood cultures with inoculation from subcultures in 50 isolates. The result was 100 % correct identifications for the standard method and 62 % (31/5) correct identifications for direct inoculation. Similar results have been reported by Kerremans et al. [32] who analyzed 161 isolates; 90 % (145/161) of the isolates were correctly identified by subculture and 80 % (129/161) by direct inoculation from blood cultures.

The identification of Gram-positive cocci by the automated VITEK® 2 system showed 92.6 % agreement with genotypic identification, which is compatible with the rate reported by Ligozzi et al. [33] who obtained 91.5 % (351/381) correct identifications. De Cueto et al. [24] obtained 100 % (50/50) correct identifications of the isolates. Funke and Funke-Kissling [34], Nakasone et al. [25] and Chatzigeorgiou et al. [35] reported higher rates of correct identification than those obtained in this study of 94.5 % (344/364), 96.1 % (226/235) and 97.9 % (144/147), respectively. Gherardi et al. [5] and Prod'hom et al. [6] obtained correct identifications of 75 % (36/48) and 74 % (133/180), while Lupetti et al. [36] found a rate of 89 % (49/55). These rates are lower than those observed in this study and are outside the acceptable parameter of 90 % correct identifications; however, these studies used direct inoculation from blood culture bottles.

With respect to genera of Gram-positive cocci, a difference in the efficiency of the VITEK® 2 system was observed. Agreement was 91.7 % (11/12) for the genus *Enterococcus*, similar to the rates reported by Nakasone et al. [25] and Jin et al. [37]. Lower efficiencies of 77.8, 83.1, 87.5, 72 and 77.8 % correct identifications of strains of this genus have been observed by Ligozzi et al. [33], d'Azevedo et al. [38], Moore et al. [39] and Paim et al. [42], respectively. In the case of *Staphylococcus*, a higher rate of incorrect identifications was observed for CoNS isolates (91.9 %), in agreement with Ligozzi et al. [33]

Table 7 Sensitivity and specificity of the conventional phenotypic methods and of the automated VITEK® 2 system in the identification of microorganisms

Microorganism	VITEK® 2 system		Phenotypic methods	
	Sensitivity (%)	Specificity (%)	Sensitivity (%)	Specificity (%)
Enterococcus faecalis	87.5	100	100	100
Staphylococcus capitis	94.4	99.5	100	100
Staphylococcus cohnii	100	99.0	100	100
Staphylococcus epidermidis	87.6	100	100	98.5
Staphylococcus haemolyticus	98.0	96.5	96.0	100
Staphylococcus hominis	91.4	98.3	94.2	100
Staphylococcus warneri	100	99.5	100	99.0

(86 %), Funke and Funke-Kissling [34] (93.7 %), Kim et al. [40] (87.5 %), Delmas et al. [41] (78.8 %), and Paim et al. [42] (72.9 %). These unsatisfactory results are due to the fact that automated identification systems are unable to perform a fully reliable differentiation between different CoNS species because of the variable expression of phenotypic characteristics in these microorganisms [43]. The slow metabolism of certain species leads to ambiguous results in their identification, a fact observed by Ligozzi et al. [33]. All *Staphylococcus aureus* isolates were correctly identified (17/17), as also reported in the studies of Delmas et al. [41] (6/6), Chatzigeorgiou et al. [35] (52/52), Paim et al. [42] (11/11), and Funke and Funke-Kissling [34] (45/45). Ligozzi et al. [33], who evaluated a larger number of isolates, found 99 % agreement (99/100). These rates of correct identification demonstrate a satisfactory performance of the VITEK® 2 system for the identification of *Staphylococcus aureus*.

The failure of the ANC card to identify Gram-positive bacilli can be explained by the variability in the genera and species of these microorganisms and the consequent difficulty in developing cards that contain variable biochemical tests necessary for correct identification. These microorganisms were not identified by conventional phenotypic methods since this identification is infeasible in routine clinical microbiology because it requires numerous expensive and time-consuming biochemical tests.

The better performance of the conventional methods for CoNS identification was responsible for the higher sensitivity of these methods compared to the VITEK® 2 system. This finding can be explained by the fact that the conventional methods used consisted of specific tests for each CoNS species and by the incubation period of 72 h, which is necessary for this correct identification since some species have a slower metabolism on some substrates.

Conclusions

The kappa values indicate reliability of the results obtained with the VITEK® 2 system. Analysis of specificity showed a performance higher than 90 % as required for commercial systems in clinical microbiology, demonstrating that this system is suitable for the identification of microorganisms isolated in routine clinical microbiology laboratories.

Authors' contributions

ACMM conceived and designed the study, performed the tests, analyzed and interpreted the data, and wrote the manuscript. CMCBF substantially contributed to the conception of the study and performed the statistical analyses. AMF collected the blood cultures and performed the automated identification. RSC participated in the data collection and analysis. EB identified the yeast isolates. MLRSC participated in the conception of the study, data analysis, and writing and revision of the manuscript. All authors read and approved the final manuscript.

Author details

[1] Departamento de Microbiologia e Imunologia, Instituto de Biociências de Botucatu, UNESP–Univ. Estadual Paulista, Distrito de Rubião Junior, s/n, Botucatu, SP CEP: 18618-970, Brazil. [2] Departamento de Doenças Tropicais, Faculdade de Medicina de Botucatu, UNESP–Univ. Estadual Paulista, Distrito de Rubião Junior, s/n, Botucatu, SP CEP: 18618-970, Brazil. [3] Laboratório de Análises Clínicas do Hospital das Clínicas de Botucatu, Faculdade de Medicina de Botucatu, UNESP–Univ. Estadual Paulista, Distrito de Rubião Junior, s/n, Botucatu, SP CEP: 18618-970, Brazil. [4] Comissão de Controle de Infecção Relacionada à Assistência à Saúde, Hospital das Clínicas, Faculdade de Medicina de Botucatu, UNESP–Univ. Estadual Paulista, Distrito de Rubião Junior, s/n, Botucatu, SP CEP: 18618-970, Brazil. [5] Departamento de Clínica Médica, Faculdade de Medicina de Botucatu, UNESP–Univ. Estadual Paulista, Distrito de Rubião Junior, s/n, Botucatu, SP CEP: 18618-970, Brazil.

Acknowledgements

We thank Fundação de Amparo à Pesquisa do Estado de São Paulo (FAPESP) for financial support (Grant 2012/1566-8).

Competing interests

The authors declare that they have no competing interests.

Funding

Fundação de Amparo à Pesquisa do Estado de São Paulo (FAPESP)—Grant 2012/1566-8.

References

1. Instituto Latino Americano para Estudos da Sepse. Sepse: um problema de saúde pública. Brasília: CFM; 2015.
2. Diament D, Salomão R, Rigatto O, Gomes B, Silva E, Carvalho NB, Machado FR. Guidelines for the treatment of severe sepsis and septic shock—management of the infectious agent—diagnosis. Rev Bras Ter Intensiva. 2011;23(2):134–44.
3. Weinstein MP, Murphy JR, Reller LB, Lichtenstein KA. The clinical significance of positive blood cultures: a comprehensive analysis of 500 episodes of bacteremia and fungemia in adults. II. Clinical observations, with special reference to factors influencing prognosis. Rev Infect Dis. 1983;5(1):54–70.
4. Barenfanger J, Drake C, Kacich G. Clinical and financial benefits of rapid bacterial identification and antimicrobial susceptibility testing. J Clin Microbiol. 1999;37(5):1415–8.
5. Gherardi G, Angeletti S, Panitti M, Pompilio A, Di Bonaventura G, Crea F, Avola A, Fico L, Palazzo C, Sapia GF, Visaggio D, Dicuonzo G. Comparative evaluation of the VITEK-2 Compact and Phoenix systems for rapid identification and antibiotic susceptibility testing directly from blood cultures of Gram-negative and Gram-positive isolates. Diagn Microbiol Infect Dis. 2012;72(1):20–31.
6. Prod'hom G, Durussel C, Greub G. A simple blood-culture bacterial pellet preparation for faster accurate direct bacterial identification and antibiotic susceptibility testing with the VITEK 2 system. J Med Microbiol. 2013;62(5):773–7.
7. Cunha MLRS, Sinzato YK, Silveira LVA. Comparison of methods for the identification of coagulase negative staphylococci. Mem Inst Oswaldo Cruz. 2004;99(8):855–60.
8. Winn WC Jr, Allen SD, Janda WM, Koneman EW, Procop GW, Schreckenberger PC, Woods GL. Koneman. Diagnóstico microbiológico: texto e altlas colorido. 6th ed. Rio de Janeiro: Editora Guanabara Koogan; 2010.

9.　Hogg GM, McKenna JP, Ong G. Rapid detection of methicillin-susceptible and methicillin-resistant *Staphylococcus aureus* directly from positive BacT/Alert blood culture bottles using real-time polymerase chain reaction: evaluation and comparison of 4 DNA extraction methods. Diagn Microbiol Infect Dis. 2008;61(4):446–52.

10.　Fredericks DN, Relman DA. Improved amplification of microbial DNA from blood cultures by removal of the PCR inhibitor sodium polyanetholesulfonate. J Clin Microbiol. 1998;36(10):2810–6

11.　McCullough MJ, Di Salvo AF, Clemons KV, Park P, Stevens DA. Molecular epidemiology of *Blastomyces dermatitidis*. Clin Infect Dis. 2000;30(2):328–35.

12.　Barry T, Colleran G, Glennon M, Dunican LK, Gannon F. The 16S/23S ribosomal spacer region as a target for DNA probes to identify eubacteria. PCR Methods Appl. 1991;1(1):51–6.

13.　Couto I, Pereira S, Miragaia M, Sanches IS, Lencastre H. Identification of clinical staphylococcal isolates from humans by internal transcribed spacer PCR. J Clin Microbiol. 2001;39(9):3099–103.

14.　Khamis A, Raoult D, La Scola B. rpoB gene sequencing for identification of *Corynebacterium* species. J Clin Microbiol. 2004;42(9):3925–31.

15.　Gouveia C, Asensi MD, Zahner V, Rangel EF, Oliveira SM. Study on the bacterial midgut microbiota associated to different Brazilian populations of *Lutzomyia longipalpis* (Lutz & Neiva) (Diptera: Psychodidae). Neotrop Entomol. 2008;37(5):597–601.

16.　Kurtzman CP, Robnett CJ. Identification of clinically important ascomycetous yeasts based on nucleotide divergence in the 59 end of the large-subunit (26S) ribosomal DNA gene. J Clin Microbiol. 1997;35(5):1216–23.

17.　Fletcher RH, Fletcher SW, Wagner EH. Diagnóstico. In: Fletcher RH, Fletcher SW, Wagner EH, editors. Epidemiologia Clínica. 3rd ed. Porto Alegre: Artes Médicas; 1991. p. 68–107.

18.　Landis JR, Koch GG. The measurement of observer agreement for categorical data. Biometrics. 1977;33(1):159–74.

19.　Fontanals D, Salceda F, Hernández J, Sanfeliu I, Torra M. Evaluation of wider system for direct identification and antimicrobial susceptibility testing of gram-negative bacilli from positive blood culture bottles. Eur J Clin Microbiol Infect Dis. 2002;21(9):693–5.

20.　Waites KB, Brookings ES, Moser SA, Zimmer BL. Direct bacterial identification from positive BacT/Alert blood cultures using MicroScan overnight and rapid panels. Diagn Microbiol Infect Dis. 1998;32(1):21–6.

21.　Alipour M, Hajiesmaili R, Talebjannat M, Yahyapour Y. Identification and antimicrobial resistance of *Enterococcus* spp. isolated from the river and coastal waters in northern Iran. Scientific World Journal. 2014; 2014:287458.

22.　Waites KB, Brookings ES, Moser SA, Zimmer BL. Direct susceptibility testing with positive BacT/Alert blood cultures by using MicroScan overnight and rapid panels. J Clin Microbiol. 1998;36(7):2052–6.

23.　Wallet F, Loïez C, Renaux E, Lemaitre N, Courcol RJ. Performances of VITEK 2 colorimetric cards for identification of Gram-positive and Gram-negative bacteria. J Clin Microbiol. 2005;43(9):4402–6.

24.　De Cueto M, Ceballos E, Martinez-Martinez L, Perea EJ, Pascual A. Use of positive blood cultures for direct identification and susceptibility testing with the VITEK 2 system. J Clin Microbiol. 2004;42(8):3734–8.

25.　Nakasone I, Kinjo T, Yamane N, Kisanuki K, Shiohira CM. Laboratory-based evaluation of the colorimetric VITEK-2 Compact system for species identification and of the Advanced Expert System for detection of antimicrobial resistances: VITEK-2 Compact system identification and antimicrobial susceptibility testing. Diagn Microbiol Infect Dis. 2007;58(2):191–8.

26.　Graf B, Adam T, Zill E, Göbel UB. Evaluation of the VITEK 2 system for rapid identification of yeast and yeast-like organisms. J Clin Microbiol. 2000;38(5):1782–5.

27.　Won EJ, Shin JH, Kim MN, Choi MJ, Joo MY, Kee SJ, Shin MG, Suh SP, Ryang DW. Evaluation of the BD Phoenix system for identification of a wide spectrum of clinically important yeast species: a comparison with VITEK 2-YST. Diagn Microbiol Infect Dis. 2014;79(4):477–80.

28.　Funke G, Monnet D, de Bernardis C, von Graevenitz A, Freney J. Evaluation of the VITEK 2 system for rapid identification of medically relevant Gram-negative rods. J Clin Microbiol. 1998;36(7):1948–52.

29.　Ling TKW, Tam PC, Liu ZK, Cheng AFB. Evaluation of VITEK 2 rapid identification and susceptibility testing system against Gram-negative clinical isolates. J Clin Microbiol. 2001;39(8):2964–6.

30.　Ling TK, Liu ZK, Cheng AF. Evaluation of the VITEK 2 system for rapid direct identification and susceptibility testing of Gram-negative bacilli from positive blood cultures. J Clin Microbiol. 2003;41(10):4705–7.

31.　Bruins MJ, Bloembergen P, Ruijs GJ, Wolfhagen MJ. Identification and susceptibility testing of Enterobacteriaceae and *Pseudomonas aeruginosa* by direct inoculation from positive BACTEC blood culture bottles into VITEK 2. J Clin Microbiol. 2004;42(1):7–11.

32.　Kerremans JJ, Goessens WH, Verbrugh HA, Vos MC. Accuracy of identification and susceptibility results by direct inoculation of VITEK 2 cards from positive BACTEC cultures. Eur J Clin Microbiol Infect Dis. 2004;23(12):892–8.

33.　Ligozzi M, Bernini C, Bonora MG, De Fatima M, Zuliani J, Fontana R. Evaluation of the VITEK 2 system for identification and antimicrobial susceptibility testing of medically relevant Gram-positive cocci. J Clin Microbiol. 2002;40(5):1681–6.

34.　Funke G, Funke-Kissling P. Performance of the new VITEK 2 GP card for identification of medically relevant Gram-positive cocci in a routine clinical laboratory. J Clin Microbiol. 2005;43(1):84–8.

35.　Chatzigeorgiou KS, Siafakas N, Petinaki E, Argyropoulou A, Tarpatzi A, Bobola M, Paniara O, Velegraki A, Zerva L. Identification of staphylococci by Phoenix: validation of a new protocol and comparison with VITEK 2. Diagn Microbiol Infect Dis. 2010;68(4):375–81.

36.　Lupetti A, Barnini S, Castagna B, Capria AL, Nibbering PH. Rapid identification and antimicrobial susceptibility profiling of Gram-positive cocci in blood cultures with the VITEK 2 system. Eur J Clin Microbiol Infect Dis. 2010;29(1):89–95.

37.　Jin WY, Jang SJ, Lee MJ, Park G, Kim MJ, Kook JK, Kim DM, Moon DS, Park YJ. Evaluation of VITEK 2, MicroScan, and Phoenix for identification of clinical isolates and reference strains. Diagn Microbiol Infect Dis. 2011;70(4):442–7.

38.　D'Azevedo PA, Cantarelli VV, Inamine E, Superti S, Dias CAG. Evaluation of an automated system for the identification of enterococci. J Bras Patol Med Lab. 2004;40(4):237–9.

39.　Moore DF, Zhowandai MH, Ferguson DM, McGee C, Mott JB, Stewart JC. Comparison of 16S rRNA sequencing with conventional and commercial phenotypic techniques for identification of enterococci from the marine environment. J Appl Microbiol. 2006;100(6):1272–81.

40.　Kim M, Heo SR, Choi SH, Kwon H, Park JS, Seong MW, Lee DH, Park KU, Song J, Kim EC. Comparison of the MicroScan, VITEK 2, and Crystal GP with 16S rRNA sequencing and MicroSeq 500 v2.0 analysis for coagulase-negative Staphylococci. BMC Microbiol. 2008;23(8):233–9.

41.　Delmas J, Chacornac JP, Robin F, Giammarinaro P, Talon R, Bonnet R. Evaluation of the VITEK 2 system with a variety of *Staphylococcus* species. J Clin Microbiol. 2008;46(1):311–3.

42.　Paim TGS, Cantarelli VV, D'Azevedo PA. Performance of the VITEK 2 system software version 5.03 in the bacterial identification and antimicrobial susceptibility test: evaluation study of clinical and reference strains of Gram-positive cocci. Rev Soc Bras Med Trop. 2013;47(3):377–81.

43.　Weinstein MP, Mirrett S, Pelt LV, McKinnon M, Zimmer L, Kloos W, Reller LB. Clinical importance of identifying coagulase-negative Staphylococci isolated from blood cultures: evaluation of MicroScan rapid and dried overnight gram-positive panels versus a conventional reference method. J Clin Microbiol. 1998;36(7):2089–92.

44.　Turton JF, Woodford N, Glover J, Yarde S, Kaufmann ME, Pitt TL. Identification of *Acinetobacter baumannii* by detection of the blaOXA-51-like carbapenemase gene intrinsic to this species. J Clin Microbiol. 2006;44(8):2974–6.

45.　Turton JF, Hyde R, Martin K, Shah J. Genes encoding OXA-134-like enzymes are found in *Acinetobacter lwoffii* and *A. schindleri* and can be used for identification. J Clin Microbiol. 2012;50(3):1019–22.

46.　Stumpf AN, Roggenkamp A, Hoffmann H. Specificity of enterobacterial repetitive intergenic consensus and repetitive extragenic palindromic polymerase chain reaction for the detection of clonality within the *Enterobacter cloacae*. Diagn Microbiol Infect Dis. 2005;53(1):9–16.

47.　Williams JM, Trope M, Caplan DJ, Shugars DC. Detection and quantitation of *E. faecalis* by real-time PCR (qPCR), reverse transcription-PCR (RT-PCR) and cultivation during endodontic treatment. J Endod. 2006;32(8):715–21.

48. Doumith M, Day MJ, Hope R, Wain J, Woodford N. Improved multiplex PCR strategy for rapid assignment of the four major *Escherichia coli* phylogenetic groups. J Clin Microbiol. 2012;50(9):3108–10.

49. Chander Y, Ramakrishnan MA, Jindal N, Hanson K, Goyal SM. Differentiation of *Klebsiella pneumoniae* and *K. oxytoca* by multiplex polymerase chain reaction. Int J Appl Res Vet Med. 2011;9(2):138–42.

50. Kim SH, An H, Visessanguan W, Benjakul S, Morrissey MT, Su YC, Pitta TP. Molecular detection of a histamine former, *Morganella morganii*, in Albacore, Mackrel, Sardine, and a processing plant. JFS. 2003;68(2):453–7.

51. Belas R, Schneider R, Melch M. Characterization of *Proteus mirabilis* precocious swarming mutants: identification of rsbA, encoding a regulator of swarming behavior. J Bacteriol. 1998;180(23):6126–39.

52. Jeong ES, Lee KS, Heo SH, Seo JH, Choi YK. Triplex PCR for the simultaneous detection of *Pseudomonas aeruginosa*, *Helicobacter hepaticus* and *Salmonella typhimurium*. Exp Anim. 2011;60(1):65–70.

53. Polson SW, Higgins JL, Woodley CM. PCR-based assay for detection of four coral pathogens. In: Proceedings of the 11th international coral reef symposium, Ft. Lauderdale. Florida. 2008. p. 247-51.

54. Martineau F, Picard FJ, Roy PH, Ouellette M, Bergeron MG. Species-specific and ubiquitous-DNA-based assays for rapid identification of *Staphylococcus aureus*. J Clin Microbiol. 1998;6(3):618–23.

55. *Stenotrophomonas maltophilia* MLST Databases. http://pubmlst.org/ smaltophilia/info/primers.shtml. Accessed 6 Apr 2016.

7

Antimicrobial resistance and virulence characterization of *Staphylococcus aureus* and coagulase-negative staphylococci from imported beef meat

Kamelia Osman[1], Avelino Alvarez-Ordóñez[2], Lorena Ruiz[3], Jihan Badr[4], Fatma ElHofy[5], Khalid S. Al-Maary[6], Ihab M. I. Moussa[6], Ashgan M. Hessain[7], Ahmed Orabi[1], Alaa Saad[4] and Mohamed Elhadidy[8,9]*

Abstract

Background: The objectives of this study were to characterize the diversity and magnitude of antimicrobial resistance among *Staphylococcus* species recovered from imported beef meat sold in the Egyptian market and the potential mechanisms underlying the antimicrobial resistance phenotypes including harboring of resistance genes (*mecA*, *cfr*, *gyrA*, *gyrB*, and *grlA*) and biofilm formation.

Results: The resistance gene *mecA* was detected in 50% of methicillin-resistant non-*Staphylococcus aureus* isolates (4/8). Interestingly, our results showed that: (i) resistance genes *mecA*, *gyrA*, *gyrB*, *grlA*, and *cfr* were absent in *Staphylococcus hominis* and *Staphylococcus hemolyticus* isolates, although *S. hominis* was phenotypically resistant to methicillin (MR-non-*S. aureus*) while *S. hemolyticus* was resistant to vancomycin only; (ii) *S. aureus* isolates did not carry the *mecA* gene (100%) and were phenotypically characterized as methicillin- susceptible *S. aureus* (MSS); and (iii) the resistance gene *mecA* was present in one isolate (1/3) of *Staphylococcus lugdunensis* that was phenotypically characterized as methicillin-susceptible non-*S. aureus* (MSNSA).

Conclusions: Our findings highlight the potential risk for consumers, in the absence of actionable risk management information systems, of imported foods and advice a strict implementation of international standards by different venues such as CODEX to avoid the increase in prevalence of coagulase positive and coagulase negative *Staphylococcus* isolates and their antibiotic resistance genes in imported beef meat at the Egyptian market.

Keywords: Coagulase-positive staphylococci, Coagulase-negative staphylococci, Antibiotic resistance genes, Imported beef meat

Background

Contamination of meat with foodborne pathogens represents a major public health threat. The increasing volume of trade and travel is considered as a potential risk factor facilitating the global transport and dissemination of pathogenic bacteria in food. Imported animal products are considered as a clear example, and risk analyses have been previously applied to characterize these

products [1]. This risk analyses strategy have been implemented following the World Trade Organization (WTO) creation. The application of sanitary and phytosanitary measures in response to the sanitary and phytosanitary measures agreement (SPS Agreement) [2] requires the WTO members to remove barriers on the trade of agricultural products, except in situations where such trade can potentially create risk to the animal, human or plant health in the importing country.

Staphylococcus aureus is one of the most common foodborne pathogens causing food poisoning outbreaks worldwide [3]. Other than *S. aureus*, the clinical and

---
*Correspondence: mm_elhadidy@mans.edu.eg
[8] Department of Bacteriology, Mycology and Immunology, Faculty of Veterinary Medicine, Mansoura University, Mansoura 35516, Egypt
Full list of author information is available at the end of the article

veterinary importance of coagulase-positive staphylococci (CPS) and coagulase-negative staphylococci (CNS) have often been neglected. In recent years, the risk of CPS and CNS has been highlighted by recent reports [4–6] with special reference to the CNS that have been commonly found in food [7, 8]. CNS have been recorded as conveying vector for virulence genes and have been implicated in some cases of food poisoning [9]. Furthermore, food-related staphylococci could act as dissemination vectors for antibiotic resistance genes to other potentially pathogenic microorganisms causing immediate threat to the public health. The *mecA*-harboring CNS (MRCNS) have been reported to have a reservoir in animal farm facilities and in meat products, with the ability to be conveyed to *S. aureus* [10–12].

The remarkable global concern of antibiotic- resistant pathogens in the food chain and the potential for these resistant pathogens to spread through the food chain prompted the Codex Alimentarius Commission to establish an *ad hoc* Intergovernmental Task Force on antimicrobial resistance. The main task of this commission is to apply a complete risk assessment strategy on the use of antimicrobials belonging to both clinical and veterinary classes. While domestic control over antimicrobial usage policies and monitoring is achievable, negligible information is available for imported food [13], with special reference to beef meat that has been incriminated to contribute to the emergence of multidrug resistance among humans through the dispersion of resistance genes carried by resistant pathogens transmitted by contaminated meat [14, 15].

Livestock-associated methicillin-resistant *S. aureus* (LA-MRSA) have acquired a number of novel and unusual antimicrobial resistance genes including multi-resistance genes such as the *cfr* gene, that confers resistance to phenicols, lincosamides, oxazolidinones, pleuromutilins, and streptogramin A [16]. Oxazolidinones are last resort antimicrobial agents for the control of serious infections caused by MRSA and vancomycin-resistant enterococci in humans. MRSA is also notoriously difficult to treat due to resistance to β-lactams (including penicillin, oxacillin, and methicillin) represent a class of antibiotics generally prescribed as the first line of defense against clinical infections caused by staphylococci, which include drugs like penicillin, oxacillin, and methicillin. This resistance was attributed to the carriage of *mecA*. The *mecA* gene encodes a different form of penicillin-binding protein, PBP2a, which β-lactam drugs cannot inactivate.

Therefore, the objectives of this study were to characterize the diversity of *Staphylococcus* strains recovered from imported meat sold in the Egyptian market and to assess recovered isolates as potential dispersion vectors for the spread of antimicrobial resistance. To achieve that aim, *Staphylococcus* isolates were tested for the presence of antimicrobial resistance phenotypes and genetic determinants (*mecA*, *cfr*, *gyrA*, *gyrB*, and *grlA*) and for their biofilm formation.

Methods
Imported beef meat samples
A total of 100 imported frozen meat samples were delivered to the Department of Poultry Diseases, Animal Health Research, Institute, Dokki, Egypt, as a routine microbiological analysis check for foodborne pathogens. Samples were collected by the food hygiene officials in ice-boxes from different supermarket chains as well as butcher shops located in the Great Cairo Zone. The meat samples (25 g) were suspended in 225 ml sterile phosphate buffered saline (PBS, pH 7.4) and homogenized in a stomacher (Lab-Blender 400, PBI, Milan, Italy) for 10 min. A total of 25 ml of the homogenate were added to 10 ml of Giolitti-Cantoni broth (BD Diagnostics, Franklin Lakes, NJ, USA). The tubes were incubated at 37 °C for 18–24 h with shaking at 200 rpm. Ten microliter aliquots of the enriched cultures were seeded on Baird Parker agar (BD Diagnostics, Franklin Lakes, NJ, USA), supplemented with egg yolk tellurite emulsion. The plates were incubated at 37 °C for 18–24 h and recovered single colonies were streaked onto blood agar plates (TSA with 5% sheep blood), and further incubated at 37 °C for 12–18 h. Characteristic staphylococci colonies (black, with or without a halo) were further identified based on Gram stain, catalase assay, tube coagulase test and further biochemical identification tests referred in standard diagnostic tables [17].

Determination of virulence factors
Production of hemolysins
Production of α-, β- and γ-hemolysins was detected by streaking each staphylococcal isolate on blood agar plates containing 5% sheep red blood cells following the protocol previously developed [18].

Vero cell cytotoxicity assay
The ability of the isolated staphylococci to initiate degeneration of Vero cells was microscopically evaluated following the validated methodology described elsewhere [19] with minor modifications. The cytotoxicity assay was carried out using Vero (African green monkey kidney) cells in 96-well microtiter trays. Suspensions of each tested strain in distilled water were adjusted to 0.5 McFarland standard. Then, 20 μl of bacterial suspensions were added to 3.5 ml of brain heart infusion broth (BBL, Becton–Dickinson Microbiology Systems). The tubes were incubated 2 days at 35 °C, and thereafter for

2 days at room temperature. After centrifugation of bacterial broth cultures, 20 μl of supernatants were added in triplicate to 180 μl of cell culture medium. After incubation at 37 °C, in a humid atmosphere and 5% CO_2, the cytotoxic effect of each staphylococcal strain on the Vero monolayer morphology was microscopically perceived up to 5 days.

Phenotypic determination of the antibiotic resistance profile

The disk diffusion method was used to investigate the antibiotic resistance phenotype of the 23 *Staphylococcus* spp. recovered from the imported beef meat on Mueller–Hinton agar plates as previously described [20]. *Escherichia coli* NCIMB 50034 and *S. aureus* ATCC 25923 were included as controls. The antibiotics tested were selected from two categories, as follows [21]: (i) Critically important antibiotics: ampicillin-sulbactam (20 μg), methicillin (5 μg), oxacillin (1 μg), penicillin (10 μg), ciprofloxacin (5 μg), erythromycin (15 μg), gentamicin (10 μg), vancomycin (30 μg) and (ii) Highly important antibiotics: chloramphenicol (30 μg), clindamycin (2 μg), tetracycline (30 μg), and sulfamethoxazole/trimethoprim (25 μg).

Molecular characterization

Overnight cultures of all *Staphylococcus* isolates were subjected to the boiling method for the preparation of cell lysates to be used for DNA templates. Genus-specific confirmation was carried out through PCR using the 16S rRNA gene *Staphylococcus*-genus-specific primers and cycling conditions previously described [22]. *S. aureus* ATCC 43300 and *E. coli* NCIMB 50034 were used as positive and negative controls, respectively. All confirmed staphylococci were submitted to further molecular analyses for the detection of the *mecA* gene, that is considered as the gold-standard for MRSA confirmation [23]. Four additional antimicrobial resistance markers frequently reported in *S. aureus* were screened by PCR, including the *gyrA*, *gyrB*, and *grlA* genes that are responsible for quinolone resistance and the *cfr* gene (chloramphenicol-florfenicol resistance gene), conferring resistance to several classes of antibiotics (phenicols, lincosamides, oxazolidinones, pleuromutilins, and streptogramin A; known as the PhLOPSA phenotype). PCR amplifications were carried out with a GeneAmp PCR System 2400 (Perkin-Elmer, Weiterstadt, Germany) using the primers and the cycling conditions previously described [8]. Two microliters of template DNA were added to 23 μl of master mix containing 1 μM of each primer and 3U of Taq polymerase. The amplicons were screened by gel-electrophoresis on 1.5% (w/v) agarose gels in TBE buffer and visualized following ethidium bromide staining. *S. aureus* reference strains EMRSA-15 and ATCC 25923 were used was used as a positive controls for the *mecA* and the *cfr* genes, respectively.

Biofilm formation

The tube method (TM) and Congo red agar (CRA) method previously described [24] were followed to assess the ability for biofilm and slime formation by the 23 *Staphylococcus* isolates using the following international reference strains as controls: the non-biofilm producers *Staphylococcus epidermidis* ATCC 12228 and *Staphylococcus warneri* ATCC 10209 (negative controls), and the biofilm producers *S. epidermidis* ATCC 35983, *Staphylococcus simulans* ATCC 27851 and *Staphylococcus xylosus* ATCC 29979 (positive controls). For the TM, adherence was observed as a ring formation on the inside walls of the test tube when stained with crystal violet. Regarding the interpretation of the TM results, strains were classified as strongly adherent (+) or negative (−). Results of the CRA method were interpreted as follows: very black, black and almost black colonies were considered to be strong biofilm formers, while very red, red and bordeaux colonies were classified as negative strains for biofilm formation.

Correlation analyses

Pearson's correlation was used to analyze the association between all studied phenotypic and genotypic features. Univariate analyses (Chi square test, $p < 0.05$) were performed to identify variables significantly associated. The p values < 0.05 were considered statistically significant. Statistical analysis and data representation were done using R software (3.3.2).

Results

Isolation and characterization of *Staphylococcus* spp. from imported beef meat samples

In this study, a total of 23 staphylococcal isolates were recovered from 100 imported meat samples (23%), including CPS strains (12/23) and CNS strains (11/23) (Table 2). The 23 *Staphylococcus* spp. (*S. aureus*, n = 3; *S. hyicus*, n = 6; *S. intermedius*, n = 3; *S. epidermidis*, n = 1; *S. hemolyticus*, n = 1; *S. hominis*, n − 1; *S. lugdunensis*, n = 3; *S. simulans*, n = 1; and *S. scuri*, n = 4) isolates were cytotoxic to Vero cells. The three types of hemolysis were manifested as α-, β- and γ-hemolysins at a percentage of 17.4, 47.8, and 34.8%, respectively (Table 1).

Biofilm formation phenotype

Using the tube method (TM), a total of 18 isolates (78.3%) were classified as positive for biofilm formation ability, while 5 isolates (21.7%) were considered negative. Using CRA method, 7 of the 23 *Staphylococcus* spp.

Table 1 Phenotypic (antibiotic resistance, haemolytic activity and biofilm formation ability) and genotypic (antibiotic resistance genes) profile of all *Staphylococcus* spp. strains isolated from imported meat

Isolate	Species	Antibiotic resistance genes					Antibiotic resistance profile												Biofilm formation		Haemolysis			Virulence
		mecA	gyrA	grlA	gyrB	Cfr	Ampicillin-sulbactam	Chloramphenicol	Ciprofloxacin	Clindamycin	Erythromycin	Gentamycin	Methicillin	Oxacillin	Penicillin	Sulfamethoxazole/trimethoprim	Tetracycline	Vancomycin	Congo Red Agar	Tube method	α	β	δ	Vero cell
1	S. aureus	–	+	–	–	–	R	S	R	R	R	S	S	R	R	R	S	S	–	+	–	–	+	+
2	S. aureus	–	+	–	–	–	S	S	S	S	S	S	S	S	R	R	S	S	–	+	–	+	–	+
3	S. aureus	–	–	–	+	–	S	S	S	S	S	S	S	S	R	R	S	S	–	+	–	+	+	+
4	S. hyicus	+	–	+	–	–	S	S	S	R	S	R	R	R	R	R	S	R	+	+	–	+	+	+
5	S. hyicus	–	+	–	–	–	S	S	S	S	S	S	S	S	R	R	S	S	–	+	–	+	–	+
6	S. hyicus	–	–	+	–	–	S	S	S	S	S	S	S	S	R	R	S	S	–	+	–	+	–	+
7	S. hyicus	+	+	+	+	–	S	S	R	R	S	R	R	R	R	R	R	R	+	+	+	–	–	+
8	S. hyicus	+	–	–	–	–	S	S	R	R	S	R	R	R	R	R	S	R	+	+	–	–	–	+
9	S. hyicus	–	+	+	–	–	S	S	S	R	S	R	S	S	R	R	S	R	–	–	–	–	+	+
10	S. intermedius	–	+	–	–	–	S	S	S	R	R	R	S	S	R	R	S	S	–	–	–	+	–	+
11	S. intermedius	–	+	+	+	–	S	S	S	R	R	R	R	R	R	R	S	R	+	+	–	–	+	+
12	S. intermedius	+	–	+	+	–	S	S	R	R	R	R	R	R	R	R	R	R	+	+	–	–	+	+
13	S. epidermidis	–	+	+	–	–	S	R	R	R	R	R	S	R	R	R	S	S	–	+	–	+	–	+
14	S. hemolyticus	–	–	–	–	–	S	S	S	S	S	S	S	S	S	S	S	R	+	+	–	+	–	+
15	S. hominus	–	–	–	–	–	R	S	S	R	R	R	R	R	R	R	R	R	–	–	–	+	–	+
16	S. lugdunensis	+	–	–	–	–	S	S	R	R	S	R	R	R	R	R	R	R	+	–	–	+	+	+
17	S. lugdunensis	–	–	–	–	–	S	S	S	S	S	S	S	S	R	R	S	S	+	+	–	+	–	+
18	S. lugdunensis	–	+	+	+	–	S	S	S	S	S	S	S	S	R	R	S	S	–	+	–	+	–	+
19	S. simulans	–	+	+	–	–	S	S	R	R	S	R	S	R	R	R	R	S	–	+	–	+	–	+
20	S. sciuri	–	+	+	+	–	R	S	R	R	S	R	R	R	R	R	R	S	+	+	–	+	–	+
21	S. sciuri	–	+	–	–	–	R	S	S	R	S	R	S	S	R	R	S	S	–	+	–	–	–	+
22	S. sciuri	–	–	–	–	–	R	S	S	R	S	R	S	R	R	R	S	S	–	+	–	–	–	+
23	S. sciuri	–	–	–	–	–	R	S	S	S	S	S	S	R	R	R	S	S	–	+	–	–	–	+

isolates (30.4%) showed black colonies with shriveled lucent texture whereas 16 (69.6%) isolates showed pink colored colonies with mucoid appearance on the CRA plates that were interpreted as negative for biofilm formation (Table 1).

Antibiotic resistance phenotypic profile

The diversity in occurrence of antibiotic resistance among the tested *Staphylococcus* spp. isolates is outlined in Tables 1 and 2 . The 23 isolates were resistant to at least one antibiotic. Less than 50% of the isolates exhibited resistance to the β-lactams ampicillin (6/23) and methicillin (8/23), erythromycin (6/23), chloramphenicol (1/23), ciprofloxacin (7/23), vancomycin (9/23), and tetracycline (6/23) (Table 2). Ninety six percent of the isolates (22/23) were resistant to penicillin and sulfamethoxazole/trimethoprim, while only one isolate was resistant to chloramphenicol (Table 1). MDR, defined as resistance to ≥3 antimicrobial classes, was observed in 16 *Staphylococcus* isolates. Fifteen multidrug resistance (MDR) combination patterns were observed (Table 2). The penicillin/sulfamethoxazole/trimethoprim (P/SXT) resistance phenotype was evident in 14/15 of these combinations.

Antimicrobial resistance genes

From the 23 screened isolates, five isolates (3/6 *S. hyicus*; 1/3 *S. intermedius*; 1/3 *S. lugdunensis*) were identified as positive for *mecA* (5/23). Four of the 13 oxacillin-resistant isolates harbored the *mecA* gene, while 4 of the

8 methicillin resistant isolates carried the *mecA* gene (Table 3).

Interestingly, the following three observations were recorded: (i) although *S. hominis* and *S. hemolyticus* isolates were resistant to methicillin and vancomycin, respectively, the resistance genes *mecA*, *gyrA*, *gyrB*, *grlA* and *cfr* were absent. (ii) three *S. aureus* isolates did not carry the *mecA* gene (100%) and were phenotypically characterized as MSS; and (iii) one *S. lugdunensis* isolate was observed to harbor the *mecA* resistance gene but was phenotypically characterized as methicillin-susceptible non-*S. aureus* (MSNSA). The resistance gene *mecA* was detected in 4/8 (50%) methicillin-resistant non-*S. aureus* (MRNSA) isolates (Table 3). Of the three MSSA isolates, two carried the *gyrA* gene (66.66%) and one carried the *gyrB* gene (33.33%) (Table 1). The *cfr* gene was absent in all *Staphylococcus* isolates. The non-*cfr*-conveying CNS showed extensive resistance to several antimicrobials irrespective of those incorporated in the *cfr*-transmitted PhLOPSA phenotype (conferring resistance to several classes of antibiotics (phenicols, lincosamides, oxazolidinones, pleuromutilins, and streptogramin A; PhLOPSA phenotype) (Table 1). Phenotypically, 40% (8/20) of NSA (non *Staphylococcus aureus*) isolates were methicillin resistant, while the *mecA* gene was detected in only 25% (5/20) of isolates.

Correlation analyses

Correlation analyses showed that presence of *mecA* was directly correlated with resistance to ciprofloxacin, gentamicin, methicillin, oxacillin, and vancomycin (Pearson's correlation coefficients of 0.50, 0.42, 0.72, 0.46 and 0.66, respectively) (Fig. 1). There were several instances of co-occurrence of resistance to various antibiotics. Indeed, resistance to various antibiotics was directly correlated. For instance, resistance to methicillin was significantly associated with resistance to ciprofloxacin (Pearson's correlation coefficient of 0.43), clindamycin (Pearson's correlation coefficient of 0.53), gentamicin (Pearson's correlation coefficient of 0.59), oxacillin (Pearson's correlation coefficient of 0.64), tetracycline (Pearson's correlation coefficient of 0.61) and vancomycin (Pearson's correlation coefficient of 0.72). Similarly, a high correlation between resistances to several other antibiotics was found (Fig. 1). In addition, biofilm formation, as assessed by the CRA tests, was directly correlated with *mecA* presence (Pearson's correlation coefficient of 0.66), methicillin resistance (Pearson's correlation coefficient of 0.72) and vancomycin resistance (Pearson's correlation coefficient of 0.63).

Discussion

Globally, an increasing recognizable concern exists on the status of antimicrobial resistant microbial contaminants in the food chain and their capacity to be widely

Table 2 Antimicrobial resistance patterns among *Staphylococcus* spp. strains isolated from imported beef meat

Antibiotics	Number of antibiotics	Total number of isolates	%
VA	1	1/23	4
P, SXT	2	6/23	26
P, TE, VA, SXT	4	1/23	4
P, CN, E, DA, SXT	5	2/23	9
P, OX, CN, DA, SXT			
P, OX, SAM, CN, DA, SXT	6	3/23	13
P, OX, MET, CN, DA, SXT			
P, OX, E, DA, C, SXT, CIP	7	5/23	22
P, CN, DA, TE, VA, SXT, CIP			
P, OX, CN, DA, TE, SXT, CIP			
P, OX, MET, CN, DA, VA, SXT			
P, OX, MET, CN, DA, VA, SXT, CIP	8	2/23	9
P, OX, MET, CN, E, DA, TE, VA, SXT	9	3/23	13
P, OX, MET, CN, E, DA, VA, SXT, CIP			
P, OX, MET, SAM, E, DA, TE, VA, SXT			

C chloramphenicol, *CIP* ciprofloxacin, *CN* gentamycin, *DA* clindamycin, *E* erythromycin, *MET* methicillin, *OX* oxacillin, *P* penicilin, *SAM* ampicillin-sulbactam, *SXT* sulfamethoxazole/trimethoprim, *TE* tetracycline, *VA* vancomycin

Table 3 Prevalence of the *mecA* gene in imported beef samples

Staphylococcus spp. (n = number of isolates)	n = of MRS	Presence of *mecA* gene		n = of MSS	Precence of *mecA* gene	
		n=	%		n=	%
S. aureus (n = 3)	0	0	0	3	0	0
S. hyicus (n = 6)	3	3	100	3	0	0
S. intermedius (n = 3)	2	1	50	1	0	0
S. epidermidis (n = 1)	0	0	0	1	0	0
S. hemolyticus (n = 1)	0	0	0	1	0	0
S. hominus (n = 1)	1	0	0	0	0	0
S. lugdunensis (n = 3)	1	0	0	2	1	50
S. simulans (n = 1)	0	0	0	1	0	0
S. scuri (n = 4)	1	0	0	3	0	0
Total	8	4	50	15	1	6.7

MRS methicillin resistant *Staphylococcus*, *MSS* methicillin susceptible *Staphylococcus*

dispersed through the international trade of food. This prompted the Codex Alimentarius Commission to establish an ad hoc Intergovernmental Task Force on Antimicrobial Resistance in 2007, bearing in mind the occurrence of national and regional diversity in antimicrobial misuse, human subjection to resistant microorganisms and determinants and their prevalence in foodborne pathogens. Egypt imports different meat types to fill the gaps in animal protein supply. According to the U.S. Meat Export Federation (USMEF) that examines key statistics and trends in beef and pork trade from 2008 to 2017, Egypt's projection for beef-importing in 2017 would reach about 332,000 metric tons of meat imports and this is supposed to grow to 2025 by 52.28% [25]. While the importation of beef meat in Egypt is crucial to close the gap in animal protein requirements, monitoring the frequency of antimicrobial resistance in imported meat must assure that quality and safety standards are met.

The spread of MRSA is a serious public health concern for both human and veterinary medicine. Due to the occurrence of MRSA, methicillin and other β-lactamic antibiotics have become useless for clinical therapy, leaving the term MRSA to be used to describe *S. aureus* strains resistant to effectively all β-lactamase-resistant penicillins and harboring the *mecA* gene [23]. Although the development and spread of multiple antibiotic-resistant MRSA have gained much attention over the past years, yet the role of imported meat has not been given much attention. In a Danish study, Agersø et al. reported that MRSA was found in 18% of the imported broiler meat and 7.5% of the imported pork [26]. MRSA are often resistant to other antimicrobials different to methicillin, highlighting the necessity for new and effective antimicrobials. Attributed to their extended antimicrobial spectra, fluoroquinolone compounds such as ciprofloxacin and norfloxacin were recommended as useful candidates for eradicating MRSA [27]. Nonetheless, due to the misuse of these compounds in the clinical practice, resistance of MRSA to these compounds has been observed [28]. For this reason ciprofloxacin is not recommended to be used in empirical therapy against MRSA infections. Furthermore, the use of other fluoroquinolones is only allowed following accurate antimicrobial susceptibility testing. Nonetheless, vancomycin remains the drug of choice to treat MRSA infections [29].

Identification of methicillin resistant staphylococci in the laboratory is often problematic due to difficulty in detecting heterogeneous methicillin-oxacillin resistance in staphylococci [30, 31]. Moreover, Standard interpretive breakpoints for oxacillin susceptibility reporting published by the CLSI (formerly the National Committee for Clinical and Laboratory Standards) were changed in 2004, and NSA isolates of veterinary origin are now more likely than in previous years to be deemed resistant by testing laboratories that use those guidelines [32].

In this study, the susceptibility of 23 *Staphylococcus* spp. strains isolated from imported meat to 12 antibiotics from different classes was evaluated. An extreme resistance was found against penicillin and sulfamethoxazole/ trimethoprim as compared to other tested antibiotics, which could be attributed to the extensive use of these antibiotics in treating mastitis cases and/or as growth promoters in animal feed in the countries from which the beef meat was imported. Resistance to other clinically important antibiotics, including β-lactamic antibiotics (such as ampicillin-sulbactam, methicillin, oxacillin), fluoroquinolones (ciprofloxacin), macrolides (erythromycin), aminoglycosides (gentamicin), glycopeptides

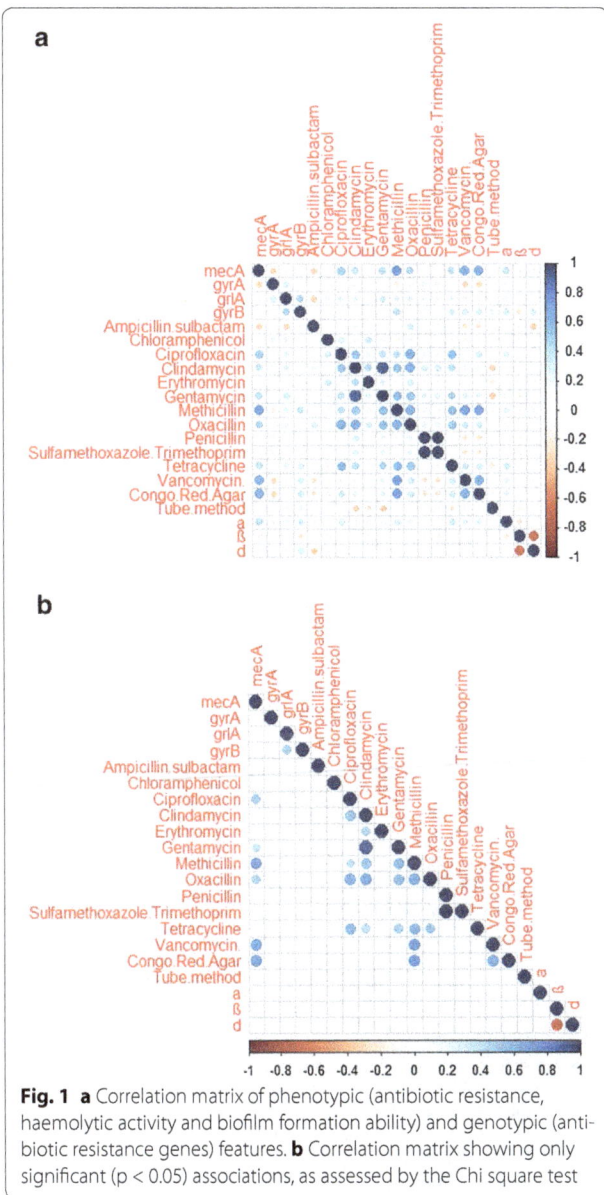

Fig. 1 a Correlation matrix of phenotypic (antibiotic resistance, haemolytic activity and biofilm formation ability) and genotypic (antibiotic resistance genes) features. **b** Correlation matrix showing only significant (p < 0.05) associations, as assessed by the Chi square test

oxacillin, tetracycline and vancomycin). The colonization ability in conjunction with the occurrence of MDR highlights the hazardous nature of the *Staphylococcus* spp. isolated from imported beef meat.

The antimicrobial resistance determinants *mecA*, *gyrA*, *gyrB*, *grlA* and *cfr*, frequently reported in *S. aureus* strains were also screened in recovered isolates. The emergence of the multiple drug resistance gene *cfr* in staphylococci is of global clinical and veterinary importance that has been previously investigated in staphylococci [34] and has been identified as a phenicol and lincosamide resistance gene [35]. In this study, the absence of the *cfr* gene among imported beef meat isolates suggests a decreased potential risk as an outcome of harboring the gene in the food chain through imported meat. Furthermore, the absence of the gene *cfr* poses a significant and interdisciplinary public health positive factor to the Egyptian consumers. One isolate showed chloramphenicol resistance but was negative for the *cfr* gene. This observation might be attributed to a possible heterogeneous expression of the *cfr* gene [36] or to different potential chloramphenicol resistance mechanisms.

The *mecA* gene confers methicillin resistance. It encodes the penicillin binding protein 2a, an enzyme that has low affinity for beta-lactams, and has been reported to lead to resistance to ciprofloxacin, gentamycin, methicillin, oxacillin and vancomycin [37]. In our study, the *mecA* gene was carried by 5 out of 23 *Staphylococcus* spp. isolates, and, as expected, presence of *mecA* was directly correlated with resistance to ciprofloxacin, gentamycin, methicillin, oxacillin, and vancomycin. Nevertheless, not all methicillin or oxacillin resistant isolates were *mecA* positive. It was previously indicated that some isolates missing the *mecA* gene could be identified as phenotypically resistant to oxacillin (MRSA) [38]. These results suggests that other potential resistance mechanisms might exist. Molecular investigations of a *S. aureus* isolate, which was found to be phenotypically resistant to methicillin but negative for the *mecA* gene, were able to identify the presence of a novel *mecA* homologue, which was found to be associated with cattle [39], suggesting the existence of a zoonotic MRSA reservoir [40]. In 2012, the International Working Group on the Classification of Staphylococcal Cassette Chromosome elements (IWCC) renamed the *mecA* variant, *mecC* [41]. Methicillin-resistant *S. aureus* strains carrying the *mecC* gene have been shown to cause a range of infections in humans and appear to be predominantly community associated [40]. The prevalence of *mecC* in CNS has been recently reported for 13 European countries, where it has been isolated from 14 different host species (Holmes et al. 42), and an allotype of the *mecC* gene has been detected in a *S. xylosus* strain [42]. It is also worth mentioning the fact

(vancomycin), lincosamides (clindamycin) and tetracycline also occurred and, in some cases, multidrug resistance phenotypes were identified. Indeed, correlation analyses showed co-occurrence of resistance to series of antibiotics. Extended-spectrum beta-lactamases (ESBL)-producing pathogens are often resistant to fluoroquinolones and aminoglycosides since resistance mechanisms for these classes of antibiotics are often carried on the same large plasmids that contain the genetic elements for ESBL production [33]. Our results corroborate this observation. Thus, for instance, resistance to methicillin was significantly associated with resistance to ciprofloxacin and gentamycin, among others (clindamycin,

that one *S. lugdunensis* isolate was observed to harbor the *mecA* resistance gene but was phenotypically characterized as MSNSA. The phenotypic susceptibility to oxacillin, methicillin, penicillin and ampicillin (β-lactam antibiotic of the penicillin class) regardless of the *mecA* presence may be attributed to the heterogeneous expression of *mecA* [43], which is more common in CNS than that in *S. aureus* [44]. Nevertheless, it should be noted that in 2014, Bhargava and Zhang emphasized the importance of MRCNSs as important reservoirs of *mecA* that could act as precursors of MRSA [11]. In addition, temperature abuse during storage and transportation to the importing country may result in multiplication of MRS [45]. An additional important finding was introduced by the identification and characterization of another gene on the SCC element called *mecR2* that regulates and increases *mecA* expression when MRSA bacteria encounter β-lactam drugs [46].

Besides resistance genes, mutation-mediated resistance is especially common among resistances to synthetic antibacterial agents, such as fluoroquinolones and oxazolidinones in *S. aureus* and other bacterial species [47]. The primers used in this study amplified only the copies of *gyrA*, *gyrB*, and *grlA* that contained mutations in the quinolone resistance-determining regions (QRDRs). In this study, the amplification of a *grlA* and *gyrA* product represented the presence of a mutation conferring resistance. Mutations in the *gyrB* gene does not play an important role in quinolone resistance [48]. Although the presence of resistance genes are a primary reason for antibiotic resistance, the resistance phenotype and gene presence are not exclusively linked in this study. Similarly, this inconsistency was common in other classes of antibiotics, demonstrating that the presence of a certain resistance gene was not necessary an indicator of antibiotic resistance [49]. A potential explanation for this inconsistency could be the lack of expression of some of the resistance genes and the presence of other genes encoding resistance. In addition, chromosomally encoded multidrug resistance pumps have been shown to have other primary functional or structural roles [50].

The connection between microbial biofilms and antibiotic resistance is of considerable interest to biomedical researchers. Previous reports have suggested that a correlation between antibiotic resistance and biofilm formation ability exists, a phenomenon that may be responsible for a decrease in the efficaciousness of antimicrobial agents against *S. aureus* infections [51]. As a consequence of biofilm development, the capability of horizontal gene transfer is increased and may facilitate the dispersion of antibiotic resistance [52]. In the present study, MRS and MDR isolates showed a good potential to form biofilms. In fact, correlation analyses

showed that biofilm formation, as assessed by the CRA tests, was directly correlated with *mecA* presence, methicillin resistance and vancomycin resistance, and biofilm producing MRNSA showed high resistance to almost all antibiotic classes compared to non-producers, which corroborates previous observations [53].

Conclusions

Despite the alert generated by the outbreaks of foot and mouth disease and swine fever, which have been attributed to international trade of meat, little information or actionable risk management information is available yet on the dissemination of microbial hazards through retail imported meat. This study reveals that imported meat can act as a transmission vector for MRSA or MRNSA harboring the *mecA* gene, which may represent a risk for both human and veterinary medicine. The data obtained on the resistance of *Staphylococcus* spp. to antimicrobials, may be used for implementing an antimicrobial resistance spread monitoring and prevention program.

Abbreviations

ESBL: extended-spectrum beta-lactamases; CNS: coagulase-negative staphylococci; CPS: coagulase-positive staphylococci (CPS); LA-MRSA: livestock-associated methicillin-resistant *Staphylococcus aureus*; MDR: multiple drug resistance; MRNSA: methicillin-resistant non-*Staphylococcus aureus*; MRSA: methicillin-resistant *Staphylococcus aureus*; MSNSA: methicillin-susceptible non-*Staphylococcus aureus*; NSA: non *Staphylococcus aureus*; QRDRs: quinolone resistance-determining regions.

Authors' contributions

KO conceived, designed the experiments, analyzed the data and wrote the paper; AAO, LR and ME conducted the data analysis and contributed to the writing of the manuscript. FE, KAM, IM and AH contributed with their scientific advice during the work and revision of the manuscript; AO and AS contributed with reagents/materials/analysis tools and performed the experiments. All authors read and approved the final manuscript.

Author details

[1] Department of Microbiology, Faculty of Veterinary Medicine, Cairo University, Giza, Egypt. [2] Department of Food Hygiene and Technology and Institute of Food Science and Technology, University of León, León, Spain. [3] Department of Nutrition, Bromatology and Food Technology, Universidad Complutense de Madrid, Madrid, Spain. [4] Department of Poultry Diseases, Animal Health Research, Institute, Giza, Egypt. [5] Department of Bacteriology, Immunology and Mycology, Faculty of Veterinary Medicine, Benha University, Moushtohor, Egypt. [6] Department of Botany and Microbiology, College of Science, King Saud University, Riyadh, Kingdom of Saudi Arabia. [7] Department of Health Science, College of Applied Studies and Community Service, King Saud University, Riyadh, Kingdom of Saudi Arabia. [8] Department of Bacteriology, Mycology and Immunology, Faculty of Veterinary Medicine, Mansoura University, Mansoura 35516, Egypt. [9] Foodborne Pathogens, Scientific Institute of Public Health, Juliette Wytsmanstraat 14, 1050 Brussels, Belgium.

Acknowledgements

The authors extend their appreciation to the Deanship of Scientific Research at King Saud University for funding the work through the research group Project No.: RGP-162.

Competing interests

The authors declare that they have no competing interests.

References

1. MacDiarmid SC. Risk analysis and the importation of animals and animal products. Rev Sci Tech. 1993;12:1093–107.
2. WTO 2016. World Trade Organization. Sanitary and phytosanitary measures: text of the agreement. The WTO Agreement on the Application of Sanitary and Phytosanitary Measures (SPS Agreement). Centre William Rappard, 154 rue de Lausanne, Geneva, Switzerland.
3. Hennekinne JA, De Buyser ML, Dragacci S. Staphylococcus aureus and its food poisoning toxins: characterization and outbreak investigation. FEMS Microbiol Rev. 2012;36:815–36.
4. Bhumbra S, Mahboubi M, Blackwood RA. Staphylococcus lugdunensis: novel organism causing cochlear implant infection. Infect Dis Rep. 2014;6:5406.
5. Giormezis N, Kolonitsiou F, Foka A, Drougka E, Liakopoulos A, Makri A, Papanastasiou AD, Vogiatzi A, Dimitriou G, Marangos M, Christofidou M, Anastassiou ED, Petinaki E, Spiliopoulou I. Coagulase-negative staphylococcal bloodstream and prosthetic-device-associated infections: the role of biofilm formation and distribution of adhesin and toxin genes. J Med Microbiol. 2014;63:1500–8.
6. Pinheiro L, Brito CI, de Oliveira A, Martins PY, Pereira VC, da Cunha Mde L. Staphylococcus epidermidis and Staphylococcus haemolyticus: molecular detection of cytotoxin and enterotoxin genes. Toxins. 2015;7:3688–99.
7. Osman KM, Abd EL-Razik KA, Marie HSH, Arafa A. Coagulase-negative staphylococci collected from bovine milk: species and antimicrobial gene diversity. J Food Saf. 2016;36:89–99.
8. Osman KM, Amer AM, Badr JM, Helmy NM, Elhelw RA, Orabi A, Bakry M, Saad AS. Antimicrobial resistance, biofilm formation and mecA characterization of methicillin-susceptible S. aureus and non-S. aureus of beef meat origin in Egypt. Front Microbiol. 2016;7:222.
9. Veras JF, Carmo LS, Tong LC, Shupp JW, Cummings C, Dos Santos DA, Cerqueira MM, Cantini A, Nicoli JR, Jett M. A study of the enterotoxigenicity of coagulase-negative and coagulase-positive staphylococcal isolates from food poisoning outbreaks in Minas Gerais, Brazil. Int J Infect Dis. 2008;12:410–5.
10. Chajęcka-Wierzchowska W, Zadernowska A, Nalepa B, Sierpińska M, Łaniewska-Trokenheim Ł. Coagulase-negative staphylococci (CoNS) isolated from ready-to-eat food of animal origin–phenotypic and genotypic antibiotic resistance. Food Microbiol. 2015;46:222–6.
11. Bhargava K, Zhang Y. Characterization of methicillin-resistant coagulase-negative staphylococci (MRCoNS) in retail meat. Food Microbiol. 2014;42:56–60.
12. Tulinski P, Fluit AC, Wagenaar JA, Mevius D, van de Vijver L, Duim B. Methicillin-resistant coagulase-negative staphylococci on pig farms as a reservoir of heterogeneous staphylococcal cassette chromosome mec elements. Appl Environ Microbiol. 2012;78:299–304.
13. Doyle MP, Loneragan GH, Scott HM, Singer RS. Antimicrobial resistance: challenges and perspectives. Comp Rev Food Sci Food Saf. 2013;12:234–48.
14. Alabi SA, Frielinghaus L, Grobusch MP, Köck R, Becker K, Issifou S, Kremsner PG, Peters G, Mellmann A. The risk to import ESBL-producing Enterobacteriaceae and Staphylococcus aureus through chicken meat trade in Gabon. BMC Microbiol. 2014;14:286.
15. Card R, Vaughan K, Bagnall M, Spiropoulos J, Cooley W, Strickland T, Davies R, Anjum MF. Virulence characterization of Salmonella enterica isolates of differing antimicrobial resistance recovered from UK livestock and imported meat samples. Front Microbiol. 2016;7:640.
16. Long KS, Poehlsgaard J, Kehrenberg C, Schwarz S, Vester B. The Cfr rRNA methyltransferase confers resistance to phenicols, lincosamides, oxazolidinones, pleuromutilins, and streptogramin A antibiotics. Antimicrob Agents Chemother. 2006;50:2500–5.
17. Bannerman T. Staphylococcus, Micrococcus, and other catalase positive cocci that grow aerobically. In: Murray PR, Baron EJ, Jorgensen JH, et al., editors. Manual of clinical microbiology. Washington, DC: ASM Press; 2003. p. 384–404.
18. Futagawa-Saito K, Ba-Thein W, Sakurai N, Fukuyasu T. Prevalence of virulence factors in Staphylococcus intermedius isolates from dogs and pigeons. BMC Vet Res. 2006;2:4.
19. Tao M, Yamashita H, Watanabe K, Nagatake T. Possible virulence factors of Staphylococcus aureus in a mouse septic model. FEMS Immunol Med Microbiol. 1999;23:135–46.
20. CLSI. Performance standards for antimicrobial susceptibility testing. Clinical and Laboratory Standards Institute 2007, CLSI M100-S17, Wayne, PA, USA.
21. WHO World Health Organization. Critically important antimicrobials for human medicine—3rd rev. WHO Press, World Health Organization, 20 Avenue Appia, 1211 Geneva 27, Switzerland; 2012.
22. Zhang K, Sparling J, Chow BL, Elsayed S, Hussain Z, Church DL, Gregson DB, Louie T, Conly JM. New quadriplex PCR assay for detection of methicillin and mupirocin resistance and simultaneous discrimination of Staphylococcus aureus from coagulase-negative staphylococci. J Clin Microbiol. 2004;42:4947–55.
23. Paterson GK, Harrison EM, Holmes MA. The emergence of mecC methicillin-resistant Staphylococcus aureus. Trends Microbiol. 2014;22:42–7.
24. Mathur T, Singhal S, Khan S, Upadhyay DJ, Fatma T, Rattan A. Detection of biofilm formation among the clinical isolates of staphylococci: an evaluation of three different screening methods. Indian J Med Microbiol. 2006;24:25–9.
25. USDA 2016 United States Department of Agriculture Foreign Agricultural Service Foreign Ag ServiceVerified account @USDAForeignAg.
26. Agersø Y, Hasman H, Cavaco LM, Pedersen K, Aarestrup FM. Study of methicillin resistant Staphylococcus aureus (MRSA) in Danish pigs at slaughter and in imported retail meat reveals a novel MRSA type in slaughter pigs. Vet Microbiol. 2012;157:246–50.
27. Gilbert MJ, Boscia A, Kobasa WD, Kaye D. Enoxacin compared with vancomycin for the treatment of experimental methicillin-resistant Staphylococcus aureus endocarditis. Antimicrob Agents Chemother. 1986;29:461–3.
28. Pai V, Rao VI, Rao SP. Prevalence and antimicrobial susceptibility pattern of methicillin-resistant Staphylococcus aureus [MRSA] isolates at a tertiary care hospital in Mangalore, South India. J Lab Phys. 2010;2:82–4.
29. Gade ND, Qazi MS. Fluoroquinolone therapy in Staphylococcus aureus infections: where do we stand? J Lab Phys. 2013;5:109–12.
30. Tenover FC, Goering RV. Methicillin-resistant Staphylococcus aureus strain USA300: origin and epidemiology. J Antimicrob Chemother. 2009;64:441–6.
31. Brown DFJ. Detection of methicillin/oxacillin resistance in staphylococci. J Antimicrob Chemother. 2002;48(S1):65–70.
32. NCCLS National Committee for Clinical Laboratory Standards. Performance standards for antimicrobial disk and dilution susceptibility tests for bacteria isolated from animals; informational supplement. 2004, Document M31-S1. Wayne, Pa: NCCLS; 2004.
33. Karam G, Chastre J, Wilcox MH, Vincent J. Antibiotic strategies in the era of multidrug resistance. Crit Care. 2016;20:136.
34. Wang Y, He T, Schwarz S, Zhao Q, Shen Z, Wu C, Shen J. Multidrug resistance gene cfr in methicillin-resistant coagulase-negative staphylococci from chickens, ducks, and pigs in China. Int J Med Microbiol. 2013;303:84–7.
35. Witte W, Cuny C. Emergence and spread of cfr-mediated multiresistance in staphylococci: an interdisciplinary challenge. Future Microbiol. 2011;6:925–31.
36. Terlizzi V, Carnovale V, Castaldo G, Castellani C, Cirilli N, Colombo C, Corti F, Cresta F, D'Adda A, Lucarelli M, Lucidi V, Macchiaroli A, Madarena E, Padoan R, Quattrucci S, Salvatore D, Zarrilli F, Raia V. Clinical expression of patients with the D1152H CFTR mutation. J Cyst Fibros. 2015;14:447–52.
37. Lee JH. Methicillin (oxacillin)-resistant Staphylococcus aureus strains isolated from major food animals and their potential transmission to humans. Appl Environ Microbiol. 2003;69:6489–94.

38. Lee JH, Jeong JM, Park YH, Choi SS, Kim YH, Chae JS, Moon JS, Park H, Kim S, Eo SK. Evaluation of the methicillin-resistant *Staphylococcus aureus* (MRSA)-screen latex agglutination test for detection of MRSA of animal origin. J Clin Microbiol. 2004;42:2780–2.

39. García-Álvarez L, Holden MT, Lindsay H, Webb CR, Brown DF, Curran MD, Walpole E, Brooks K, Pickard DJ, Teale C, Parkhill J, Bentley SD, Edwards GF, Girvan EK, Kearns AM, Pichon B, Hill RL, Larsen AR, Skov RL, Peacock SJ, Maskell DJ, Holmes MA. Methicillin-resistant *Staphylococcus aureus* with a novel *mec*A homologue in human and bovine populations in the UK and Denmark: a descriptive study. Lancet Infect Dis. 2011;11:595–603.

40. Petersen A, Stegger M, Heltberg O, Christensen J, Zeuthen A, Knudsen LK, Urth T, Sorum M, Schouls L, Larsen J, Skov R, Larsen AR. Epidemiology of methicillin-resistant *Staphylococcus aureus* carrying the novel mecC gene in Denmark corroborates a zoonotic reservoir with transmission to humans. Clin Microbiol Infect. 2013;19:E16–22.

41. Ito T, Hiramatsu K, Tomasz A, de Lencastre H, Perreten V, Holden MT, Coleman DC, Goering R, Giffard PM, Skov RL, Zhang K, Westh H, O'Brien F, Tenover FC, Oliveira DC, Boyle-Vavra S, Laurent F, Kearns AM, Kreiswirth B, Ko KS, Grundmann H, Sollid JE Jr, John JF, Daum R, Soderquist B, Buist G, and International Working Group on the Classification of Staphylococcal Cassette Chromosome Elements (IWG-SCC). Guidelines for reporting novel *mec*A gene homologues. Antimicrob Agents Chemother. 2012;56:4997–9.

42. Holmes M, Zadoks R. Methicillin resistant *S. aureus* in human and bovine mastitis. Mammary Gland Biol Neoplasia. 2011;16:373–82.

43. Stegger M. Rapid detection, differentiation and typing of methicillin-resistant *Staphylococcus aureus* harbouring either *mec*A or the new *mec*A homologue *mec*A (LGA251). Clin Microbiol Infect. 2012;18:395–400.

44. Stepanovic S, Hauschild T, Dakic I, Al-Doori Z, Svabic-Vlahovic M, Ranin L, Morrison D. Evaluation of phenotypic and molecular methods for detection of oxacillin resistance in members of the *Staphylococcus sciuri* group. J Clin Microbiol. 2006;44:934–7.

45. de Boer E, Zwartkruis-Nahuis JT, Wit B, Huijsdens XW, de Neeling AJ, Bosch T, van Oosterom RA, Vila A, Heuvelink AE. Prevalence of methicillin-resistant *Staphylococcus aureus* in meat. Int J Food Microbiol. 2009;134:52–6.

46. Arêde P, Milheiriço C, de Lencastre H, Oliveira DC. The anti-repressor *MecR2* promotes the proteolysis of the *mec*A repressor and enables optimal expression of β-lactam resistance in MRSA. PLoS Pathog. 2012;8:e1002816.

47. Aldred KJ, Kerns RJ, Osheroff N. Mechanism of quinolone action and resistance. Biochemistry. 2014;53:1565–74.

48. Sierra JM, Marco F, Ruiz J, Jime´nez de Anta MT, Vila J. Correlation between the activity of different fluoroquinolones and the presence of mechanisms of quinolone resistance in epidemiologically related and unrelated strains of methicillin-susceptible and –resistant *Staphylococcus aureus*. Clin Microbiol Infect. 2002;8:781–90.

49. Xu J, Shi C, Song M, Xu X, Yang P, Paoli G, Shi X. Phenotypic and genotypic antimicrobial resistance traits of foodborne *Staphylococcus aureus* isolates from Shanghai. J Food Sci. 2014;79:M635–42.

50. Kosmidis C, Schindler BD, Jacinto PL, Patel D, Bains K, Seo SM, Kaatz GW. Expression of multidrug resistance efflux pump genes in clinical and environmental isolates of *Staphylococcus aureus*. Intl J Antimicrob Agents. 2012;40:204–9.

51. Gu¨ndog¨an N, Citak S, Turan E. Slime production, DNAse activity and antibiotic resistance of *Staphylococcus aureus* isolated from raw milk, pasteurized milk and ice cream samples. Food Control. 2006;17:389–92.

52. Lee HW, Koh YM, Kim J, Lee JC, Lee YC, Seol SY, Cho DT, Kim J. Capacity of multidrug-resistant clinical isolates of *Acinetobacter baumannii* to form biofilm and adhere to epithelial cell surfaces. Clin Microbiol Infect. 2008;14:49–54.

53. Donlan RM, Costerton W. Biofilms: survival mechanisms of clinically relevant microorganisms. Clin Microbiol Rev. 2002;15:167–93.

8

Extended-spectrum beta-lactamase-producing *Pseudomonas aeruginosa* in camel in Egypt: potential human hazard

Mahmoud Elhariri[1], Dalia Hamza[2*], Rehab Elhelw[1] and Sohad M. Dorgham[3]

Abstract

Background: The rapid increase of extended-spectrum beta-lactamase (ESBL) producing bacteria are a potential health hazard. Development of antimicrobial resistance in animal pathogens has serious implications for human health, especially when such strains could be transmitted to human. In this study, the antimicrobial resistance due to ESBL producing *Pseudomonas aeruginosa* in the camel meat was investigated.

Methods: In this study meat samples from 200 healthy camels at two major abattoirs in Egypt (Cairo and Giza) were collected. Following culture on cetrimide agar, suspected *P. aeruginosa* colonies were confirmed with a Vitek 2 system (bioMe´rieux). *P. aeruginosa* isolates were phenotypically identified as ESBL by double disk synergy test. Additionally antimicrobial susceptibility testing of ESBL producing *P. aeruginosa* isolates were done against 11 antimicrobial drugs and carried out by disk diffusion method. The ESBL genotypes were determined by polymerase chain reaction according to the presence of the bla_{PER-1}, bla_{CTX-M}, bla_{SHV}, and bla_{TEM}.

Results: *Pseudomonas aeruginosa* was isolated from 45 camel meat sample (22.5%). The total percentage of ESBL producing *P. aeruginosa* was 45% (21/45) from camel meat isolates. Antibiogram results revealed the highest resistance was for c, ceftriaxone and rifampicin followed by cefepime and aztreonam. The prevalence rates of β-lactamase genes were recorded (bla_{PER-1} 28.5%, bla_{CTX-M} 38%, bla_{SHV} 33.3% and bla_{TEM} 23.8%).

Conclusions: This study illustrates the presence of high rates of ESBL-*P. aeruginosa* in camels that represents an increasing alarming for the risk of transmission to human and opens the door for current and future antibiotics therapy failure. Livestock associated ESBL-*P. aeruginosa* is a growing disaster, therefore, attention has to be fully given to livestock associated ESBL-bacteria which try to find its way to human beings.

Keywords: Camel, ESBL, *P. aeruginosa*, Resistance genes, Livestock, Egypt

Background

The increasing resistance of potentially pathogenic bacteria to multiple conventional antibiotics is an urgent problem in global public health [1]. *Pseudomonas aeruginosa* is one of the major causes of diseases such as otitis, mastitis, endometritis, hemorrhagic pneumonia and urinary tract infections in both livestock and companion animals [2–4]. The multiple-drug-resistant (MDR) *Pseudomonas* can be transmitted from different sources to humans and also to the environment through horizontal gene, the emergence and occurrence of MDR *P. aeruginosa* strains are growing in the world, leading to limited therapeutic options [5, 6].

The prevalence of MDR enterobacteriaceae in slaughterhouses, including swine and poultry environments, has been reported in several studies building a growing alarm about their effect on animal and human health

---

*Correspondence: daliahamza@cu.edu.eg
[2] Department of Zoonoses, Faculty of Veterinary Medicine, Cairo University, PO Box 12211, Giza, Egypt
Full list of author information is available at the end of the article

[7, 8]. Recently encountered the emergence of livestock associated ESBL-producing *P. aeruginosa* in cow, poultry and pigs [9, 10].

In Middle East region, camels are important in the livestock economy by their adaptability to adverse environmental conditions and naturally resistant to most of the diseases commonly affecting livestock [11]. Camels provide milk, meat, wool, hides, and skin, and their dung is used for fires [12]. They are acting one of major and good sources of protein and income for developing countries.

Transmission of ESBL-producing gram-negative bacteria between food-producing animals and humans via direct contact or meat is supposed [13]. Accordingly, livestock associated ESBL-producing gram-negative bacteria become new alarm for emerging infectious pathogens to human and animals.

This study aimed to investigate the role of camels as a risky reservoir and disseminating carrier of ESBL producing *P. aeruginosa* especially as this micro-organism has the ability of producing multidrug resistant enzymes that could be easily disseminated in the community via livestock products, particularly through direct contact and/or consumption of meat as well as other infected animal products.

Methods
Camel meat samples
This study was carried out on 200 apparently healthy camels. These camels were selected from two major abattoirs (Cairo and Giza) from April to September 2015. Meat samples from slaughtered camels in the abattoirs were collected in sterile containers and sent on ice to the microbiology department laboratory.

Meat samples preparation
Twenty-five grams of the collected meat samples were weighed and transferred to sterile flasks containing 100 ml of phosphate buffer saline (PBS). Samples were homogenized using a meat grinder under aseptic conditions.

Isolation and identification of *P. aeruginosa*
Two hundred meat samples were cultured into cetrimide agar, the plates were incubated aerobically at 37 °C for 24 h. The putative colonies were examined for their colonial morphology and microscopically according to Quinn et al. [14], the purified isolates of *P. aeruginosa* were finally confirmed with a Vitek 2 system (bioMe´rieux) which is rapid and reliable identification method.

Phenotypic detection of ESBL by double-disk synergy test method (DDST)
ESBL production in *P. aeruginosa* was identified by the double disk synergy test (DDST) as described by Jarlier

[15]. Mueller–Hinton agar was inoculated with standardized inoculum (corresponding to 0.5 McFarland tube) using a sterile cotton swab. An Augmentin (20 μg amoxicillin and 10 μg of clavulanic acid-AMC) disk was inserted in the center of the plate and test disks of 3rd generation cephalosporins (ceftazidime-CAZ 30 μg, ceftriaxone-CRO 30 μg, cefotaxime-CTX 30 μg) and aztreonam (ATM 30 μg) disks were placed at 20 mm distance (center to center) from the amoxicillin clavulanic acid disk. The plate was incubated overnight at 37 °C. Enhancement of the zone of inhibition of any one of the four drug disks toward amoxicillin–clavulanic acid suggested the presence of extended-spectrum beta-lactamases.

Escherichia coli 25922 was used as a negative control for the ESBL and *P. aeruginosa* ATCC 27853 was used as a control strain for a positive ESBL.

Antimicrobial susceptibility testing
Antibiotic susceptibility tests were performed for ESBL producing *P. aeruginosa* isolates by using the standard disc diffusion method (Kirby–Bauer) on Mueller–Hinton agar plates. The standard procedures of the CLSI, 2015 and British Society for Antimicrobial Chemotherapy (BSAC) disc diffusion method were strictly followed [16, 17], accordingly the antimicrobial susceptibility of *P. aeruginosa* strains were tested against 11 antimicrobial drugs: aztreonam (30 μg), ceftazidime (30 μg), ceftriaxone (30 μg), cefepime (30 μg), amikacin (30 μg), gentamicin (10 μg), ciprofloxacin (5 μg), rifamycin (30 μg), imipenem (10 μg), meropenem (1 μg) and sulphamethoxazole/trimethoprim (25 μg). *E. coli* ATCC 25922 and *P. aeruginosa* ATCC 27853 were used as quality controls.

DNA extraction
The whole genomic DNA from ESBL resistant *P. aeruginosa* strains totaling 21 was extracted using QIAamp Mini Kit (QIAGEN, Hombrechtikon, Switzerland) according to the manufacturer's instructions.

Molecular detection of ESBL-encoding genes
PCRs for detection of the bla_{PER-1}, bla_{CTX-M}, bla_{SHV} and bla_{TEM} genes. Specific primers for amplifying the selected genes by PCR are shown in Table 1.

The reaction mixture consisted of 25 μl Platinum™ Hot Start PCR Master Mix (Invitrogen™), 1 μl DNA extract, 0.5 μl of each primer in the concentration of (20 pmol) and nuclease free water up to 50 μl. The cycling conditions included denaturation for 10 min at 95 °C, amplification for 30 cycles of 30 s at 95 °C, 1 min at 55 °C, and 1 min at 72 °C, and extension for 10 min at 72 °C. The PCR products were resolved by electrophoresis on 1.5% (wt/vol) agarose gels (QIAGEN, Hombrechtikon, Switzerland).

Table 1 Primers used for detection of resistance genes

Target gene	Primer sequence (5′–3′)	Product size (bp)	References
bla_{PER-1}	F: ATGAATGTCATTATAAAAGC	926	[18]
	R: TTAATTTGGGCTTAGGG		
bla_{CTX-M}	F: GCGATGGGCAGTACCAGTAA	392	
	R: TTACCCAGCGTCAGATTCCG		
bla_{SHV}	F: TCAGCGAAAAACACCTTG	472	[19]
	R: TCCCGCAGATAAATCACCA		
bla_{TEM}	F: ATGAGTATTCAACATTTCCG	861	[20]
	R: TTACCAATGCTTAATCAGTGAG		

One uni plex PCR for detection of bla_{TEM} gene and two multiplex PCR were conducted for the (bla_{PER-1} and bla_{CTX-M}) and another one for (bla_{SHV}) gene

Results

Isolation and identification of P. aeruginosa

Forty-five isolates (22.5%) from meat samples of 200 camels were produced characteristic growth features of *Pseudomonas* species on the cetrimide agar medium. The isolates were obtained as one specific colony per camel meat sample. The isolates were confirmed as by Vitek 2 system (bioMe´rieux).

Phenotypic detection of ESBL by double-disk synergy test method (DDST)

Phenotypic detection of ESBL by DDST revealed that 21 *P. aeruginosa* isolates. Accordingly, a total percentage of ESBL was detected in overall, 45% (21/45) from camel meat isolates.

Antimicrobial susceptibility testing

The results of the antimicrobial susceptibility testing for the 21 ESBL *P. aeruginosa* shows a high-level resistance (100%) to ceftazidime, ceftriaxone and rifampicin followed by cefepime (95.2%) and aztreonam (76.1%). The susceptibilities of the isolates to meropenem, amikacin, imipenem, gentamicin and ciprofloxacin were 85.8, 81.0, 76.2, 71. 4 and 66.7 respectively (Table 2).

Molecular detection of ESBL-encoding genes

PCR screening of genes encoding ESBL revealed the amplification of bla_{PER-1}, bla_{CTX-M}, bla_{SHV} and bla_{TEM} genes in all tested isolates except three isolates coded p-4, -11, and -18 did not harbor any of ESBL genes (Table 3).

Furthermore, eight out of 21 ESBL-positive isolates had the bla_{CTX-M} (38%), seven had bla_{SHV} gene (33.3), and six carried bla_{TEM} and bla_{PER} genes (28.5).

Discussion

Extended-spectrum beta lactamase-producing bacteria are one of the fastest emerging resistance problems worldwide. ESBL-producing bacteria were observed in human medical practice, the observation of these

Table 2 Antibiotic resistance pattern of 21 *Pseudomonas aeruginosa* isolates

Antibiotic	No (%) resistant	No (%) sensitive
Amikacin (30 μg)	4 (19.0)	17 (81.0)
Imipenem (10 μg)	5 (23.8)	16 (76.2)
Gentamicin (10 μg)	6 (28.5)	15 (71.4)
Ciprofloxacin (5 μg)	7 (33.3)	14 (66.7)
Sulphamethoxazole/trimethoprim (25 μg)	8 (38.0)	13 (61.9)
Rifampicin (30 μg)	21 (100)	–
Ceftriaxone (30 μg)	21 (100)	–
Cefepime (30 μg)	20 (95.2)	1 (4.7)
Aztreonam (30 μg)	15 (76.1)	6 (28.5)
Meropenem (1.0 μg)	3 (14.2)	18 (85.8)
Ceftazidime (30 μg)	21 (100)	–

bacteria in companion animals and the increase in livestock has initiated monitoring studies concentrating on livestock [13, 21].

Livestock may be an important vehicle for the community-wide dissemination of antimicrobial-resistant *Enterobacteriaceae*, also *P. aeruginosa* especially ESBL-producing type isolates have been found in increasing numbers in food-producing animals [9, 10, 22].

Accordingly to the hypothesis that animals might become infection sources or even natural persistent sources acting as risky reservoirs of infection leading to the spread of these bacteria specifically multidrug resistant types in community [23]. There are essential needs for monitoring or surveillance studies incorporating veterinary medicine to identify transmissible pathogens to human and its risk factors.

The dromedary camel is a good source of meat, especially in areas where the climate adversely affects the performance of other meat animals. This is because of the unique physiological characteristics of camels [24]. The interest for camel meat seems by all accounts to be expanded because of wellbeing reasons, as it contains

Table 3 ESBL resistance genes percent and antibiotic pattern of multiple drug resistant strains

Isolates	Resistance gene pattern				Antimicrobial resistance	Antibiotic pattern
	bla_{PER-1}	bla_{CTX-M}	bla_{SHV}	bla_{TEM}		
P-1		+		+	CAZ, CRO, RD, FEP, ATM, AK, CN, CIP	MDR
P-2	+	+	+		CAZ, CRO, RD, FEP, ATM, MEM	MDR
P-3		+		+	CAZ, CRO, RD, FEP, ATM, CIP	MDR
P-4					CAZ, CRO, RD, FEP, ATM, CN	MDR
P-5		+			CAZ, CRO, RD, FEP, IPM	MDR
P-6	+				CAZ, CRO, RD, FEP, ATM, SXT	MDR
P-7		+	+		CAZ, CRO, RD, FEP, ATM, IPM	MDR
P-8		+		+	CAZ, CRO, RD, FEP, ATM,AK, CIP	MDR
P-9	+		+		CAZ, CRO, RD, FEP, ATM, MEM, CIP, SXT	MDR
P-10	+				CAZ, CRO, RD, FEP, CN, CIP	MDR
P-11					CAZ, CRO, RD, FEP, ATM, CIP	MDR
P-12				+	CAZ, CRO, RD, FEP, AK, CIP	MDR
P-13	+	+			CAZ, CRO, RD, FEP, CN	MDR
P-14			+		CAZ, CRO, RD, FEP, IPM, SXT	MDR
P-15				+	CAZ, CRO, RD, FEP, AK, CN	MDR
P-16		+			CAZ, CRO, RD, FEP, ATM, SXT	MDR
P-17		+	+		CAZ, CRO, RD, FEP, ATM, SXT	MDR
P-18					CAZ, CRO, RD, FEP, IPM, CN	MDR
P-19				+	CAZ, CRO, RD, FEP, SXT	MDR
P-20	+				CAZ, CRO, RD, FEP, ATM, IPM, SXT	MDR
P-21			+		CAZ, CRO, RD, MEM, SXT	MDR
%	(6/21) 28.5	(8/21) 38	(7/21) 33.3	(6/21) 28.5		

MDR Multiple drug resistant

less fat and in addition less cholesterol and generally high polyunsaturated unsaturated fats than other animal's meat [25].

To the best of our knowledge, this is the first time that an attempt has been made to determine ESBL *P. aeruginosa* resistance in camel meat. In this study, the prevalence of *P. aeruginosa* in camel was determined about 22.5% (45/200). This percent is so higher to the encountered investigations on fish and cow in Switzerland and Nigeria [9, 26]. Even though *P. aeruginosa* is ubiquitous, the prevalence of its isolation among camel isolates in this study was lower compared to the presence rate of *E. coli* that isolated from camel in Saudi Arabia with 26.0% [27].

Class A (ESBLs) are typically identified in *P. aeruginosa* isolates and showing resistance to the extended-spectrum cephalosporin (ESCs) [28], this resistance is often due to the production of β-lactamases. Clinically, ESBLs are generally encoded by plasmid-mediated *bla* genes; three major clinically relevant β-lactamase genes are bla_{SHV}, bla_{TEM} and $bla_{CTX-M 2, 4}$ [29].

The total percentage of ESBL producing *P. aeruginosa* was 45% (21/45) from camel meat isolates by DDST, accordingly, the most frequently β-lactamase-genes detected in this isolates were bla_{CTX-M} (38%), followed by bla_{SHV} (33.3%) and bla_{TEM}, bal_{PER-1} (28.5%).

CTX-M enzymes have now become the most widespread type of ESBL worldwide and represent the wide dissemination of particular plasmids or bacterial clones [30]. On the other hand, bla_{PER-1} were found to be the most prevalent type of β-lactamase-encoding genes in *Acinetobacter baumannii* in Egypt [31] and this suggests the horizontal transfer of this gene.

In the present study antibiogram of ESBL producing *P. aeruginosa* showed high-level resistance (100%) to ceftazidime, ceftriaxone and rifampicin followed by cefepime (95.2%) and aztreonam (76.1%).The susceptibilities of the isolates to meropenem, amikacin, imipenem, gentamicin, ciprofloxacin and amikacin were 85.8, 81.0, 76.2, 71.5 and 67% respectively (Table 2).

Pseudomonas aeruginosa and other gram negative bacteria with ESBLs contain other β-lactamases that makes difficult the phenotypic detection of ESBL [32], this issue need further investigation.

Many investigators focus on MDR *P. aeruginosa* from human. *P. aeruginosa* are multi-drug resistant to amikacin (17.25%), ciprofloxacin (27.59%), ceftriaxone varied from 51.00 to 73.00% and all the strains were susceptible to imipenem (20.69%) [33]. High resistance to amino-glycosides had been reported in Malaysia [34]. Similarly higher rates of resistance to fluoroquinolones such as ciprofloxacin (40.5%) had been reported in a study done in India. Lesser rate of resistance to ceftriaxone (40%) had been reported in Andhra Pradesh, India [35].

The presence of high resistance profile by camel *P. aeruginosa* isolates my attributed antibiotics used in management of this animals or natural resistance of camel that suites it as a risk reservoir for such pathogens.

Conclusion
The present study demonstrates, for the first time in Egypt, the presence a high rate of ESBL-*P. aeruginosa* in camels, The abundance MDR *P. aeruginosa* from camel meat in this study suggests a potential risk of human susceptibility to such pathogen group which remodels the epidemiology of antibiotic resistance. Urgent control measures are necessary to be applied to restrict the continuous abuse of antibiotics, especially in livestock production.

Abbreviations
ESBL: extended-spectrum beta-lactamase; MBL: metallo-β-lactamases; DDST: double disk synergy test; AST: antimicrobial susceptibility testing; PCR: polymerase chain reaction; MDR: multiple-drug-resistant; HGT: horizontal gene transfer; DDST: double-disk synergy test method; CLSI: the National Committee for Clinical Laboratory Standards; CAZ: ceftazidime; AK: amikacin; CRO: ceftriaxone; FEP: cefepime; ATM: aztreonam; MEM: meropenem; CIP: ciprofloxacin; SXT: sulphamethoxazole/trimethoprim; IPM: imipenem; CN: gentamicin; RD: rifampicin.

Authors' contributions
All authors contributed to the collection of samples, isolation of strains, performing the microbiological examinations, antimicrobial susceptibility testing and molecular detection of target genes, analysis and interpretation of the data as well as writing the manuscript. All authors read and approved the final manuscript.

Author details
[1] Department of Microbiology, Faculty of Veterinary Medicine, Cairo University, PO Box 12211, Giza, Egypt. [2] Department of Zoonoses, Faculty of Veterinary Medicine, Cairo University, PO Box 12211, Giza, Egypt. [3] Department of Microbiology and Immunology, National Research Centre, Giza, Egypt.

Acknowledgements
Not applicable.

Competing interests
The authors declare that they have no competing interests.

Funding
The authors declare that they did not have any funding source or grant to support their research work.

References
1. Strauß LM, Dahms C, Becker K, Kramer A, Kaase M, Mellmann A. Development and evaluation of a novel universal β-lactamase gene subtyping assay for bla$_{SHV}$, bla$_{TEM}$ and bla$_{CTX-M}$ using clinical and livestock-associated *Escherichia coli*. J Antimicrob Chemother. 2015;70(3):710–5.
2. Kidd TJ, Ritchie SR, Ramsay KA, Grimwood K, Bell SC, Rainey PB. *Pseudomonas aeruginosa* exhibits frequent recombination, but only a limited association between genotype and ecological setting. PLoS ONE. 2012;7(9):e44199.
3. Poonsuk K, Chuanchuen R. Contribution of the MexXY multidrug efflux pump and other chromosomal mechanisms on aminoglycoside resistance in *Pseudomonas aeruginosa* isolates from canine and feline infections. J Vet Med Sci. 2012;74(12):1575–82.
4. Salomonsen CM, Themudo GE, Jelsbak L, Molin S, Høiby N, Hammer AS. Typing of *Pseudomonas aeruginosa* from hemorrhagic pneumonia in mink (Neovison vison). Vet Microbiol. 2013;163(1):103–9.
5. Breidenstein EB, de la Fuente-Núñez C, Hancock RE. *Pseudomonas aeruginosa*: all roads lead to resistance. Trends Microbiol. 2011;19(8):419–26.
6. Tavajjohi Z, Moniri R, Khorshidi A. Detection and characterization of multidrug resistance and extended-spectrum-beta-lactamase-producing (ESBLS) *Pseudomonas aeruginosa* isolates in teaching hospital. Afr J Microbiol Res. 2011;5(20):3223–8.
7. Miko A, Pries K, Schroeter A, Helmuth R. Molecular mechanisms of resistance in multidrug-resistant serovars of *Salmonella enterica* isolated from foods in Germany. J Antimicrob Chemother. 2005;56(6):1025–33.
8. Schwaiger K, Huther S, Hölzel C, Kämpf P, Bauer J. Prevalence of antibiotic-resistant enterobacteriaceae isolated from chicken and pork meat purchased at the slaughterhouse and at retail in Bavaria, Germany. Int J Food Microbiol. 2012;154(3):206–11.
9. Odumosu BT, Ajetunmobi O, Dada-Adegbola H, Odutayo I. Antibiotic susceptibility pattern and analysis of plasmid profiles of *Pseudomonas aeruginosa* from human, animal and plant sources. SpringerPlus. 2016;5(1):1381.
10. Zurfluh K, Hindermann D, Nüesch-Inderbinen M, Poirel L, Nordmann P, Stephan R. Occurrence and features of chromosomally encoded carbapenemases in gram-negative bacteria in farm animals sampled at slaughterhouse level. Schweiz Arch Tierheilkd. 2016;158(6):457–60.
11. Ismail M, El-Deen NE, El-Hariri M. Bacteriological examination of respiratory tract of apparently healthy camels in Egypt. Int J. 2014;5(1):65–8.
12. Fadlelmula A, Al-Hamam NA, Al-Dughaym AM. A potential camel reservoir for extended-spectrum β-lactamase-producing *Escherichia coli* causing human infection in Saudi Arabia. Trop Anim Health Prod. 2016;48(2):427–33.
13. Smet A, Martel A, Persoons D, Dewulf J, Heyndrickx M, Herman L, Haesebrouck F, Butaye P. Broad-spectrum β-lactamases among Enterobacteriaceae of animal origin: molecular aspects, mobility and impact on public health. FEMS Microbiol Rev. 2010;34(3):295–316.
14. Quinn PJ, Carter ME, Markey B, Carter GR. Enterobacteriaceae. Clinical veterinary microbiology. London: Wolfe Publishing; 1994. p. 209–36.
15. Jarlier V, Nicolas MH, Fournier G, Philippon A. Extended spectrum β-lactamases conferring transferable resistance to newer β-lactam agents in Enterobacteriaceae: hospital prevalence and susceptibility patterns. Rev Infect Dis. 1988;10:867–78.
16. Clinical and Laboratory Standards Institute (CLSI). M100-S25 Performance standards for antimicrobial susceptibility testing: 25th informational supplement. Wayne: CLSI; 2015.
17. Andrews JM, for the BSAC Working Party on Susceptibility Testing. BSAC standardized disc susceptibility testing method (version 8). J Antimicrob Chemother. 2009;64:454–89.

18. Neyestanaki DK, Mirsalehian A, Rezagholizadeh F, Jabalameli F, Taheri-kalani M, Emaneini M. Determination of extended spectrum beta-lactamases, metallo-beta-lactamases and AmpC-beta-lactamases among carbapenem resistant *Pseudomonas aeruginosa* isolated from burn patients. Burns. 2014;40(8):1556–61.

19. M'Zali FH, Gascoyne-Binzi DM, Heritage J, Hawkey PM. Detection of mutations conferring extended-spectrum activity on SHV β-lactamases using polymerase chain reaction single strand conformational polymorphism (PCR-SSCP). J Antimicrob Chemother. 1996;37(4):797–802.

20. Celenza G, Pellegrini C, Caccamo M, Segatore B, Amicosante G, Perilli M. Spread of *bla*CTX-M-type and *bla*PER-2 β-lactamase genes in clinical isolates from Bolivian hospitals. J Antimicrobl Chemother. 2006;57(5):975–8.

21. Ewers C, Grobbel M, Bethe A, Wieler LH, Guenther S. Extended-spectrum beta-lactamases-producing gram-negative bacteria in companion animals: action is clearly warranted. Berl Munch Tierarztl Wochenschr. 2011;124(3/4):4–101.

22. Mir RA, Weppelmann TA, Johnson JA, Archer D, Morris JG Jr, Jeong KC. Identification and characterization of cefotaxime resistant bacteria in beef cattle. PLoS ONE. 2016;11(9):e0163279.

23. Watkins RR, Bonomo RA. Overview: global and local impact of antibiotic resistance. Infect Dis Clin North Am. 2016;30(2):313–22.

24. Kadim IT, Mahgoub O, Purchas RW. A review of the growth, and of the carcass and meat quality characteristics of the one-humped camel (*Camelus dromedaries*). Meat Sci. 2008;80(3):555–69.

25. Abdelhadi OM, Babiker SA, Bauchart D, Listrat A, Rémond D, Hocquette JF, Faye B. Effect of gender on quality and nutritive value of dromedary camel (*Camelus dromedarius*) longissimus lumborum muscle. J Saudi Soc Agri Sci. 2015. doi:10.1016/j.jssas.2015.08.003.

26. Boss R, Overesch G, Baumgartner A. Antimicrobial resistance of *Escherichia coli, enterococci, Pseudomonas aeruginosa*, and *Staphylococcus aureus* from raw fish and seafood imported into Switzerland. J Food Prot. 2016;79(7):1240–6.

27. Fadlelmula A, Al-Hamam NA, Al-Dughaym AM. A potential camel reservoir for extended-spectrum β-lactamase-producing *Escherichia coli* causing human infection in Saudi Arabia. Trop Anim Health Prod. 2016;48(2):427–33.

28. Fadlelmula A, Al-Hamam NA, Al-Dughaym AM. A potential camel reservoir for extended-spectrum β-lactamase-producing *Escherichia coli* causing human infection in Saudi Arabia. Trop Anim Health Prod. 2016;48(2):427–33.

29. Bush K. The ABCD's of β-lactamase nomenclature. J Infect Chemother. 2013;19(4):549–59.

30. Cantón R, Novais A, Valverde A, Machado E, Peixe L, Baquero F, Coque TM. Prevalence and spread of extended-spectrum β-lactamase-producing *Enterobacteriaceae* in Europe. Clin Microbiol Infect. 2008;14(s1):144–53.

31. Al-Agamy MH, Khalaf NG, Tawfick MM, Shibl AM, El Kholy A. Molecular characterization of carbapenem-insensitive *Acinetobacter baumannii* in Egypt. Int J Infect Dis. 2014;22:49–54.

32. Manchanda V, Singh NP. Occurrence and detection of AmpC beta-lactamases among gram-negative clinical isolates using a modified three-dimensional test at Guru Tegh Bahadur Hospital, Delhi, India. J Antimicrob Chemother. 2003;51:415–8.

33. Chander A, Raza MS. Antimicrobial susceptibility patterns of *Pseudomonas aeruginosa* clinical isolates at a tertiary care hospital in Kathmandu, Nepal. Asian J Pharm Clin Res. 2013;6(3):235–8.

34. Fazlul MK, Zaini MZ, Rashid MA, Nazmul MH. Antibiotic susceptibility profiles of clinical isolates of *Pseudomonas aeruginosa* from Selayang Hospital, Malaysia. Biomed Res. 2011;22(3):263.

35. Ramana BV, Chaudhury A. Antibiotic resistance pattern of *Pseudomonas aureuginosa* isolated from healthcare associated infections at a tertiary care hospital. J Sci Soc. 2012;39(2):78.

9

Vitamin D deficiency among smear positive pulmonary tuberculosis patients and their tuberculosis negative household contacts in Northwest Ethiopia: a case–control study

Belay Tessema[1*], Feleke Moges[1], Dereje Habte[2], Nebiyu Hiruy[2], Shewaye Yismaw[3], Kassahun Melkieneh[2], Yewulsew Kassie[4], Belaineh Girma[5], Muluken Melese[2] and Pedro G. Suarez[6]

Abstract

Background: Vitamin D is a fat-soluble vitamin that increases the immunity against tuberculosis (TB), decreases the re-activation of latent TB and reduces the severity of active TB disease. Epidemiological studies on the prevalence of vitamin D deficiency, and its association with TB showed inconsistent results in different countries. This study was aimed to determine the prevalence of vitamin D deficiency and its association with TB in Northwest Ethiopia.

Methods: A case–control study was conducted among smear positive pulmonary tuberculosis patients and their household contacts without symptoms suggestive of TB. Study participants were recruited at 11 TB diagnostic health facilities in North and South Gondar zones of Amhara region between May 2013 and April 2015. The spot-morning-spot sputum samples and 5 ml blood sample were collected prior to commencing TB treatment for the diagnosis of TB and serum vitamin D assay, respectively. The diagnosis of TB was performed using smear microscopy and GeneXpert. Serum vitamin D level was analyzed using VIDAS 25 OH Vitamin D Total testing kits (Biomerieux, Marcy l'Etoile, France) on mini VIDAS automated immunoassay platform. Vitamin D status was interpreted as deficient (<20 ng/ml), insufficient (20–29 ng/ml), sufficient (30–100 ng/ml) and potential toxicity (>100 ng/ml).

Results: Of the total study participants, 134 (46.2%) were vitamin D deficient, and only 56 (19.3%) had sufficient vitamin D level. A total of 59 (61.5%) TB patients and 75 (38.7%) non TB controls were vitamin D deficient. Results of multivariate logistic regression analyses showed a significantly higher vitamin D deficiency among tuberculosis cases (p < 0.001), females (p = 0.002), and urban residents (p < 0.001) than their respective comparison groups. Moreover, age groups of 35–44 (p = 0.001), 45–54 (p = 0.003) and ≥55 (p = 0.001) years had significantly higher vitamin D deficiency compared with age group <15 years.

Conclusions: Vitamin D deficiency is highly prevalent among TB patients and non TB controls in Ethiopia where there is year round abundant sunshine. Study participants with tuberculosis, females, older age groups, and urban residents had significantly higher prevalence of vitamin D deficiency. These findings warrant further studies to investigate the role of vitamin D supplementation in the prevention and treatment of tuberculosis in high TB burden countries like Ethiopia.

Keywords: Vitamin D deficiency, Tuberculosis, Household contacts

*Correspondence: bt1488@yahoo.com
[1] Department of Medical Microbiology, College of Medicine and Health Sciences, University of Gondar, Gondar, Ethiopia
Full list of author information is available at the end of the article

Background

Tuberculosis (TB) remains one of the deadliest communicable diseases in the world. According to World Health Organization (WHO) global TB report 2014, Ethiopia ranked 7th among the 22 high TB burden countries and 15th among the 27 high Multi-Drug Resistant Tuberculosis (MDR-TB) burden countries in the world. Ethiopia had an estimated 211 prevalent TB case per 100,000 population and a total of 30,000 TB related deaths. Among patients with notified pulmonary TB cases in the year 2013, there was an estimated 1400 MDR-TB cases in the country [1].

Vitamin D is a fat-soluble vitamin that plays important role against infectious diseases including tuberculosis [2]. The two most likely ways by which vitamin D controls the immune system in the fight against *M. tuberculosis* are: (1) Vitamin D decreases the viability of *M. tuberculosis* by increasing the fusion of the phagosome and lysosome in infected macrophages [3]; (2) It may improve the production of LL-37, an antimicrobial peptide of the cathelicidin family [3–6]. Defensin and cathelicidin are some of the antimicrobial peptides that involve as a first line of defenses in the inhibition of infections with infectious diseases such as TB. The vitamin D in neutrophils and macrophages controls the hCAP-18 gene that codes for LL-37, hence, vitamin D may increase the host body defenses to control TB [3–7]. The use of vitamin D to treat TB patients has a long history even before Robert Koch discovered the etiologic agent of TB [3].

Vitamin D can be present naturally in very few foods, as dietary supplements, and produced endogenously when ultraviolet rays from sunlight strike the skin and trigger vitamin D synthesis, however, vitamin D deficiency has been shown to be common in low-income countries, including those in equatorial Africa [8–10].

Inadequate vitamin D level, vitamin D insufficiency or deficiency, is a global problem. It was estimated that one billion people globally have inadequate level of vitamin D [11]. Previous studies have shown that vitamin D deficiency is a problem in Africa [12–16]. Higher prevalence of vitamin D deficiency was observed among untreated pulmonary TB patients compared to the non-TB healthy controls [17]. Vitamin D deficiency among TB patients have been reported in different African countries with the prevalence ranging from 8.5 to 62.7% [8, 10, 14–16]. A study conducted in the central part of Ethiopia showed a prevalence of 42% vitamin D deficiency among school children [18]. Another study conducted in Israel among adult Ethiopian women immigrants showed that all women (five) with hypocalcaemia were also vitamin D deficient [19].

Previous reports showed that inadequate vitamin D status is a public health problem globally. However, there are discrepancies in the prevalence of vitamin D deficiency, and the association between vitamin D deficiency and TB among studies conducted in different countries. The lack of consistency of results may be due to the fact that the level of vitamin D in human is affected by several factors such as race, latitude, exposure to sunlight, socioeconomic status, nutrition, and traditional/cultural traits [20]. As far as our knowledge is concerned, there are quite few reports, one on the prevalence of vitamin D deficiency among children and the other on Ethiopian women immigrants, but no data on the association between vitamin D deficiency and tuberculosis in Ethiopia. Therefore, this study was aimed to determine the prevalence of vitamin D deficiency and the association between vitamin D deficiency and tuberculosis among smear positive pulmonary tuberculosis patients and their household contacts without symptoms suggestive of TB in Northwest Ethiopia.

Methods
Study design, settings and study period

A prospective case–control study was conducted among smear positive pulmonary tuberculosis patients and their household contacts without symptoms suggestive of TB (controls). A total of 290 study participants were included in this study. Of them, 96 participants are TB patients and 194 are non TB controls. Study participants were recruited at 11 TB diagnostic health facilities in North and South Gondar zones of Amhara region between May 2013 and April 2015. The 11 TB diagnostic health facilities included in this study are Gondar Health Center (HC), Marakie HC, Woleka HC, Gebriel HC, Azezo HC, Kola Duba HC, Tseda HC, Maksegnit HC, Enferanze HC, Addis Zemen HC, and Woreta HC.

Based on the 2007 census conducted by the central statistical agency of Ethiopia (CSA) [21], Amhara region has a total population of 17,221,976, of whom, 8,641,580 are males and 8,580,396 are females. It is the second populous region in the country. The Amhara region extends from 9° to 13° 45′ N and 36° to 40° 30′ E. It covers approximately 161,828.4 sq km in area. This is 11% of Ethiopia's total area. This land consists of three major geographical zones. These are highlands (above 2300 m above sea level), semi-highlands (1500–2300 m above sea level) and lowlands (below 1500 m above sea level) accounting 20, 44 and 28%, respectively. The Amhara region, like the rest of the country, is located within the tropics where there is no significant variation in day length and the angle of the sun throughout the year. As a result, the average annual temperatures in the region are high. The region has three climatic zones such as hot dry tropical (800–1830 m above sea level), sub tropical (1830–2440 m above sea level), cool temperature (over 2440 m above sea level) with average annual temperatures 27, 22 and 16 °C, respectively. In all climatic zones there is sunshine throughout the year.

Recruitment of the study participants

All smear positive TB patients diagnosed during the study period and their household contacts without symptoms suggestive of TB, volunteered to participate were enrolled in this study. Clinical screening of contacts was conducted using the WHO screening criteria [22] in 2 weeks time after the index case diagnosed. For all study subjects, information on the socio-demographic data was collected using structured questionnaire. The spot-morning-spot sputum samples and 5 ml venous blood sample were collected prior to commencing TB treatment. Sputum and serum specimens were stored at −20 °C until transported to University of Gondar and Felege Hiwot hospitals using cold box. Sputum samples transported to University of Gondar Hospital for GeneXpert testing while serum samples transported to Felege Hiwot Hospital, Bahir Dar for serum Vitamin D assay.

Laboratory diagnosis of tuberculosis

The spot- morning-spot sputum samples collected from presumptive TB patients were examined using either Zihel Neelsen microscopy or light emitting diode (LED) fluorescence microscopy (FM) for acid fast bacilli (AFB) at respective health facilities following the manufacturer's procedures (Zeiss, Germany). Split sputum samples of all smear positive TB patients were further examined using the Gene Xpert MTB/RIF (Cepheid, USA) following the standard procedure to confirm TB positive study participants.

Study participants were considered TB positive, if their sputum samples are positive for TB by GeneXpert or both GeneXpert and smear microscopy. Study subjects were considered TB negative controls, if household contacts of smear positive TB cases had no symptoms suggestive of TB. TB negative study participants were included in this study as a control to compare the association between TB and vitamin D deficiency.

Measurement of serum vitamin D concentration

Serum samples were separated by centrifugation and frozen immediately at −20 °C. Serum 25 OH Vitamin D levels were measured using a VIDAS 25 OH Vitamin D Total testing kits (Biomerieux, Marcy I'Etoile, France) on mini VIDAS automated immunoassay platform. VIDAS 25 OH Vitamin D Total is a quantitative test using Enzyme Linked Fluorescent Assay (ELFA) technology. The vitamin D status of study participants was interpreted based on the serum 25-(OH) Vitamin

D concentration following the manufacturer's instructions as deficient (<20 ng/ml), insufficient (20–29 ng/ml), sufficient (30–100 ng/ml) and potential toxicity (>100 ng/ml). The VIDAS 25-OH Vitamin D Total assay showed excellent performance with correlation of r = 0.93 compared with the reference standard liquid chromatography/mass spectrometry methods (LC–MS/MS) [23].

Quality control of laboratory methods

The reliability of the study findings was guaranteed by implementing quality control measures throughout the whole process of the laboratory work. All materials, equipment and procedures were adequately controlled.

Statistical analysis

The data analysis was made using SPSS version 16 software (SPSS Inc., Chicago, IL) after the data was entered and properly cleared. The Chi square test was used to compare the categorical variables. The two important outcome variables assessed using logistic regression analysis model were TB and Vitamin D deficiency. The odds ratios (OR) and 95% confidence intervals (CI) were calculated for demographic and epidemiologic variables by using logistic regression analysis. A multivariate binary logistic regression analysis was used to identify independent risk factors associated with TB and vitamin D deficiency in the study participants. P value <0.05 was considered statistically significant.

Results
General characteristics of study participants

A total of 290 study participants (141 males and 149 females) were included in this study. The study included 96 TB patients (57 males and 39 females) and 194 non TB controls (84 males and 110 females). Majority, 180 (62.1%) of the study participants were urban residents. Eighty one of the study participants (27.9%) were children, <15 years of age. The proportion of children among controls was 35.1% compared to the 13.5% children among TB cases. The mean age (SD) of the study subjects was 27.1 (16.7) years (Table 1).

Serum vitamin D levels

Of the total study participants, 134 (46.2%) were vitamin D deficient, 100 (34.5%) had insufficient vitamin D and only 56 (19.3%) study participants had sufficient vitamin D level. In the TB positive cases, 59 patients (61.5%) were vitamin D deficient and 20 (20.8%) had insufficient vitamin D. While, 75 study participants (38.7%) in the non TB controls were vitamin D deficient and 80 (41.2%) had insufficient vitamin D (Table 2).

Table 1 Socio-demographic and clinical characteristics of study participants (N = 290)

Characteristics	TB patients (N = 96) N (%)	Non TB controls (N = 194) N (%)	Total (N = 290)
Gender			
Male	57 (59.4)	84 (43.3)	141 (48.6)
Female	39 (40.6)	110 (56.7)	149 (51.4)
Residence			
Rural	34 (35.4)	76 (39.2)	110 (37.9)
Urban	62 (64.6)	118 (60.8)	180 (62.1)
Age group in years			
<15	13 (13.5)	68 (35.1)	81 (27.9)
15–24	27 (28.1)	33 (17.0)	60 (20.7)
25–34	30 (31.2)	33 (17.0)	63 (21.7)
35–44	10 (10.4)	27 (13.9)	37 (12.8)
45–54	6 (6.2)	17 (8.8)	23 (7.9)
55+	10 (10.4)	16 (8.2)	26 (9.0)

N number, *TB* tuberculosis

Risk factors associated with tuberculosis

As shown in Table 3, tuberculosis cases had significantly higher rate of vitamin D deficiency (AOR 3.3; 95% CI 1.8–6.0; p < 0.001) than non TB controls. Significantly higher number of males had active TB compared with females (AOR 2.5; 95% CI 1.4–4.3; p = 0.001). Furthermore, study participants in the age groups of 15–24 (AOR 4.5; 95% CI 2.0–10.2; p < 0.001) and 25–34 (AOR 4.3; 95% CI 1.9–96; p < 0.001) years had significantly higher proportion of active TB compared with age group <15 years of age.

Risk factors associated with vitamin D deficiency

Results of multivariate logistic regression analyses showed that females had significantly higher prevalence of vitamin D deficiency than males (AOR 2.3; 95% CI 1.3–3.9; p = 0.002). Urban residents had significantly higher proportion of vitamin D deficiency compared with rural residents (AOR 3.0; 95% CI 1.7–5.3; p < 0.001). Moreover, study subjects in the age groups of 35–44 (AOR 4.5; 95% CI p = 0.001), 45–54 (AOR 5.8; 95% CI 0 1.8–18.6; p = 0.003) and ≥55 (AOR 7.5; 95% CI 2.3–24.2; p = 0.001) years had significantly higher proportion of vitamin D deficiency compared with age group <15 years of age (Table 4).

Discussion

In this study, a high prevalence of vitamin D deficiency, 46.2% was observed among the total study participants. This finding is in agreement with a previous report from the central part of Ethiopia with the total prevalence of 42% vitamin D deficiency among school children [18]. This finding shows that vitamin D deficiency is highly prevalent among the general community in Ethiopia.

Table 2 Vitamin D levels among study participants (n = 290)

Characteristics	Vitamin D levels			Total N
	Deficient (<20 ng/ml) N (%)	Insufficient (20–29 ng/ml) N (%)	Sufficient (30–100 ng/ml) N (%)	
Total	134 (46.2)	100 (34.5)	56 (19.3)	290
TB status				
Positive	59 (61.5)	20 (20.8)	17 (17.7)	96
Negative	75 (38.7)	80 (41.2)	39 (20.1)	194
Gender				
Male	56 (39.7)	49 (34.8)	36 (25.5)	141
Female	78 (52.3)	51 (34.2)	20 (13.4)	149
Residence				
Rural	36 (32.7)	42 (38.2)	32 (29.1)	110
Urban	98 (54.4)	58 (32.2)	24 (13.3)	180
Age group				
<15	25 (30.9)	37 (45.7)	19 (23.5)	81
15–24	22 (36.7)	21 (35.0)	17 (28.3)	60
25–34	32 (50.8)	19 (30.2)	12 (19.0)	63
35–44	20 (54.1)	14 (37.8)	3 (8.1)	37
45–54	15 (65.2)	5 (21.7)	3 (13.0)	23
55+	20 (76.9)	4 (15.4)	2 (7.7)	26

N number, *TB* tuberculosis

Table 3 Risk factors associated with tuberculosis (n = 290)

Characteristics	Total	TB status		Univariate analysis		Multivariate analysis	
		TB patients (N = 96) N (%)	Controls (N = 194) N (%)	COR (95% CI)	p values	AOR (95% CI)	p values
Vit D deficient							
Yes	96	59 (61.5)	37 (38.5)	2.5 (1.5–4.2)	<0.001	3.3 (1.8–6.0)	<0.001
No	194	75 (38.7)	119 (61.3)	1			
Gender							
Male	141	57 (40.4)	84 (59.6)	1.9 (1.2–3.2)	0.010	2.5 (1.4–4.3)	0.001
Female	149	39 (26.2)	110 (73.8)	1			
Residence							
Rural	110	34 (30.9)	76 (69.1)	1			
Urban	180	62 (34.4)	118 (65.6)	1.2 (0.7–2.0)	0.535	0.8 (0.4–1.4)	0.427
Age group							
<15	81	13 (16.0)	68 (84.0)	1			
15–24	60	27 (45.0)	33 (55.0)	4.3 (2.0–9.4)	<0.001	4.5 (2.0–10.2)	<0.001
25–34	63	30 (47.6)	33 (52.4)	4.8 (2.2–10.3)	<0.001	4.3 (1.9–9.6)	<0.001
35–44	37	10 (27.0)	27 (73.0)	1.9 (0.8–4.9)	0.167	1.4 (0.5–3.8)	0.475
45–54	23	6 (26.1)	17 (73.9)	1.8 (0.6–5.6)	0.276	1.3 (0.4–4.2)	0.662
55+	26	10 (38.5)	16 (61.5)	3.3 (1.2–8.8)	0.019	2.0 (0.7–5.6)	0.203

N number, TB tuberculosis, COR crude odds ratio, AOR adjusted odds ratio, Vit D vitamin D, CI confidence interval

The prevalence of vitamin D deficiency among TB patients (61.5%) reported in our study is comparable to that reported in South Africa (62.7%) [16]. On the contrary, lower prevalence of vitamin D deficiency was reported in Tanzania (10.6%) [8], Guinea Bissau (8.5%) [10] and Uganda (7%) [14] compared to our study. These discrepancies among different reports might be due to the differences in the laboratory assay methods used to measure vitamin D level, definition of vitamin D deficiency, dietary habits of the study population, latitude of the study sites and frequencies of co-morbidities in the study population of different studies. The different

Table 4 Risk factors associated with vitamin D deficiency (n = 290)

Characteristics	Total	Vit D deficiency		Univariate analysis		Multivariate analysis	
		Deficient (<20 ng/ml) N (%)	Not deficient (20–100 ng/ml) N (%)	COR (95% CI)	p values	AOR (95% CI)	p values
Total	290	134 (46.2)	156 (53.8)				
Gender							
Male	141	56 (39.7)	85 (60.3)	1			
Female	149	78 (52.3)	71 (47.7)	1.7 (1.0–2.7)	0.03	2.3 (1.3–3.9)	0.002
Residence							
Rural	110	36 (32.7)	74 (67.3)	1			
Urban	180	98 (54.4)	82 (45.6)	2.5 (1.5–4.0)	<0.001	3.0 (1.7–5.3)	<0.001
Age group							
<15	81	25 (30.9)	56 (69.1)	1			
15–24	60	22 (36.7)	38 (63.3)	1.5 (0.8–2.9)	0.227	1.0 (0.5–2.1)	0.995
25–34	63	32 (50.8)	31 (45.2)	2.0 (1.0–4.1)	0.054	1.6 (0.7–3.4)	0.252
35–44	37	20 (54.1)	17 (45.9)	3.9 (1.7–9.2)	0.002	4.5 (1.8–11.3)	0.001
45–54	23	15 (65.2)	8 (34.8)	4.9 (1.7–14.2)	0.004	5.8 (1.8–18.6)	0.003
55+	26	20 (76.9)	6 (23.1)	7.6 (2.5–22.9)	<0.001	7.5 (2.3–24.2)	0.001

N number, COR crude odds ratio, AOR adjusted odds ratio, Vit D vitamin D, CI confidence interval

techniques used to measure serum vitamin D concentrations in the studies done in Uganda [14], Guinea Bissau [10] and Tanzania [8] were a semi-automated solid phase extraction reverse phase high performance liquid chromatography assay, isotope-dilution liquid chromatography–tandem mass spectrometry on an API3000 mass spectrometer and Radio Immuno Assay (RIA) with ^{125}I-labeled 25(OH) D $[^{125}I$-25(OH)D] as tracer using a kit from Immunodiagnostic-Systems, respectively.

In this study, multivariate logistic regression analysis showed a significant association between vitamin D deficiency and tuberculosis ($p < 0.001$). The possible association between vitamin D deficiency and active tuberculosis was first reported more than 20 years ago [24], however, several studies reported conflicting results. Similar to our study, many studies have reported a significant association between vitamin D deficiency and TB. Studies in West Africa [10], Australia [12], Kenya [17], Vietnam [25], Tanzania [26] and India [27] have reported higher levels of vitamin D deficiency in patients with TB compared with non TB controls. A meta-analysis by Nnoaham et al. also showed that serum vitamin D levels were 0.68 standard deviation lower in TB patients compared to controls [20]. However, studies from Indonesia [28], China [29], Hong Kong [30] and Korea [31] have reported no significant difference in serum vitamin D levels between TB patients and controls. The discrepancies between these studies may be due to differences in cultural characteristics, ethnic, sunlight exposure, skin color or dietary practices. Although there is good evidence to suggest that a decrease in serum vitamin D levels compromises immunity and leads to the re-activation of latent tuberculosis [32], the low serum vitamin D levels may also result from tuberculosis itself.

In the present study, it was noted that a significantly higher level of vitamin D deficiency was observed among females compared with males ($p = 0.002$). Similarly, a report from Pakistan showed that vitamin D deficiency was significantly higher in females than males [33]. Possible reasons for this female preponderance might be due to poorer nutritional status than their male counterparts, inadequate exposure to sunlight because of the culture of most females to stay at home, and pregnancy experiences.

Increasing age was found to be significantly associated with vitamin D deficiency in our study. Similar findings have also been observed in reports from Uganda [34], and in the USA [35]. Older people are prone to develop vitamin D deficiency because of various risk factors: decreased dietary intake, diminished sunlight exposure, reduced skin thickness, impaired intestinal absorption, and impaired hydroxylation in the liver and kidneys [36–38].

In this study, urban residence was found to be a significant risk factor for vitamin D deficiency compared with rural residence. Our finding was in agreement with the findings of the previous studies in the central part of Ethiopia [18] and in Peru [39] that showed significant association between vitamin D deficiency and urban environment. This might be due to lifestyle changes associated with urbanization that may lead to less time spent outdoors which in turn can be associated with being vitamin D deficient.

The major limitations of our study include dietary intake, biochemical variables (calcium, parathyroid hormone), HIV status and latent TB infections, all of which could affect vitamin D deficiency, were not considered in this study. However, the effect of these factors on the level of vitamin D among TB patients was controlled using tight control groups from the same household who did not have TB diseases. As the cases and controls shared similar environment and household, the cases and controls are likely to have similar risk factors exposures including dietary intake.

Conclusions

Vitamin D deficiency is highly prevalent among TB patients and non TB controls in Ethiopia where there is year round abundant sunshine. This study confirms a significant association between vitamin D deficiency and tuberculosis in Ethiopia. Vitamin D deficiency was also significantly higher in females, older age groups, and urban residents. The findings of this study warrant further studies first to resolve the chicken–egg dilemma of the association between vitamin D deficiency and TB using cohort study and then to determine whether vitamin D supplementation can have a role in the prevention and treatment of tuberculosis in high TB burden countries like Ethiopia.

Authors' contributions
BT conceived the study, involved in proposal writing and design, data collection, analysis, interpretation and draft manuscript writing. FM, BG and MM involved in proposal writing and design and reviewed the manuscript. DH, NH and SY involved in data analysis, interpretation of results and reviewed the manuscript. KM, YK and PGS reviewed the manuscript. All authors read and approved the final manuscript.

Author details
[1] Department of Medical Microbiology, College of Medicine and Health Sciences, University of Gondar, Gondar, Ethiopia. [2] Management Sciences for Health, Help Ethiopia Address the Low Performance of Tuberculosis (HEAL TB) Project, Addis Ababa, Ethiopia. [3] Department of Chemistry, College of Natural and Computational Sciences, University of Gondar, Gondar, Ethiopia. [4] USAID/Ethiopia, Addis Ababa, Ethiopia. [5] Monitoring and Evaluation TA, National Tuberculosis Program, Lilongwe, Malawi. [6] Management Sciences for Health, Health Programs Group, Arlington, VA, USA.

Acknowledgements

The authors would like to thank data collectors and study participants from all study areas in Northwest Ethiopia. Authors also express their appreciation to Fikerte Estefanus and Workeneh Ayalew for their kind assistance during serum vitamin D level measurement at Felege Hiwot Hospital Laboratory, and Asnakew Belete and Kefyalew Negerie for their assistance during TB diagnosis using GeneXpert assay at University of Gondar. Authors would also like to acknowledge Degu Jerene for his contribution to review the manuscript.

Competing interests

The authors declare that they have no competing interests.

Consent for publication

All authors read and approved the final manuscript for submission for publication.

Funding

The United States Agency for International Development (USAID) supported this work through HEAL TB, under cooperative agreement number AID-663-A-11-00011. The contents of the article are the responsibility of the authors alone and do not necessarily reflect the views of USAID or the United States government.

References

1. World Health Organization. Global tuberculosis report. Geneva: WHO; 2014.
2. Hewison M. Vitamin D and the immune system: new perspectives on an old theme. Endocrinol Metab Clin North Am. 2010;39:365–79.
3. Chocano-Bedoya P, Ronnenberg AG. Vitamin D and tuberculosis. Nutr Rev. 2009;67:289–93.
4. Martineau AR, Wilkinson KA, Newton SM, Floto RA, Norman AW, et al. IFN-gamma- and TNF-independent vitamin D-inducible human suppression of mycobacteria: the role of cathelicidin LL-37. J Immunol. 2007;178:7190–8.
5. Ralph AP, Kelly PM, Anstey NM. L-arginine and vitamin D: novel adjunctive immunotherapies in tuberculosis. Trends Microbiol. 2008;16:336–44.
6. Campbell GR, Spector SA. Vitamin D inhibits human immunodeficiency virus type 1 and *Mycobacterium tuberculosis* infection in macrophages through the induction of autophagy. PLoS Pathog. 2012;8:1523–5.
7. Liu PT, Stenger S, Li H, Wenzel L, Tan BH. Toll-like receptor triggering of a vitamin D-mediated human antimicrobial response. Science. 2006;311:1770–3.
8. Friis H, Range N, Pedersen ML, Mølgaard C, Changalucha J, et al. Hypovitaminosis D is common among pulmonary tuberculosis patients in Tanzania but is not explained by the acute phase response. J Nutr. 2008;138:2474–80.
9. Fischer PR, Thacher TD, Pettifor JM. Pediatric vitamin D and calcium nutrition in developing countries. Rev Endocr Metab Disord. 2008;9:181–92.
10. Wejse C, Olesen R, Rabna P, Kaestel P, Gustafson P, et al. Serum 25- hydroxyvitamin D in a West African population of tuberculosis patients and unmatched healthy controls. Am J Clin Nutr. 2007;86:1376–83.
11. Holick MF. Vitamin D deficiency. N Engl J Med. 2007;357:266–81.
12. Gibney K, MacGregor L, Leder K, et al. Vitamin D deficiency is associated with tuberculosis and latent tuberculosis infection in immigrants from sub-Saharan Africa. Clin Infect Dis. 2008;46:443–6.
13. van der Meer M, Middelkoop B, Boeke A, Lips P. Prevalence of vitamin D deficiency among Turkish, Moroccan, Indian and sub-Sahara African populations in Europe and their countries of origin: an overview. Osteoporos Int. 2011;22:1009–21.
14. Nansera D, Graziano F, Friedman D, et al. Vitamin D and calcium levels in Ugandan adults with human immunodeficiency virus and tuberculosis. Int J Tuberc Lung Dis. 2011;15:1522–7.
15. Banda R, Mhemedi B, Allain T. Prevalence of vitamin D deficiency in adult tuberculosis patients at a central hospital in Malawi. Int J Tuberc Lung Dis. 2011;15:408–10.
16. Martineau A, Nhamoyebonded S, Onic T, et al. Reciprocal seasonal variation in vitamin D status and tuberculosis notifications in Cape Town, South Africa. Proc Natl Acad Sci. 2011;108:19013–7.
17. Davies P, Church H, Brown R, et al. Raised serum calcium in tuberculosis patients in Africa. Eur J Respir Dis. 1987;71:341–4.
18. Wakayo T, Belachew T, Vatanparast H, Whiting SJ. Vitamin D deficiency and its predictors in a country with thirteen months of sunshine: the case of school children in central Ethiopia. PLoS ONE. 2015;10(3):e0120963. doi:10.1371/journal.pone.0120963.
19. Fogelman Y, Rakover Y, Luboshitzky R. High prevalence of vitamin D deficiency among Ethiopian women immigrants to Israel: exacerbation during pregnancy and lactation. Isr J Med Sci. 1995;31(4):221–4.
20. Nnoaham KE, Clarke A. Low serum vitamin D levels and tuberculosis: a systematic review and meta-analysis. Int J Epidemiol. 2008;37:113–9.
21. Central Statistical Agency (CSA) of Ethiopia. Summary and statistical report of the 2007 population and housing census. Addis Ababa: CSA; 2008.
22. World Health Organization. Global Tuberculosis Control 2010. WHO/HTM/TB/2010.7. Geneva: WHO; 2010.
23. Moreau E, Bacher S, Mery S, Le Goff C, Piga N, Vogeser M, Hausmann M, Cavalier E. Performance characteristics of the VIDAS® 25-OH Vitamin D Total assay—comparison with four immunoassays and two liquid chromatography-tandem mass spectrometry methods in a multicentric study. Clin Chem Lab Med. 2015. doi:10.1515/cclm-2014-1249.
24. Bartley J. Vitamin D: emerging roles in infection and immunity. Expert Rev Anti Infect Ther. 2010;8:1359–69.
25. Ho-Pham LT, Nguyen ND, Nguyen TT, et al. Association between vitamin D insufficiency and tuberculosis in a Vietnamese population. BMC Infect Dis. 2010;10:306.
26. Tostmann A, Wielders JPM, Kibiki GS, Verhoef H, Boeree MJ. Serum 25-hydroxy-vitamin D3 concentrations increase during tuberculosis treatment in Tanzania. Int J Tuberc Lung Dis. 2010;14:1147–52.
27. Wilkinson RJ, Llewelyn M, Toossi Z, et al. Influence of vitamin D deficiency and vitamin D receptor polymorphisms on tuberculosis among Gujarati Asians in West London: a casecontrol study. Lancet. 2000;355:618–21.
28. Grange JM, Davies PD, Brown RC, Woodhead JS, Kardjito T. A study of vitamin D levels in Indonesian patients with untreated pulmonary tuberculosis. Tubercle. 1985;66:187–91.
29. Chan TY, Poon P, Pang J, et al. A study of calcium and vitamin D metabolism in Chinese patients with pulmonary tuberculosis. J Trop Med Hyg. 1994;97:26–30.
30. Chan TY. Differences in vitamin D status and calcium intake: possible explanations for the regional variations in the prevalence of hypercalcemia in tuberculosis. Calcif Tissue Int. 1997;60:91–3.
31. Koo HK, Lee JS, Jeong YJ, et al. Vitamin D deficiency and changes in serum vitamin D levels with treatment among tuberculosis patients in South Korea. Respirology. 2012;17:808–13.
32. Rook GAW. The role of vitamin D in tuberculosis. Am Rev Respir Dis. 1988;138:768–70.
33. Raheel I, Sultan MK, Adnan Q, Ehtesham H, Hassan BU. Vitamin D deficiency in patients with tuberculosis. J Coll Phys Surg Pak. 2013;23:780–3.

34. Davis K, Edrisa M, Richard S, William W, Harriet MK. Vitamin D deficiency among adult patients with tuberculosis: a cross sectional study from a national referral hospital in Uganda. BMC Res Notes. 2013; 6:293. http://www.biomedcentral.com/1756-0500/6/293.

35. Gloth FM, Gundberg CM, Hollis BW, Haddad JG, Tobin JD. Vitamin D deficiency in homebound elderly persons. JAMA. 1995;274:1683–6.

36. Omdahl JL, Garry PJ, Hunsaker LA, Hunt WC, Goodwin JS. Nutritional status in a healthy elderly population: vitamin D. Am J Clin Nutr. 1982;36:1225–33.

37. McKenna MJ. Differences in vitamin D status between countries in young adults and the elderly. Am J Med. 1992;93:69–77.

38. Holick MF. Environmental factors that influence the cutaneous production of vitamin D. Am J Clin Nutr. 1995;61:638S–45S.

39. Checkley W, Robinson CL, Baumann LM, et al. 25-hydroxy vitamin D levels are associated with childhood asthma in a population-based study in Peru. Clin Exp Allergy. 2015;45:273–82.

10

Genetic elements associated with antimicrobial resistance among avian pathogenic *Escherichia coli*

Amal Awad[1], Nagah Arafat[2] and Mohamed Elhadidy[1,3*]

Abstract

Background: Avian-pathogenic *Escherichia coli* (APEC) are pathogenic strains of *E. coli* that are responsible for one of the most predominant bacterial disease affecting poultry worldwide called avian colibacillosis. This study describes the genetic determinants implicated in antimicrobial resistance among APEC isolated from different broiler farms in Egypt.

Methods: A total of 116 APEC were investigated by serotyping, antimicrobial resistance patterns to 10 antimicrobials, and the genetic mechanisms underlying the antimicrobial-resistant phenotypes.

Results: Antibiogram results showed that the highest resistance was observed for ampicillin, tetracycline, nalidixic acid, and chloramphenicol. The detected carriage rate of integron was 29.3% (34/116). Further characterization of gene cassettes revealed the presence gene cassettes encoding resistance to trimethoprim (*dfrA1, dfrA5, dfrA7, dfrA12*), streptomycin/spectinomycin (*aadA1, aadA2, aadA5, aadA23*), and streptothricin (*sat2*). To our knowledge, this the first description of the presence of *aadA23* in APEC isolates. Analysis of other antimicrobial resistance types not associated with integrons revealed the predominance of resistance genes encoding resistance to tetracycline (*tetA* and *tetB*), ampicillin (*bla*$_{TEM}$), chloramphenicol (*cat1*), kanamycin (*aphA1*), and sulphonamide (*sul1* and *sul2*). Among ciprofloxacin-resistant isolates, the S83L mutation was the most frequently substitution observed in the quinolone resistance-determining region of *gyrA* (56.3%). The *bla*$_{TEM}$ and *bla*$_{CTX-M-1}$ genes were the most prevalent among APEC isolates producing extended-spectrum beta-lactamase (ESβL).

Conclusions: These findings provided important clues about the role of integron-mediated resistance genes together with other independent resistance genes and chromosomal mutations in shaping the epidemiology of antimicrobial resistance in *E. coli* isolates from poultry farms in Egypt.

Keywords: Antimicrobial resistance, *E. coli*, Poultry, Integron, Genes

Background

Avian colibacillosis is an extraintestinal infection associated with upper respiratory tract infection typically air saculitis that can evolve into multiple lesions in different organs as polyserositis, cellulitis, salpingitis, perihepatitis, peritonitis, septicaemia, and death. These cause severe economic losses in the poultry industry due to the remarkable number of morbidities, mortalities, slaughter condemnation, and reduced productivity of the affected birds [1].

To reduce the high incidence and mortalities caused by avian colibacillosis in poultry farms, antimicrobials are considered as one of the gold choices among veterinarians in the poultry industry. However, in Egypt and other developing countries, antimicrobials are not only used for therapeutic reasons but also for prophylactic purposes in disease prevention and growth promotion. Such overuse and/or misuse contribute to the development and spread of antimicrobial resistance (AMR) among poultry flocks, leading to emergence of multiple drug

*Correspondence: mm_elhadidy@mans.edu.eg
[1] Department of Bacteriology, Mycology and Immunology, Faculty of Veterinary Medicine, Mansoura University, Mansoura 35516, Egypt
Full list of author information is available at the end of the article

resistance (MDR) pathogens [2]. These MDR profiles can be transmitted to human through the food chain adding serious burden to human health. In addition, several studies supported the growing evidence that antimicrobial resistance can occur in the absence of selective pressure, highlighting the crucial role of antibiotic resistance genes in the development of MDR bacteria [3]. The acquisition and dissemination of these antibiotic resistance genes is mainly mediated by horizontal gene transfer in which several mobile genetic elements facilitate this process, including plasmids, transposons, integrons, and bacteriophages [4]. Integron is one of the major genetic elements by which bacteria can capture or excise one or more resistance gene cassettes by site-specific recombination. The mobilization of integron through transposons, plasmids, or other mobile genetic elements enables the spread of integrated resistance genes. This potentially facilitate the integration of almost all antimicrobial agents through the integron and increase the diversity of integrons in isolates from different sources, including human, avian, livestock, and environmental isolates [4–6].

The aim of this study was to determine the antibiotic susceptibility phenotypes of APEC isolated from different broiler farms in Egypt and to evaluate the association of observed phenotypes with the acquisition of integron mediated resistance gene cassettes or other resistance genes and chromosomal mutations located outside the integron.

Methods

Bacterial isolates

In total, 116 APEC isolates recovered from 400 different samples were assayed. Samples were obtained from liver, lungs, air sacs and spleen from chicken with typical lesions of colisepticemia and were collected from 28 different broiler farms located in different geographic areas of Dakahlia Governorate in 2014 and 2015. Samples were cultured onto eosin methylene blue (EMB) agar (Oxoid, Basingstoke, UK) and incubated for 18–24 h at 37 °C. Typical colonies were subcultured onto MacConkey agar (Oxoid, Basingstoke, UK) and were biochemically confirmed using API 20E system (BioMérieux, Marcy-l'Étoile, France). Once identified, the isolates were preserved at −70 °C in brain heart infusion broth containing 20% glycerol (vol/vol) for further studies. Serotyping of *E. coli* isolates was performed using rapid diagnostic *E. coli* antisera sets (Denka Seiken Co., Japan) using 8 polyvalent, 43 monovalent somatic, and 22 flagellar antisera. Bacterial DNA for PCR analysis was prepared by boiling a bacterial culture in 300 μl of distilled water for 10 min, followed by centrifugation for 5 min at 10,000×g. A

volume of 1 μl of the supernatant was used as a template for each 25 μl PCR mixture.

Antimicrobial susceptibility testing and detection of ESβL

The susceptibility of isolates to 10 different antimicrobial agents was determined by disc diffusion assay as described by Clinical and Laboratory Standards Institute (CLSI) [7]. According to the measurement of inhibition zones, tested strains were evaluated as susceptible or resistant. The following antimicrobial discs (Oxoid, Basingstoke, UK) were used: gentamicin (GN, 10 μg), kanamycin (KAN, 30 μg), ampicillin (AMP, 10 μg), cefotaxime (CTX, 30 μg), nalidixic acid (NA, 30 μg), ciprofloxacin (CIP, 5 μg), tetracycline (TET, 30 μg), sulfamethoxazole-trimethoprim (STX, 25 μg), chloramphenicol (C, 30 μg), and streptomycin (S, 10 μg). The isolates were defined as multidrug-resistant APEC if they exhibited resistance to at least one agent in three or more antimicrobial categories [8]. *Escherichia coli* strain ATCC 25922 was used as a reference strain for susceptibility test. All cefotaxime-resistant isolates were confirmed for the production of extended-spectrum beta-lactamase (ESβL) by using the double-disk synergy test (DDST) following recommendation and interpretations of CLSI standards [7].

Detection of integrons and characterization of associated gene cassettes

The presence of integrons among APEC isolates was assayed using primers hep35 and hep36 that amplify conserved regions of integron-encoded integrase genes *intI1*, *intI2*, and *intI3* using published PCR protocols [9]. Integron-positive isolates were characterized for the integron class using integron class-specific primers and PCR conditions previously described [10]. Further characterization of gene cassette content within integron classes was determined using primers 5′CS/3′CS and hep74/hep51 for amplification of gene cassettes within integron classes 1 and 2, respectively as published [11, 12]. Samples with similar amplicon size were further subjected to restriction enzyme *HinfI* or *RsaI* [12] following manufacturer instructions (New England Biolabs, UK) and fragments obtained were separated on a 2.5% agarose gel. Isolates with similar polymorphism patterns were considered to harbor similar gene cassettes. Amplification products of samples with unique amplification products and one representative sample from samples with similar restriction patterns were purified from the agarose gel using QIA quick Gel Extraction Kit (Qiagen, USA) and sequenced using ABI Prism 377 automated sequencer (Applied Biosystems). All sequence results were compared with the available sequences in GenBank (http://www.ncbi.nlm.nih.gov/BLAST).

Detection of antimicrobial resistance genes outside the integron cassettes

Different PCR protocols were applied to detect specific genetic determinants corresponding to the resistance phenotype using Applied Biosystems 96-well thermal cycler and PCR conditions suggested by the referenced authors. These determinants included those encoding resistance to tetracycline (*tetA*, *tetB*, *tetC*, *tetD*, *tetE*, and *tetG*) [13], chloramphenicol (*cat1*, *cat2*, *cat3*, *cmlA*, and *cmlB*) [14], streptomycin (*strA-strB*) [15], Kanamycin (*aphA1* and *aphA2*) [16], and sulfonamide including *sul1*, *sul2* [17], and *sul3* [18]. The PCR amplification products were separated by agarose gel electrophoresis and visualized by ethidium bromide staining. Resistance to ciprofloxacin was assayed by determining mutations in DNA gyrase subunit A (*gyrA*) and topoisomerase IV subunit C (*ParC*) in the quinolone resistance determining region (QRDR) using protocol previously described [19]. The resulting PCR amplicons were purified using QIA quick Gel Extraction Kit (Qiagen, USA) and bi-directionally sequenced using same primers. Strains that exhibited negative results for mutations in QRDR were screened for plasmid-mediated quinolone resistance (PMQR) including *qnrA*, *qnrB*, *qnrS* [20], *qnrD* [21], and *aac (6')-Ib-cr* [22]. Ampicillin-resistant isolates were screened for the β-Lactamases genes *bla*$_{TEM}$ and *bla*$_{SHV}$, and *bla*$_{OXA-1}$ using multiplex PCR protocol published [23]. The later protocol was used to screen potential ESβL-producing *E. coli* isolates that initially exhibited resistance to cefotaxime. These isolates were further screened for *bla*$_{CTX-M}$ five phylogenetic groups (groups 1, 2, 8, 9, and 25) using multiplex PCR protocol previously described [24].

Pulsed-field gel electrophoresis (PFGE)

PFGE was performed to determine that isolates exhibiting similar antibiogram resistance profile and similar serotype are non-identical. PFGE for tested APEC isolates was performed using XbaI restriction enzyme according to the PulseNet protocol from the Centers for Disease Control and Prevention [25]. At least one band difference was required to distinguish between pulsotypes.

Statistical analysis

Differences in the occurrence of integrons in resistant and susceptible APEC strains were tested using the Chi square (χ^2) test. Differences among means with $P < 0.05$ were considered as statistically significant. For the statistical analysis, intermediate resistant strains were considered as resistant.

Results

APEC serotypes

A total of 116 *E. coli* isolates were recovered from 400 samples from diseased chicken. Serotyping recovered isolates identified 15 different *E. coli* serotypes (Table 1). All isolates exhibiting similar serotype and antimicrobial resistance patterns were confirmed to be non-duplicates as confirmed by PFGE. Among identified serotypes, O78 was found to be the most prevalent serotype (27.6%).

Antimicrobial resistance patterns and ESβL phenotype

Antibiotic susceptibility of 116 APEC isolates against 10 different antimicrobial drugs is presented in Table 2. The highest frequencies of resistance detected were those against ampicillin (100%), tetracycline (93.1%), nalidixic acid (84.5%), chloramphenicol (84.5%), kanamycin (69.0%), sulfamethoxazole-trimethoprim (58.6%), cefotaxime (58.6%), streptomycin (50.0%), gentamicin (48.3%), and ciprofloxacin (41.4%). A diversity of resistance patterns observed among tested *E. coli* isolates is shown in Table 1. Screening the potential ESβL producers confirmed that all cefotaxime-resistant isolates to be ESβL producers (68/68, 100%).

Distribution of integrons and associated gene cassettes

Of the 116 isolates tested, 34 isolates (29.3%) representing six serotypes were integron positive (Table 1). All integron-harboring *E. coli* isolates were multidrug resistant. Integron-positive isolates were significantly more resistant to streptomycin, kanamycin, gentamicin, and sulfamethoxazole-trimethoprim than integron-negative isolates (P < 0.05). Among integron-positive isolates, class 1 integrons were detected in 30 isolates (25.9%) and class 2 in four isolates (3.4%) (Table 1). None of the isolates possessed the combination of class 1 and class 2 integrons. Class 3 was absent in tested APEC isolates. Further characterization of gene cassettes by PCR, restriction digestion, and sequencing revealed eight different cassette arrangements within class 1 integron and a single cassette arrangement within class 2 integron. Among class 1 integron, the gene cassettes included those encoding resistance to trimethoprim (*dfrA1*, *dfrA5*, *dfrA7*, and *dfrA12*) and streptomycin (*aadA1*, *aadA2*, *aadA5*, and *aadA23*). A total of seven isolates harbored *aadA1* + *dfrA1* (20.6%); six isolates carried *dfrA7* (17.6%); five isolates had *aadA1* (14.7%); four isolates carried *aadA5* (11.8%); three isolates (8.8%) contained *dfrA5*; two isolate (5.8%) carried *aadA2* + *dfrA12*, two isolate (5.8%) carried *aadA23*, and one (2.9%) had *dfrA1*. All class 2 integron-carrying isolates possessed the gene cassette array *dfrA1-sat2-aadA1* that encode resistance to trimethoprim, streptothricin, and streptomycin (Table 3).

Distribution of antimicrobial resistance genes outside the integron cassettes

Different frequencies of genes encoding resistance to tetracycline, chloramphenicol, ampicillin, streptomycin,

Table 1 Overview and characteristics (MDR strains, integron presence, and antibiotic resistance) of the APEC strains classified per serotype

Serotype	No. of strains	No. of MDR strains[a]	No. of different antibiotic resistance profiles	No. isolates carrying integrons		
				Class 1	Class 2	Total
O1:H7	14 (12.1%)	6	14	2	0	2 (14.3%)
O2:H6	18 (15.5%)	14	18	6	0	6 (33.3%)
O8	2 (1.7%)	2	2	0	0	0 (0%)
O111:H2	4 (3.4%)	4	4	2	2	4 (100%)
O26:H11	6 (5.2%)	6	6	4	0	4 (66.7%)
O44:H18	2 (1.7%)	2	2	0	0	0 (0%)
O55:H7	10 (8.6%)	8	6	0	0	0 (0%)
O78	32 (27.6%)	28	24	16	0	16 (50.0%)
O119:H6	6 (5.2%)	4	6	0	0	0 (0%)
O124	4 (3.4%)	4	4	0	0	0 (0%)
O126:H2	6 (5.2%)	6	6	0	0	0 (0%)
O127:H6	6 (5.2%)	4	6	0	2	2 (33.3%)
O128:H2	2 (1.7%)	2	2	0	0	0 (0%)
O142:H6	2 (1.7%)	0	2	0	0	0 (0%)
O158	2 (1.7%)	0	2	0	0	0 (0%)
Total	116	90 (77.6%)		30 (25.9%)	4 (3.4%)	34 (29.3%)

[a] *MDR strains* multidrug-resistant strains that exhibited resistance to 3 or more different classes of antimicrobials

kanamycin, ciprofloxacin, cefotaxime, sulfonamide, and ESβL production are reported in Table 2. Among tetracycline resistant isolates, 50 (46.3%) isolates carried *tetA* and 54 (50.0%) isolates were positive for *tetB*. Our results also showed that four isolates (3.7%) possessed both determinants. All isolates were negative for *tetC*, *tetD*, *tetE*, and *tetG*. Among the ampicillin-resistant isolates, 102 (87.9%) isolates possessed bla_{TEM}, 14 (12.1%) isolates carried bla_{oxa1}. None of these isolates carried bla_{SHV} gene. The *cat1* was the most common gene present among the chloramphenicol-resistant isolates (86/98; 87.8%). Isolates (n = 68) that were resistant for sulfamethoxazole were tested for amplification of the *sul* genes. The *sul2 and sul1* genes were present in 39 (57.3%) and 23 (33.8%) isolates, respectively. All ciprofloxacin-resistant APEC isolates were screened for mutations in QRDR of *gyrA* and *ParC* by PCR and DNA sequencing. Our sequencing results showed that a total of 56.3% (27/48) of tested isolates possessed S83L mutation in *gyrA*. Four ciprofloxacin- resistant isolates harbored double mutations of *gyrA* at residues 83 and 87 (S83L + D87 N). One APEC isolate had a single mutation in *parC* encoding Ser80Ile. The PMQR were investigated in APEC isolates with no mutations in QRDR to explore further mechanisms of resistance. The *qnrA*, *qnrB*, and *qnrS* genes were found in these isolates (10, 4 and 2 isolates, respectively). None of the isolates were positive for *qnrD* or *aac (6′)-Ib-cr* genes. The *strA-strB* genes encoding streptomycin resistance were examined to investigate

streptomycin resistance determinants other than *aadA* present in the integron cassette and both genes were detected in 34 (58.6%) isolates. The *aphA1* and *aphA2* gene markers, conferring kanamycin resistance were identified in a total of 65 (81.3%) and 11 (13.7%) isolates, respectively. The combined presence of both gene alleles was found in 4 (5%) isolates. Screening ESβL-producing *E. coli* isolates by multiplex PCR analysis revealed that 15 isolates were group in CTX-M-1 group. Group 9 enzymes were produced by two isolates. In addition, bla_{TEM} and bla_{OXA-1} genes were present in 20 (29.4%) and 7 (10.3%) ESβL-producing *E. coli* isolates, respectively. A total of 24 isolates were observed to simultaneously carry bla_{TEM} and contain alleles encoding group 1 CTX-M enzymes (Table 2).

Discussion

The emerging antimicrobial resistance among different APEC isolates has stimulated our interest in exploring the mechanisms of resistance and the frequencies of genetic determinants. In this study, the majority of recovered isolates belonged to serogroups O1, O2, O78. A similar observation was reported by other studies supporting the previous postulation that these serotypes are the most common serotypes in *E. coli* of avian origin worldwide [26].

Similar to the findings of previous studies [2, 5], most (84–100%) APEC isolates were highly resistant to ampicillin, tetracycline, nalidixic acid, and chloramphenicol.

Table 2 Molecular characterization of antimicrobial resistance genotypes among APEC isolates

Antibiotic	Antimicrobial class	Number of resistance isolates	Associated genes tested	Number of positive isolates
Ampicillin	Penicillins	116 (100%)	bla_{TEM}	102
			bla_{SHV}	0
			bla_{oxa1}	14
Chloramphenicol	Phenicols	98 (84.5%)	cat1	86
			cat2	4
			cat3	0
			cmlA	8
			cmlB	0
Streptomycin	Aminoglycosides	58 (50%)	strA-strB	34
Ciprofloxacin	Quinolones	48 (41.4%)	PMQR[a]	
			qnrA	10
			qnrB	4
			qnrS	2
			qnrD	0
			aac (6')-Ib-cr	0
			QRDR[b]	
			S83L (gyrA)	27
			S83L + D87 N (gyrA)	4
			S80I (pyrC)	1
Sulfamethoxazole-trimethoprim	Potentiated sulfonamides	68 (58.6%)	sul1	23
			sul2	39
			sul3	0
Tetracycline	Tetracyclines	108 (93.1%)	tetA	50
			tetB	54
			tetC	0
			tetD	0
			tetE	0
			tetG	0
			tetA + tetB	4
Kanamycin	Aminoglycosides	80 (69.0%)	aphA1	65
			aphA2	11
			aphA1 + aphA2	4
Cefotaxime (ESβL)	Cephalosporins	68 (58.6%)	CTX-M (group 1)	15
			CTX-M (group 2)	0
			CTX-M (group 8)	0
			CTX-M (group 9)	2
			CTX-M (group 25)	0
			bla_{TEM}	20
			bla_{SHV}	0
			bla_{oxa1}	7
			CTX-M (group 1) + bla_{TEM}	24

[a] Plasmid-mediated quinolone resistance

[b] Quinolone resistance determining region

Table 3 Distribution of class 1 and class 2 integrons among APEC isolates

Integron genotype	Integron class	Number of positive integron harboring isolates
aadA1-dfrA1	1	7
dfrA7	1	6
aadA1	1	5
aadA5	1	4
dfrA5	1	3
aadA2-dfrA12	1	2
aadA23	1	2
dfrA1	1	1
dfrA1-sat2-aadA1	2	4
Total		34

Many (41–69%) APEC isolates were resistant to streptomycin, gentamycin, kanamycin, sulfamethoxazole combined with trimethoprim, ciprofloxacin, and cefotaxime. Most of these antimicrobial agents are regularly used as prophylactic agents or as growth promoters in the poultry industry in Egypt.

In the present study, the proportion of integron carriage among APEC isolates is consistent with previous studies worldwide [10, 27]. In a study conducted in Egypt on APEC isolated from septicemic broilers, higher prevalence was reported for class 1 and 2 (46.6 and 9.6%, respectively) [5]. Our results revealed that the genes found in class 1 and class 2 integrons encode for adenyltransferase conferring resistance to streptomycin and spectinomycin (aadA) and for a dihydrofolate reductase conferring resistance to trimethoprim (dfr). These gene cassettes are the most frequently detectable genes from pathogenic and commensal E. coli from poultry farms and also from different animal, environmental, and human sources [4–6].

Among class 1 integron-harboring isolates, four different trimethoprim resistance genes (dfrA1, dfrA5, dfrA7, dfrA12) and four streptomycin/spectinomycin resistance genes (aadA1, aadA2, aadA5, aadA23) were detected as gene cassettes in class 1 integrons. The aadA23 gene cassette detected in this study was first reported in 2005 in Brazil from Salmonella Agona strains isolated from a pig carcass [28]. In Egypt, this gene cassette was previously described among E. coli strains isolated from neonatal calf diarrhea [29]. To our knowledge, the first description of aadA23 in E. coli of avian origin. All class 2 integron carrying isolates processed the gene cassette array dfrA1-sat2-aadA1 that is considered as the classical gene cassette found in class 2 integron among APEC strains [5, 30]. The absence of class 3 integron among our isolates corroborate previous studies [5, 30], suggesting the less

significant role of this integron in dissemination of antimicrobial resistance among APEC.

We further assessed the presence of other genetic determinants located outside the integron that were previously proposed to be responsible for resistance to different antimicrobial agents. Among tetracycline-resistant isolates, tetA and tetB markers were the only tet genes reported in this study either in single or combined genes. These results supported the observation that these efflux genes are the most frequent tet genes found in Enterobacteriaceae [31]. The high prevalence of these variants might be attributed to their higher association with plasmids, mainly the conjugative ones or transposons [31], suggesting that these genes are the major genes implicated in the efflux mechanism in APEC leading to the resistance phenotype. The high prevalence of cat1 among chloramphenicol-resistant isolates supports previous studies highlighting the crucial role of this allele in chloramphenicol resistance [16]. The combined presence of strA-strB determinants encoding two enzymes required for high level of streptomycin resistance [32] was assayed in this study as aadA gene observed in the integron has been proposed to confer low level of streptomycin [33]. In this study, the presence of the strA-strB gene pair among streptomycin-resistant was within the range reported among APEC strains isolated in Korea during the period 2000 to 2005 [34]. The high prevalence of aphA1 among kanamycin-resistant isolates is consistent with other studies that proposed aphA1 to be the main neomycin/kanamycin resistance marker [16, 35]. The predominance of bla_{TEM} gene (87.9%) among ampicillin-resistant isolates corroborates a previous study that suggested bla_{TEM} gene to be the most common β-lactamase responsible for ampicillin resistance [34].

Resistance to quinolone in APEC is mainly mediated by spontaneous mutations in the QRDR of gyrA and parC genes [2, 34]. Nonetheless, in a previous study conducted among APEC isolates in Egypt, these substitutions in QRDR genes were not screened and only PMQR genes were investigated [5]. Our results revealed that among ciprofloxacin-resistant isolates, the mutation in gyrA (S83L) involved in fluoroquinolone resistance was the most prevalent genetic determinant, an observation previously reported in a study conducted among quinolone-resistant APEC isolates in Korea [34].

One of the most striking findings from this study was the high prevalence of ESβL-producing isolates recovered from broilers (58.6%). This represents a serious public health threats attributed to the ability of these bacteria to hydrolyze third-generation cephalosporins that are commonly used to treat serious infections and the potential transfer and spread of these resistance genes to human through food chain, direct contact, or the environment

[36–38]. The higher frequency of CTX-M-1-group in this study supports recent reports that postulated this group to the most predominant CTX-M group among ESβL-producing APEC in Egypt or worldwide [5, 39, 40].

Conclusions

Our results reported high rates of antibiotic resistance among APEC isolates recovered from different poultry farms in Egypt, including those drugs of broad-spectrum-activity such as β-lactams, third generation cephalosporins, and quinolones. Furthermore, our findings suggested diverse genetic makeup involved in antimicrobial resistance phenotype. Indeed, integron-mediated resistance could explain only a part of the resistance profile of the isolates as other independent genes were significantly observed. This diversity in distribution of resistance determinants could be responsible for the high resistance profiles recorded and the potential spread of antimicrobial resistance determinants among APEC. These advices more restriction in antimicrobials use in poultry farms among veterinarians to prevent and control the spread of antimicrobial-resistant bacteria and their genetic determinants. Consequently, our future studies will be directed to study the clonal link and compare the overlapping characteristics of recovered APEC isolates with human ExPEC (extra-intestinal pathogenic *E. coli*) to confirm the zoonotic potential of APEC, including their potential ability to transfer antimicrobial resistance to human.

Abbreviations

APEC: avian-pathogenic *Escherichia coli*; AMR: antimicrobial resistance; CLSI: Clinical and Laboratory Standards Institute; EMB: eosin methylene blue; ESβL: extended-spectrum beta-lactamase; ExPEC: extra-intestinal pathogenic *E. coli*; MDR: multiple drug resistance; PFGE: pulsed-field gel electrophoresis; PMQR: plasmid-mediated quinolone resistance; QRDR: quinolone resistance determining region.

Authors' contributions

ME conceived and designed the study, performed the tests, analyzed and interpreted the data, and wrote the manuscript. AA and NA substantially contributed to collection of samples, isolation of strains and participated in data analysis, and revision of the manuscript. All authors read and approved the final manuscript.

Author details

[1] Department of Bacteriology, Mycology and Immunology, Faculty of Veterinary Medicine, Mansoura University, Mansoura 35516, Egypt. [2] Department of Poultry diseases, Faculty of Veterinary Medicine, Mansoura University, Mansoura 35516, Egypt. [3] Foodborne Pathogens, Scientific Institute of Public Health, Juliette Wytsmanstraat 14, 1050 Brussels, Belgium.

Acknowledgements

The authors would like to thank Dr. Eman Abo Elfadl at the Department of Animal Husbandry and Development of Animal Wealth, Faculty of Veterinary Medicine, Mansoura University for her technical help during this study. Dr. Mohamed Elhadidy is currently a visiting research fellow at Scientific Institute of Public Health in Brussels funded by Federal Science Policy Office.

Competing interests

The authors declare that they have no competing interests.

Funding

The authors declare that they did not have any funding source or grant to support their research work.

References

1. Dho-Moulin M, Fairbrother JM. Avian pathogenic *Escherichia coli* (APEC). Vet Res. 1999;30:299–316.
2. Yang H, Chen S, White DG, Zhao S, McDermott P, Walker R, Meng J. Characterization of multiple-antimicrobial-resistant *Escherichia coli* isolates from diseased chickens and swine in China. J Clin Microbiol. 2004;42:3483–9.
3. Bean DC, Livermore DM, Hall LM. Plasmids imparting sulfonamide resistance in *Escherichia coli*: implications for persistence. Antimicrob Agents Chemother. 2009;53:1088–93.
4. Karczmarczyk M, Walsh C, Slowey R, Leonard N, Fanning S. Molecular characterization of multidrug-resistant *Escherichia coli* isolates from Irish cattle farms. Appl Environ Microbiol. 2011;77:7121–7.
5. Ahmed AM, Shimamoto T, Shimamoto T. Molecular characterization of multidrug-resistant avian pathogenic *Escherichia coli* isolated from septicemic broilers. Int J Med Microbiol. 2013;303:475–83.
6. Cocchi S, Grasselli E, Gutacker M, Benagli C, Convert M, Piffaretti JC. Distribution and characterization of integrons in *Escherichia coli* strains of animal and human origin. FEMS Immunol Med Microbiol. 2007;50:126–32.
7. Clinical and Laboratory Standards Institute. Performance standards for antimicrobial susceptibility testing; 20th informational supplement M100-S20. Wayne: CLSI; 2010.
8. Magiorakos AP, Srinivasan A, Carey RB, Carmeli Y, Falagas ME, Giske CG, Harbarth S, Hindler JF, Kahlmeter G, Olsson-Liljequist B, Paterson DL, Rice LB, Stelling J, Struelens MJ, Vatopoulos A, Weber JT, Monnet DL. Multidrug-resistant, extensively drug-resistant and pandrug-resistant bacteria: an international expert proposal for interim standard definitions for acquired resistance. Clin Microbiol Infect. 2012;18(268–81):27.
9. Nagachinta S, Chen J. Integron-mediated antibiotic resistance in Shiga toxin-producing *Escherichia coli*. J Food Prot. 2009;72:21–7.
10. Povilonis J, Seputiene V, Ruzauskas M, Siugzdiniene R, Virgailis M, Pavilonis A, Suziedeliene E. Transferable class 1 and 2 integrons in *Escherichia coli* and *Salmonella enterica* isolates of human and animal origin in Lithuania. Foodborne Pathog Dis. 2010;7:1185–92.
11. Levesque C, Piche L, Larose C, Roy PH. PCR mapping of integrons reveals several novel combinations of resistance genes. Antimicrob Agents Chemother. 1995;39:185–91.
12. White PA, McIver CJ, Deng Y, Rawlinson WD. Characterisation of two new gene cassettes, aadA5 and dfrA17. FEMS Microbiol Lett. 2000;182:265–9.
13. Ng LK, Martin I, Alfa M, Mulvey M. Multiplex PCR for the detection of tetracycline resistant genes. Mol Cell Probes. 2001;15:209–15.
14. Chen S, Zhao S, White D, Schroeder CM, Lu R, Yang H, McDermott PF, Ayers S, Meng J. Characterization of multiple-antimicrobial-resistant *Salmonella serovars* isolated from retail meats. Appl Environ Microbiol. 2004;70:1–7.
15. Tamang MD, Oh JY, Seol SY, Kang HY, Lee JC, Lee YC, Cho DT, Kim J. Emergence of multidrug-resistant *Salmonella enterica* serovar Typhi associated with a class 1 integron carrying the dfrA7 gene cassette in Nepal. Int J Antimicrob Agents. 2007;30:330–5.

16. Maynard C, Fairbrother JM, Bekal S, Sanschagrin F, Levesque RC, Brousseau R, Masson L, Lariviere S, Harel J. Antimicrobial resistance genes in enterotoxigenic *Escherichia coli* O149:K91 isolates obtained over a 23-year period from pigs. Antimicrob Agents Chemother. 2003;47:3214–21.

17. Kerrn MB, Klemmensen T, Frimodt-Moller N, Espersen F. Susceptibility of Danish *Escherichia coli* strains isolated from urinary tract infections and bacteraemia, and distribution of sul genes conferring sulphonamide resistance. J Antimicrob Chemother. 2002;50:513–6.

18. Hammerum AM, Sandvang D, Andersen SR, Seyfarth AM, Porsbo LJ, Frimodt-Moller N, Heuer OE. Detection of sul1, sul2 and sul3 in sulphonamide resistant *Escherichia coli* isolates obtained from healthy humans, pork and pigs in Denmark. Int J Food Microbiol. 2006;106:235–7.

19. Everett MJ, Jin YF, Ricci V, Piddock LJV. Contribution of individual mechanisms to fluoroquinolone resistance in 36 *Escherichia coli* strains isolated from humans and animals. Antimicrob Agents Chemother. 1996;40:2380–6.

20. Cattoir V, Poirel L, Rotimi V, Soussy CJ, Nordmann P. Multiplex PCR for detection of plasmid-mediated quinolone resistance qnr genes in ESBL-producing enterobacterial isolates. J Antimicrob Chemother. 2007;60:394–7.

21. Cavaco LM, Hasman H, Xia S, Aarestrup FM. qnrD, a novel gene conferring transferable quinolone resistance in *Salmonella enterica* serovar Kentucky and Bovismorbificans strains of human origin. Antimicrob Agents Chemother. 2009;53:603–8.

22. Park CH, Robicsek A, Jacoby GA, Sahm D, Hooper DC. Prevalence in the United States of aac (6')-Ib-cr encoding a ciprofloxacin-modifying enzyme. Antimicrob Agents Chemother. 2006;50:3953–5.

23. Colom K, Pérez J, Alonso R, Fernández-Aranguiz A, Lariño E, Cisterna R. Simple and reliable multiplex PCR assay for detection of blaTEM, bla(SHV) and blaOXA-1 genes in *Enterobacteriaceae*. FEMS Microbiol Lett. 2003;223:147–51.

24. Woodford N, Fagan EJ, Ellington MJ. Multiplex PCR for rapid detection of genes encoding CTX-M extended-spectrum (beta)-lactamases. J Antimicrob Chemother. 2005;57:154–5.

25. Ribot EM, Fair MA, Gautom R, Cameron DN, Hunter SB, Swaminathan B, Barrett TJ. Standardization of pulsed-field gel electrophoresis protocols for the subtyping of *Escherichia coli* O157:H7, *Salmonella*, and *Shigella* for PulseNet. Foodborne Pathog Dis. 2006;3:59–67.

26. Ewers C, Janssen T, Kiessling S, Philipp HC, Wieler LH. Molecular epidemiology of avian pathogenic *Escherichia coli* (APEC) isolated from colisepticemia in poultry. Vet Microbiol. 2004;104:91–101.

27. Oosterik LH, Peeters L, Mutuku I, Goddeeris BM, Butaye P. Susceptibility of avian pathogenic *Escherichia coli* from laying hens in Belgium to antibiotics and disinfectants and integron prevalence. Avian Dis. 2014;58:271–8.

28. Michael GB, Cardoso M, Schwarz S. Class 1 integron-associated gene cassettes in *Salmonella enterica* subsp. enterica serovar Agona isolated from pig carcasses in Brazil. J Antimicrob Chemother. 2005;55:776–9.

29. Ahmed AM, Younis EE, Osman SA, Ishida Y, El-Khodery SA, Shimamoto T. Genetic analysis of antimicrobial resistance in *Escherichia coli* isolated from diarrheic neonatal calves. Vet Microbiol. 2009;136:397–402.

30. Cavicchio L, Dott G, Giacomelli M, Giovanardi D, Grilli G, Franciosini MP, Trocino A, Piccirillo A. Class 1 and class 2 integrons in avian pathogenic *Escherichia coli* from poultry in Italy. Poult Sci. 2015;94:1202–8.

31. Chopra I, Roberts M. Tetracycline antibiotics: mode of action, applications, molecular biology, and epidemiology of bacterial resistance. Microbiol Mol Biol Rev. 2001;65:232–60.

32. Chiou CS, Jones AL. Expression and identification of the strA-strB gene pair from streptomycin-resistant *Erwinia amylovora*. Gene. 1995;152:47–51.

33. Sunde M, Norstrom M. The genetic background for streptomycin resistance in *Escherichia coli* influences the distribution of MICs. J Antimicrob Chemother. 2005;56:87–90.

34. Kim TE, Jeong YW, Cho S, Kim SJ, Kwon HJ. Chronological study of antibiotic resistances and their relevant genes in Korean avian pathogenic *Escherichia coli* isolates. J Clin Microbiol. 2007;45:3309–15.

35. Pezzella C, Ricci A, DiGiannatale E, Luzzi I, Carattoli A. Tetracycline and streptomycin resistance genes, transposons, and plasmids in *Salmonella enterica* isolates from animals in Italy. Antimicrob Agents Chemother. 2004;48:903–8.

36. Kluytmans AJW, Overdevest ITMA, Willemsen I, Kluytmans-van den Bergh MF, van der Zwaluw K, Heck M, Rijnsburger M, Vandenbroucke-Grauls CM, Savelkoul PH, Johnston BD, Gordon D, Johnson JR. Extended-spectrum β-lactamase producing *Escherichia coli* from retail chicken meat and humans: comparison of strains, plasmids, resistance genes, and virulence factors. Clin Infect Dis. 2013;56:478–87.

37. Huijbers PMC, Graat EAM, Haenen APJ, van Santen MG, van Essen-Zandbergen A, Mevius DJ, van Duijkeren E, van Hoek AH. Extended-spectrum β-lactamase- and AmpC β-lactamase-producing *Escherichia coli* in broilers and people living and/or working on broiler farms: prevalence, risk factors, and molecular characteristics. J Antimicrob Chemother. 2014;69:2669–75.

38. Voets GM, Fluit AC, Scharringa J, Schapendonk C, van den Munckhof T, Leverstein-van Hall MA, Stuart JC. Identical plasmid AmpC beta-lactamase genes and plasmid types in *E. coli* isolates from patients and poultry meat in the Netherlands. Int J Food Microbiol. 2013;167:359–62.

39. Abdallah HM, Reuland EA, Wintermans BB, Al Naiemi N, Koek A, Abdelwahab AM, Ammar AM, Mohamed AA, Vandenbroucke-Grauls CM. Extended Spectrum β Lactamases and/or CarbapenemasesProducing *Enterobacteriaceae* isolated from retail chicken meat in Zagazig, Egypt. Plos ONE. 2015;18:e0136052.

40. Livermore DM, Hawkey PM. CTX-M: changing the face of ESBLs in the UK. J Antimicrob Chemother. 2005;56:451–4.

11

Trends in paediatric and adult bloodstream infections at a Ghanaian referral hospital: a retrospective study

Noah Obeng-Nkrumah[1†], Appiah-Korang Labi[2*†], Naa Okaikor Addison[2], Juliana Ewuramma Mbiriba Labi[3] and Georgina Awuah-Mensah[1]

Abstract

Background: Bloodstream infections (BSI) are life-threatening emergencies. Identification of the common pathogens and their susceptibility patterns is necessary for timely empirical intervention.

Methods: We conducted a 4-year retrospective analysis of blood cultures from all patients excluding neonates at the Korle-Bu Teaching hospital, Ghana, from January 2010 through December 2013. Laboratory report data were used to determine BSI, blood culture contamination, pathogen profile, and antimicrobial resistance patterns.

Results: Overall, 3633 (23.16 %) out of 15,683 blood cultures were positive for various organisms. Pathogen-positive cultures accounted for 1451 (9.3 %, 95 % CI 8.5–9.8 %). Infants recorded the highest true blood culture positivity (20.9 %, n = 226/1083), followed by the elderly (13.3 %, n = 80/601), children (8.9 %, n = 708/8000) and adults (7.2 %, n = 437/6000) ($p = 0.001$ for Marascuilo's post hoc). Overall occurrence of BSI declined with increasing age-group ($p = 0.001$) but the type of isolates did not vary with age except for *Citrobacter*, *Escherichia coli*, *Klebsiella*, *Salmonella*, and *Enterococcus* species. Gram negative bacteria predominated in our study (59.8 %, n = 867/1451), but the commonest bacterial isolate was *Staphylococcus aureus* (21.9 %, n = 318/1451)—and this trend run through the various age-groups. From 2010 to 2013, we observed a significant trend of yearly increase in the frequency of BSI caused by cephalosporin-resistant enterobacteria (Chi square for trend, $p = 0.001$). Meropenem maintained high susceptibility among all Gram-negative organisms ranging from 96 to 100 %. Among *Staphylococcus aureus*, susceptibility to cloxacillin was 76.6 %.

Conclusion: Our study shows a significantly high blood culture positivity in infants as compared to children, adults and the elderly. There was a preponderance of *S. aureus* and Gram-negative bacteria across all age-groups. Meropenem was the most active antibiotic for Gram-negative bacteria. Cloxacillin remains a very useful anti-staphylococcal agent.

Keywords: Ghana, Bloodstream, Infections, Infants, Adults, Antibiotic susceptibility

Background

Developing countries, especially in Africa, have a disproportionate burden of global bacterial bloodstream infections (BSI). This contributes significantly to morbidity, mortality, and increased health care costs [1–3]. The potential outcomes of bloodstream infections are such that treatment is often empirical, due to delays in performing and receiving blood culture results. In developing countries, this is further worsened by the unavailability of well-resourced microbiology facilities [4]. Empirical antibiotics used in such instances are usually based on international guidelines and not guided by local susceptibility data [5]. The rise in antibiotic resistance worldwide means that the likelihood of inadequate

*Correspondence: appiahl@yahoo.com
†Noah Obeng-Nkrumah and Appiah-Korang Labi contributed equally to this work
[2] Department of Microbiology, Korle-Bu Teaching Hospital, P.O. Box 77, Accra, Ghana, West Africa
Full list of author information is available at the end of the article

therapy in BSI is heightened, with increased chances of poor therapeutic outcomes [6, 7]. Knowledge of the local antibiotic resistance profile of bacteria increases the probability of selecting effective empirical therapy [2, 8]. In a recent study on the cost-effectiveness of bloodstream infection surveillance for the management of sepsis in low-resource settings, Penno et al. [5] showed that antibiotic prescribing, based on local antibiogram is able to save 534 additional lives per 100,000 patients. The finding suggests that it is crucial to monitor emerging trends in resistance at the local level to support clinical management. However, data on antimicrobial resistance, especially regarding trends in BSI, remain scarce in Ghanaian healthcare settings including Korle-Bu Teaching Hospital (KBTH).

Published data describing BSI in KBTH are limited to short study periods [9] and have mainly focused on children [10]. Using a large collection of blood culture data, we have examined trends in pediatric and adult BSI over 4 years at KBTH; determined blood culture yields and contamination rate; and analyzed the antibiotic susceptibility profiles of the associated organisms, with emphasis on multidrug resistant phenotypes of public health concern.

Methods
Study design
This was a hospital based retrospective analysis of blood culture reports from January 2010 to December 2013 at the Korle-Bu Teaching Hospital in Ghana, West Africa. We followed guidelines for the reporting of studies conducted using observational routinely-collected health data (RECORD) [11]. The KBTH is a 2000-bed tertiary teaching hospital with about 200 admissions per day [12]. The central outpatient department records about 29,757 patients per month [12]. The hospital covers all medical specialties and provides referral healthcare services to an estimated population of 24 million Ghanaians.

Study settings and population
We collated blood culture results of patients older than 28 days, from the bacteriology unit of the Microbiology Laboratory in KBTH. Data on BSI of patients ≤28 days old will be published elsewhere. The bacteriology unit of KBTH processes over 40,000 clinical cultures annually. To obtain a good representation of the repertoire of BSI isolates occurring at a tertiary health facility, we have included all blood culture results of patients primarily receiving healthcare at the KBTH (n = 15,072) or secondarily referred to the laboratory from other health facilities for microbiological investigations (n = 611). We included data for the period January 2010 to December 2013. Data

prior to this period were not properly archived and therefore difficult to access.

Selection, review and extraction of data from laboratory reports
A data entry team comprising three bacteriologists and a physician who assisted with the medical reconciliation of data conducted a manual work-through of laboratory paper records to select blood cultures conducted between 2010 and 2013. Selected blood culture reports were reviewed and extracted into a computerized database (Statistical Package for Social Sciences, Version 20.0) as the primary data source. We had no independent means of validating laboratory results, thus reports were excluded from entry on the basis of incomplete data if results regarding the positivity or otherwise of blood cultures were inconclusive. The quality of abstracted data was assessed by an independent reviewer in a standardized manner by comparing paper records to the electronic entries. Disagreements between data were resolved by consensus between the reviewer and the data entry team. Extracted information included patient demographics, bacterial and fungal isolates, BSI categorization, and antibiogram of isolates. Reports for patients aged ≤28 days were not considered for analysis. True positive cultures were those with identified bacteria plus corresponding susceptibility results, or yeast. Organisms, including *Micrococcus species*, *Bacillus species*, and diphtheroids were classified as contaminants. For the majority of patients, only a single blood culture was submitted per infection episode. Where duplicate cultures were submitted, and the same organism was isolated within 14 days of the previous culture, then the latter isolate was excluded except when there was variation in antibiotic susceptibility pattern.

Data source/methods of laboratory assessment for blood cultures
For patients with suspected sepsis, local guidelines recommended the inoculation of 1–3 mL (for paediatric patients; however, for older children, larger blood inoculums of 10 mL were encouraged) and 8–10 mL (for adults) directly into Bactec® culture vials (Becton–Dickinson, USA). Routinely at the laboratory, cultures were processed with the BACTEC 9240 blood culture system (Becton–Dickinson, NJ, USA) according to manufacturer's instructions. Where bacterial growth was detected in vials, Gram-stains were performed; and subcultures were typically made onto appropriate media based on Gram-stain results. Bacterial isolates were identified using routine biochemical methods. Bacteria speciation was done with the BBL® Crystal identification system (Becton–Dickinson, NJ, USA). For positive fungal blood cultures,

organisms were identified on the basis of morphology. As part of regular practice at the laboratory, consultant microbiologists evaluated all positive blood cultures to categorize isolates as contaminants or true pathogens. Susceptibility testing for bacterial pathogens were conducted using the Kirby-Bauer disc diffusion method with antibiotic discs; and these tests were interpreted according to guidelines by the Clinical and Laboratory Standards Institute (CLSI) [13].

Antibiotic resistance phenotypes

We assessed the occurrence of six epidemiologically important bacterial pathogens: vancomycin resistant *Enterococcus* species (VRE) [based on in vitro susceptibility to vancomycin disk (30 µg)], methicillin resistant *Staphylococcus aureus* (MRSA) [based on in vitro susceptibility to cefoxitin disk (30 µg)], penicillin resistant streptococci (PRS) [based on in vitro susceptibility to ampicillin disk (10 µg)], cephalosporin resistant enterobacteria (Ceph-R Ent) [based on in vitro susceptibility to cefotaxime disk (30 µg)], multi-drug resistant *Pseudomonas* species (MDR Ps.) and multi-drug resistant *Acinetobacter* species (MDR Act). A multidrug resistant (MDR) phenotype was defined, relative to the panel of antibiotics reported for each bacteria, as in vitro non-susceptibility to ≥1 agent in ≥3 antimicrobial classes: penicillins, cephalosporins, β-lactamase inhibitor combinations, carbapenems, tetracyclines, folate pathway inhibitors, glycopeptides, fluoroquinolones, chloramphenicol, aminoglycosides, and macrolides [14].

Data analysis

Data analysis was performed with the Statistical Package for Social Sciences, Version 20.0. The distribution of BSI and resistance profiles of bacterial isolates were assessed using descriptive methods. Blood culture positivity and contamination levels were calculated by dividing positive blood cultures and contaminants respectively by the total number of blood cultures submitted. Susceptibility tests reports were classified as resistant or susceptible, and the data expressed as the proportion of susceptible isolates out of the total valid test results for the specific antibiotic and pathogen. Missing data were excluded from analysis. Study data were compared across four patient age categories: infants (>28 days–1 year), children (>1–15 years), adults (>15–65 years), and the elderly (>65 years). The Chi square analysis with Marascuilo's post hoc tests for multiple comparisons was used to compare categorical data within patient groups. A Chi square test for linear trend was used to assess changes in categorical variables over the study period. Continuous data were compared using Students' t test with analyses of variance (ANOVA) for multiple comparisons.

Ethical considerations

During the data extraction process, we de-identified blood culture reports to ensure complete obscurity from laboratory archives. Arbitrary numbers were assigned to all reported isolates. Patients' clinical data were not reviewed for analysis. Owing to the retrospective study design, and given the anonymized nature of our data, patients' consent for use of the laboratory records could not be obtained. Ethical approval for isolates and laboratory data was not required as the study was regarded as part of routine surveillance measures for infection control. Study findings are freely available to the hospital for the formulation of guidelines for treatment of BSI.

Results

Figure 1 shows the flow diagram for data collation and outcome. Overall, a total of 15,683 blood cultures were performed for infants (n = 1082), children (n = 8003), adults (n = 5987), and the elderly (n = 601). Males comprised 53 % (n = 8312) of patients. The median age of the study population was 31.6 years (range 29 days–69 years). About 3633 (23.16 %) blood cultures were positive: 1451 (9.3 %, 95 % CI 8.5–9.8) were considered true pathogens and 2182 (13.9 %) considered contaminants. The rate of BSI was 92.5 per 1000 blood cultures submitted to the laboratory, with no significant variation across the years under review (2010, 82.4 per 1000 blood cultures; 2011, 94.2 per 1000 blood cultures; 2012, 87.2 per 1000 blood cultures; 2013, 90.3 per 1000 blood cultures: $p = 0.0841$ for Marascuilo's post hoc). The median age of patients with BSI was 13.5 years (range 29–81 years). Chi square for linear trend analysis showed that the overall occurrence of BSI declined with increasing age-group ($p = 0.001$), but most of the isolates did not vary with age (Table 1). The highest true blood culture positivity was observed among infants (20.9 %, n = 226/1083), followed by the elderly (13.3 %, n = 80/601), children (8.9 %, n = 708/8000) and adults (7.2 %, n = 437/6000) ($p = 0.001$ for Marascuilo's post hoc). The proportion of blood cultures positive for various pathogens remained similar ($p = 0.412$ for Chi square test) between patients receiving care at KBTH (9.3 %, n = 1407/15,072) and those referred to the laboratory from other health facilities (7.6 %, n = 44/611). In the proceeding analysis, we have disregarded comparing results between the two sources of blood cultures because there were few true positive cultures from the latter.

Distribution of isolates

Gram-negative bacteria accounted for 59.8 % (n = 867/1451) of BSI pathogens, whilst Gram-positives and fungi accounted for 38.8 % (n = 563/1451) and 1.4 % (n = 21/1451) respectively ($p = 0.001$ for Marascuilo's

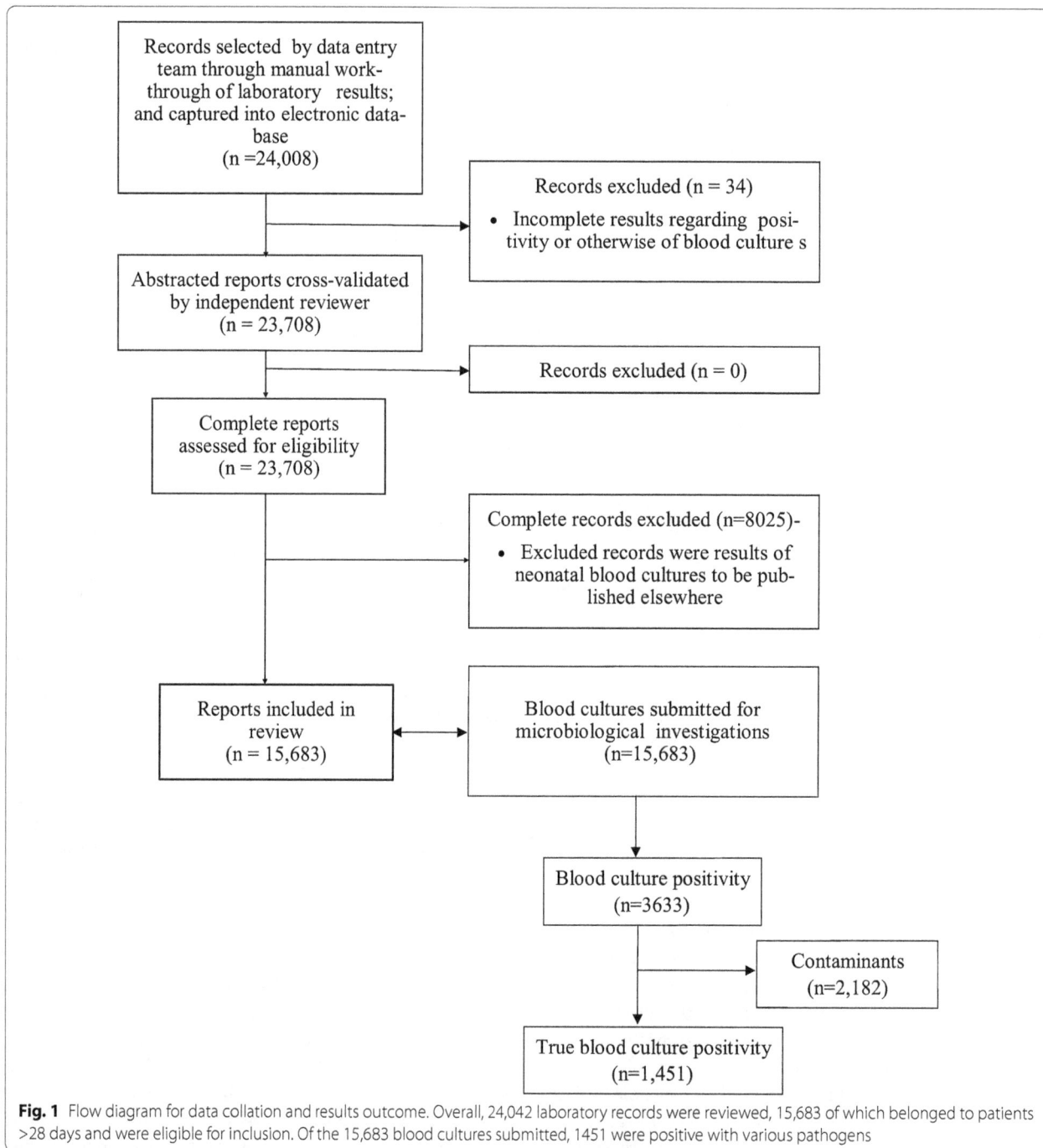

Fig. 1 Flow diagram for data collation and results outcome. Overall, 24,042 laboratory records were reviewed, 15,683 of which belonged to patients >28 days and were eligible for inclusion. Of the 15,683 blood cultures submitted, 1451 were positive with various pathogens

post hoc)—and the trend was similar within each age-group. *Staphylococcus aureus* was the most isolated organism (21.9 %, n = 318/1451). The majority of Gram-negative bacteria belonged to the family *Enterobacteriaceae* (73.9 %, n = 640/867), with *Salmonella* (11.1 %) and *Citrobacter* (10.2 %) species being the second and third most isolated pathogens (Table 1).

Antibiotic susceptibility

Our results show high levels of ampicillin resistance among Gram-negative (Table 2) and Gram-positive (Table 3) organisms. Susceptibility among the enterobacteria ranged from 0 % among *Proteus* and *Klebsiella* species to 36.1 % in *Salmonella* species. There was 100 % susceptibility among *Neisseria meningitides* isolates.

Table 1 Distribution of BSI isolates across age groups

Organism (n, %)	Infants (A) (29 days–1 year)	Children (B) (1–15 years)	Adults (C) (15–65 years)	Elderly (D) (>65 years)	Post hoc comparison	X^2 trend
GNB (n = 867, 59.8 %)	123 (54.4)	407 (57.5)	265 (65.4)	52 (65.0)	A = B = C = D	0.002
Enterobacteria (n = 640, 44.1 %)	81 (35.8)	312 (44.1)	203 (46.4)	44 (55.0)	A < D = B = C	0.001
Citrobacter sp. (n = 148, 10.2 %)	14 (6.2)	58 (8.1)	65 (13.0)	11 (13.7)	A = B = C = D	0.001
E. coli (n = 118, 8.1 %)	8 (3.5)	27 (3.8)	60 (13.7)	23 (28.7)	A = B < C = D*	0.001
Enterobacter sp. (n = 105, 7.2 %)	14 (6.2)	53 (7.5)	32 (7.3)	6 (7.5)	A = B = C = D	0.731
Klebsiella sp. (n = 63, 4.3 %)	16 (7.1)	30 (4.2)	14 (3.2)	3 (3.8)	A = B = C = D	0.037
Proteus sp. (n = 9, 0.6 %)	2 (0.8)	3 (0.4)	4 (0.9)	0	A = B = C = D	0.668
Providencia sp. (n = 4, 0.4 %)	1 (0.4)	1 (0.1)	2 (0.5)	0	A = B = C = D	0.738
P. agglomerans (n = 2, 0.1 %)	0	1 (0.1)	1 (0.2)	0	A = B = C = D	0.992
Salmonella sp. (169, 11.6 %)	23 (9.7)	127 (17.9)	18 (4.3)	1 (1.3)	B > C = A > D*	0.001
Serratia sp. (n = 1, 0.1 %)	0	0	1 (0.2)	0	A = B = C = D	0.755
Other coliform (n = −21, 1.4 %)	3 (1.3)	12 (1.7)	6 (1.4)	0	A = C = D < B	0.429
Non-fermentative bacilli (n = 223, 15.3 %)	42 (18.5)	92 (12.9)	81 (18.5)	8 (10.0)	A = B = C = D	0.818
Acinetobacter sp. (n = 120, 8.3 %)	24 (10.6)	56 (7.9)	36 (8.2)	4 (5.0)	A = B = C = D	0.173
Pseudomonas sp. (n = 101, 7.0 %)	18 (7.9)	35 (4.9)	44 (10.0)	4 (5.0)	A = B < C = D*	0.404
S. paucimobilis (n = 1, 0.1 %)	0	1 (0.1)	0	0	A = B = C = D	0.334
S. maltophilia (n = 1, 0.1 %)	0	0	1 (0.2)	0	A = B = C = D	0.759
Other gram negatives (n = 4, 0.2 %)	0	3 (0.4)	1 (0.2)	0	A = B = C = D	0.738
Chromobacter sp. (n = 1, 0.1 %)	0	0	1 (0.2)	0	A = B = C = D	0.759
N. meningitides (n = 2, 0.2 %)	0	3 (0.4)	0	0	A = B = C = D	0.350
GPB (n = 563, 36.5 %)	102 (45.1)	289 (40.7)	146 (25.9)	26 (32.5)	C < A = B = D	0.0001
Enterococcus sp. (n = 43, 0.3 %)	8	24 (3.4)	10 (22.8)	1 (1.3)	A = B = C = D	0.139
S. aureus (n = 318, 21.9 %)	60 (26.5)	148 (20.9)	99 (22.6)	11 (13.8)	A = B = C = D	0.092
S. epidermidis (n = 67, 4.6 %)	11 (4.8)	42 (5.9)	12 (2.7)	2 (2.6)	A = B = C = D	0.047
S. agalactiae (n = 1, 0.1 %)	1 (0.4)	0	0	1 (1.3)	A = B = C = D	0.984
S. pneumoniae (n = 35, 2.4 %)	6 (2.6)	23 (3.2)	3 (0.6)	3 (3.8)	A = B < C = D*	0.159
S. pyogenes (n = 3, 0.2 %)	0	1 (0.1)	1 (0.2)	1 (1.3)	A = B = C = D	0.217
S. viridans (n = 48, 3.3 %)	10 (4.4)	23 (3.2)	9 (8.9)	6 (7.5)	A = B = C = D	0.739
Other Streptococcus sp. (n = 48, 3.3 %)	7 (3.1)	28 (4.0)	12 (2.7)	1 (1.3)	A = B = C = D	0.243
Fungi (n = 21, 1.3 %)	2 (0.8)	12 (1.7)	5 (1.1)	2 (2.6)	A = B = C = D	0.596
Aspergillus sp. (n = 3, 0.2 %)	0	2 (0.2)	0	1 (1.3)	A = B = C = D	0.588
Candida sp. (n = 17, 1.2 %)	2 (0.8)	10 (1.4)	4 (0.9)	1 (1.3)	A = B = C = D	0.816
Cryptococcus sp. (n = 1, 0.1 %)	0 (0)	0	1 (0.2)	0	A = B = C = D	0.759
True blood culture positivity (n = 1451, 9.3 %)	226 (20.9 %)	708 (8.9 %)	437 (7.3 %)	80 (13.3 %)	A > D > B > C*	<0.001

Sp., species; GNB, gram negative bacteria; GPB, gram positive bacteria; E. coli, Escherichia coli; P. agglomerans, Pantoea agglomerans; S. paucimobilis, Sphingomonas paucimobilis; S. maltophilia, Stenotrophomonas maltophilia; N. meningitis, Neisseria meningitis; S. aureus, Staphylococcus aureus; S. epidermidis, Staphylococcus epidermidis; S. agalactiae, Streptococcus agalactiae; S. pneumoniae, Streptococcus pneumoniae; S. pyogenes, Streptococcus pyogenes; S. viridans, Streptococcus viridans; X^2 trend, Chi square for linear trend; Post hoc, comparison compares the proportion of bloodstream infections among age-groups

* Comparisons with significant (p < 0.05) differences

Among Gram-positive organisms, susceptibility ranged from 7.7 % in *Enterococcus* species to 100 % in *Streptococcus pyogenes*. Among the aminoglycosides, Gram-negative organisms maintained high susceptibility to amikacin than to gentamicin. For *Pseudomonas* species, susceptibility of 86.9 and 67.2 % were respectively recorded for amikacin and gentamicin, whilst for *Citrobacter* species, susceptibility of 84.7 and 33.1 % were noted. In this study, moderate to high level susceptibility of Gram-negative organisms to quinolones was recorded, exemplified by 64.9 and 69.6 % susceptibility of *Citrobacter* species, as well as 100 and 97.6 % susceptibility of *Salmonella* species, to ciprofloxacin and levofloxacin respectively. Most enterobacteria showed low to moderate (20–43 %) susceptibility to cefotaxime. High percentage susceptibility were however recorded for *Salmonella* (95.5 %). Meropenem retained high susceptibility among all Gram-negative organisms, ranging from 96 % among *Pseudomonas*

Table 2 Percentage susceptibility of gram negative pathogens

Organism	Amp	Am/cl	Gen	Amk	Cip	Lev	Cef	Ctx	Mem	Cot	Tet	Chl
Citrobacter sp.	6/120 (5)	8/33 (24.2)	44/133 (33.1)	100/118 (84.7)	46/64 (71.9)	19/27 (70.4)	34/136 (25)	46/142 (32.4)	148/148	19/113 (16.8)	15/103 (14.6)	11/96 (11.5)
Serratia sp.	0/1		1/1	1/1	1/1		1/1	1/1	1/1	0/1	1/1	1/1
E. coli	2/86 (2.3)	5/40 (12.5)	40/86 (46.5)	67/87 (77)	25/66 (37.9)	9/31 (29)	31/104 (29.8)	49/112 (43.8)	118/118 (100)	6/79 (7.6)	6/69 (8.7)	8/71 (11.3)
Enterobacter sp.	2/91 (2.2)	2/29 (6.9)	27/86 (31.4)	68/89 (76.4)	37/57 (64.9)	16/23 (69.6)	19/98 (19.4)	22/100 (22)	104/105 (99)	14/81 (17.3)	7/71 (9.9)	7/64 (10.9)
Klebsiella sp.	0/56 (0)	3/18 (16.7)	11/52 (21.2)	43/53 (81.1)	20/33 (60.1)	12/19 (63.2)	9/59 (15.3)	12/60 (20)	62/63 (98.4)	7/53 (13.2)	3/45 (6.7)	6/44 (13.6)
Proteus sp.	0/6 (0)	2/4 (50)	5/7 (71.4)	5/6 (83.3)	4/5 (80)	1/2 (50)	5/9 (5.6)	6/9 (66.7)	9/9	1/6 (16.7)	0/3 (0)	1/5 (20)
Providencia sp.	0/3		3/4 (75)	4/4	1/1		1/4 (25)	2/4 (50)	4/4	0/4	1/3 (33.3)	0/5
P. agglomerans	0/2		1/2 (50)	2/2			0/2	0/2	2/2	0/2	0/2	
Salmonella sp.	48/133 (36.1)	35/46 (76.1)	125/133 (94)	131/133 (98.5)	96/96 (100)	40/41 (97.6)	130/156 (83.3)	154/162 (95.1)	169/169	59/122 (48.3)	35/106 (33)	29/111 (26.1)
Serratia sp.	0/1 (0)		1/1	1/1	1/1		1/1	1/1	1/1	0/1	1/1	1/1
Acinetobacter sp.	4/56 (7.1)	6/16 (37.5)	25/55 (45.5)	43/57 (75.4)	18/25 (72)	10/17 (58.8)	17/66 (25.8)	16/70 (22.9)	116/120 (96.7)	12/51 (23.5)	3/50 (6)	6/50 (12)
Pseudomonas sp.			45/67 (67.2)	53/61 (86.9)	41/51 (80.4)	39/49 (79.6)			97/101 (96)			
S. maltophilia			0/1	0/1		1/1			1/1			
S. paucimobilis	1/1		1/1	1/1			1/1	1/1	1/1	0/1	0/1	
Chromobacter sp.		0/1		1/1		1/1	0/1	1/1	1/1			
N. meningitidis	1/1	1/1			2/3 (66.7)		2/3 (66.7)	3/3		0/1		0/1

Amp ampicillin, *Am/cl* amoxicillin clavulanic acid, *Gen* gentamicin, *amk* amikacin, *cip* ciprofloxacin, *Lev* levofloxacin, *Cef* cefuroxime, *ceft* cefotaxime, *Mem* meropenem, *Cot* cotrimoxazole, *Tet* tetracycline, *Chl* chloramphenicol, *sp* species, *E. coli* Escherichia coli, *P. agglomerans* Pantoea agglomerans, *S. paucimobilis* Sphingomonas paucimobilis, *S. maltophilia* Stenotrophomonas maltophilia, *N. meningitis* Neisseria meningitis

Table 3 Percentage susceptibility of gram positive pathogens

Organisms	Pen	Amp	Amc/cl	Gen	Cef	Ox	Vanc	Ery	Tet	Ctx	Cot	Chl
Staphylococcus epidermidis						3/6 (50)	4/4 (100)					
Staphylococcus aureus	20/293 (6.8)	26/260 (10)	42/60 (70)	170/250 (68)	141/291 (48.5)	226/295 (76.6)	144/144 (100)	111/182 (70)			59/242 (24.4)	89/233 (38.2)
Enterococcus sp.	1/38 (2.6)	3/39 (7.7)					15/17 (88.2)		14/33 (42.4)			
Streptococcus pyogenes	3/3 (100)	2/2 (100)	2/2 (100)		3/3 (100)		2/2 (100)	2/2 (100)		1/1 (100)		
Streptococcus viridans	4/45 (8.9)	7/42 (16.6)	5/13 (34.5)		16/40 (.4)		19/20 (95)	5/20 (25)		28/40 (70)		4/25 (16)
Streptococcus agalactiae	0/1 (0)	0/1 (0)			0/1 (0)		0/1 (0)	0/1 (0)				
Streptococcus pneumoniae	10/31 (32.5)	14/30 (46.7)	10/10 (100)		27/39 (69.2)		12/12 (100)	16/19 (84.2)		32/32 (100)		4/19 (21.1)
Streptococcus sp.	3/41 (7.3)	6/42 (14.3)	6/9 (66.7)		20/43 (46.5)		24/27 (88.9)	15/28 (53.8)		12/23 (52.2)		12/35 (34.3)

Data not available for blank cells

Pen penicillin, *Amp* ampicillin, *Am/cl* amoxicillin clavulanic acid, *Gen* gentamicin, *Cef* cefuroxime, *Cot* cotrimoxazole, *Tet* tetracycline, *Chl* chloramphenicol, *Ctx* cefotaxime, *Chl* chloramphenicol

species to 100 % among *Citrobacter* species. Among *Staphylococcus aureus*, susceptibility to cloxacillin over the period was 76.6 %, cefuroxime 48.5 %, erythromycin 70 %, co-trimoxazole 24 %, gentamicin 68 % and vancomycin 100 %. Isolates of *Streptococcus pneumoniae* were moderately susceptible to penicillin (32.5 %) and ampicillin (46.7), but highly susceptible to erythromycin (84.2 %) and vancomycin (100 %).

Trends in antibiotic susceptibility patterns

In Fig. 2, we assessed antibiotic susceptibility patterns over 4 years, looking out for significant trends. There was a significant rise in susceptibility to penicillin ($p = 0.001$), ampicillin ($p = 0.000$), cefuroxime (0.0000), cloxacillin ($p = 0.0000$), cotrimoxazole ($p = 0.012$), cefotaxime ($p = 0.0197$) and chloramphenicol ($p = 0.001$). Figure 3 shows the occurrence of some epidemiologically important antibiotic resistance phenotypes: VRE, MRSA, PRS, Cef-R Ent, MDR Ps, MDR Act, and all MDRs. From 2010 to 2013, we observed a significant trend towards increasing frequency of BSI caused by Cef-R Ent (Chi square for trend, $p = 0.001$). No other resistant phenotype varied with years.

Discussion

Bloodstream infections accounted for 9.3 % of blood cultures and varied significantly within age-groups, where the highest prevalence was recorded among patients at the extremes of ages: the elderly (13.3 %) and infants (20.9 %). The reasons for this distribution is unclear, as risk factors for developing BSI were not assessed in this study. Nevertheless, infants were significantly more likely to have BSI compared with patients aged >3 years. There may be several reasons for this association. Infants are likely to have frequent exposure to healthcare environments or participate in activities that predispose them to microbial contamination. They also have poor skin integrity and an immature immune system [15–19].

In keeping with previous studies from Ghana [20, 21], Gram-negative bacteria predominated in our study, but the majority of bacterial findings were *S. aureus*, which also predominated in other studies from Guinea-Bissau [22], Nigeria [16] and Malawi [23]. We believe that the aetiology of BSI is changing, so that BSI are due largely to Gram-negative bacteria, but with a significant contribution from Gram-positive isolates, mostly *Staphylococcus* species. Other studies in Africa have documented this phenomenon, attributing the predominance of Gram-positive bacteria (mostly *S. pneumoniae and S. aureus*) to community-acquired infections [24–26] and Gram-negative bacteria (predominantly *E. coli and K. pneumoniae*) to healthcare related infections [27]. We are unable to determine which BSI were healthcare related or community-acquired because of insufficient data on inpatient and outpatient status. The presence of *Streptococcus pneumoniae* as a cause of BSI was uncommon in our study. This could partially be attributable to pneumococcal vaccine introduced in January 2012. Immunization of infants with the vaccine has led not only to major declines in childhood invasive pneumococcal sepsis but also to a reduction in infections among adults due to herd immunity [27]. It is the experience in KBTH that *Salmonella* species constitute a prominent pathogen in

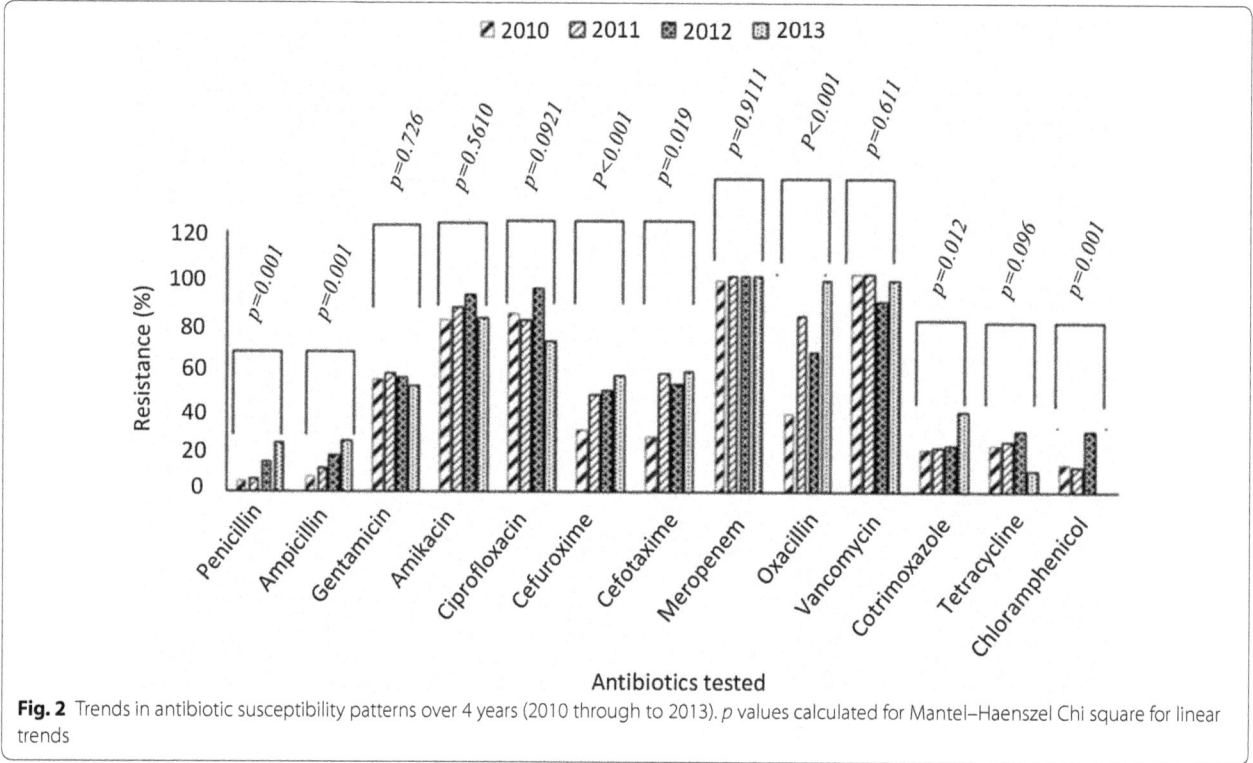

Fig. 2 Trends in antibiotic susceptibility patterns over 4 years (2010 through to 2013). *p* values calculated for Mantel–Haenszel Chi square for linear trends

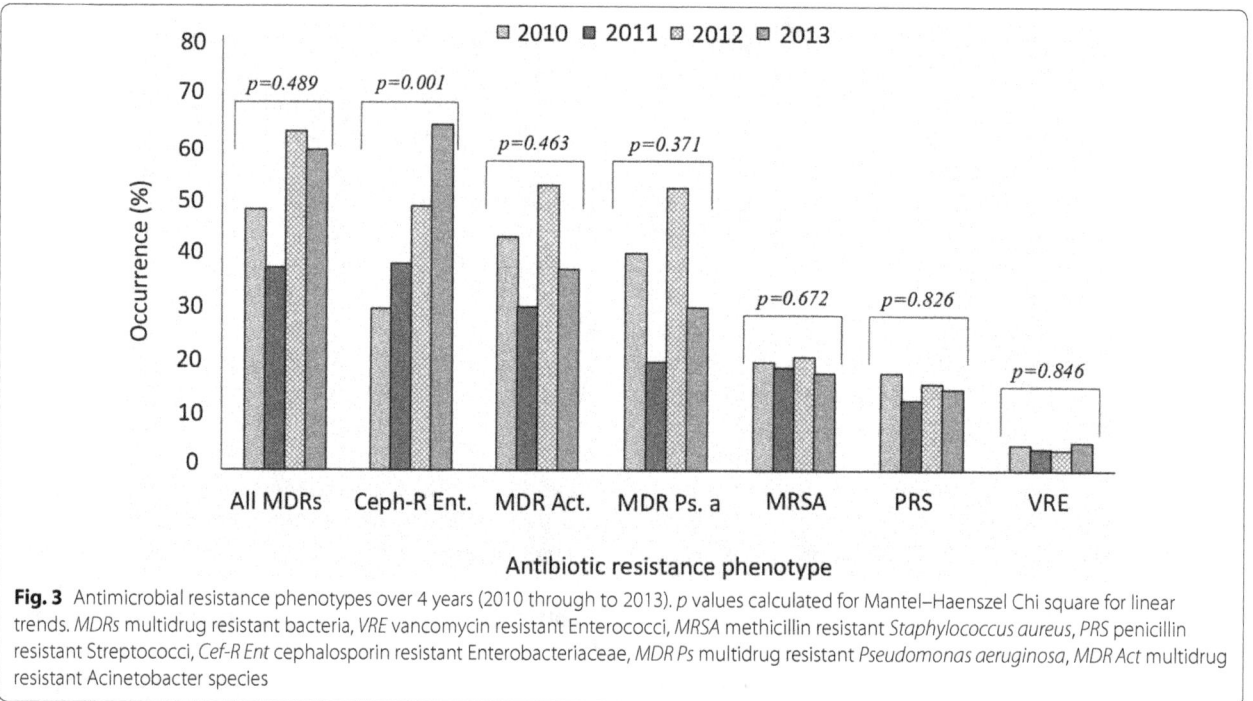

Fig. 3 Antimicrobial resistance phenotypes over 4 years (2010 through to 2013). *p* values calculated for Mantel–Haenszel Chi square for linear trends. *MDRs* multidrug resistant bacteria, *VRE* vancomycin resistant Enterococci, *MRSA* methicillin resistant *Staphylococcus aureus*, *PRS* penicillin resistant Streptococci, *Cef-R Ent* cephalosporin resistant Enterobacteriaceae, *MDR Ps* multidrug resistant *Pseudomonas aeruginosa*, *MDR Act* multidrug resistant Acinetobacter species

BSI, with a preponderance of non-typhoidal salmonellae over typhoidal salmonellae. Children under 5 years bear the brunt of the disease [28]. These observations are generally consistent with findings from other African studies, particularly in malaria-endemic regions, where *Salmonella* species have predominated in BSI [29, 30].

Favoured by of their low toxicity, broad spectrum and comparatively high effectiveness, the cephalosporin antibiotics are widely used in Ghana. A worrying observation is the increasing isolation of cephalosporin resistant *Enterobacteriaceae* over the 4-year review period. The enterobacteria constituted over 40 % of the bloodstream pathogens. Given that the variety of class C cephalosporinases (AmpCs) and extended spectrum β-lactamases (ESBLs) remain the principal mechanisms for cephalosporin resistance worldwide [31–33], the high levels of cephalosporin resistance observed in our study may be compatible with results from other studies in Ghana, demonstrating high levels of ESBLs (>45 %) among the enterobacteria [31, 34].

Based on the low frequency of fungi and the dominance of both GPB and GNB, it may be necessary for clinicians to consider suitable empiric regimens that provide adequate cover for both bacterial groups. Cefotaxime, gentamicin, ciprofloxacin and amoxicillin plus clavulanic acid, in various combinations, have been the predominant empiric therapies for bloodstream infections in Ghana [35]. We have demonstrated here and in previous studies that the general antibiogram of the GNB and GPB reveal an overall high resistance to these routinely used drugs [31, 32]. Our observations are in consonance with other studies in Ghana and at Korle-Bu teaching Hospital, which found high resistance to ampicillin, gentamicin and cefotaxime among bacteria isolates of various infections [31, 32, 36]. Carbapenem was the most active antibiotic against Gram-negative infections. Meanwhile, cloxacillin remained a very useful anti-staphylococcal agent due the relatively low prevalence of MRSA.

This study has several limitations. Being retrospective, we were unable to ascertain the standardization of techniques for blood cultures and laboratory procedures for individual patients. The study is also unable to evaluate the accuracy of bacteria isolates classified as contaminants in laboratory records. As the study lacks comprehensive clinical data or information on recent antibiotic use and/or hospitalization, our data on the occurrence of BSI should be interpreted with caution. Finally, our study was performed in a single center, and cannot be generalized to the entire patient population in Ghana. Our study nonetheless provides relevant data which may be used to guide empirical therapy, change antibiotic prescription policy in our institution or serve as a baseline for future research. We recommend future studies to ascertain the changing eligibility of our findings over time beyond the review years reported in this study.

Conclusion

Our study shows that blood culture positivity was significantly higher in infants compared to children, adults and the elderly; with a preponderance of *S. aureus* and Gram-negative bacteria in all age-groups. The findings presented here suggest the need to review empiric antibiotic options in these patient populations, given the relatively low susceptibility of the bacterial isolates to many routinely used antibiotics.

Abbreviations
µg: microgram; ANOVA: analysis of variance; BSI: blood stream infections; CI: confidence interval; CLSI: Clinical and Laboratory Standards Institute; GNB: gram-negative bacteria; GPB: gram-positive bacteria; KBTH: Korle-Bu Teaching Hospital; MDR: multidrug resistance; SPSS: statistical package for social sciences; NJ: New Jersey; USA: United States of America; VRE: vancomycin resistant *Enterococcus* species; MRSA: methicillin resistant *Staphylococcus aureus*; PRS: penicillin resistant streptococci; Ceph-R Ent: cephalosporin resistant enterobacteria; MDR: multidrug resistant; MDR Ps: multi-drug resistant *Pseudomonas* species; MDR Act: multi-drug resistant *Acinetobacter* species.

Authors' contributions
AKL conceived the study; participated in its design, coordination, and collation of laboratory data; and helped to draft the manuscript. NON participated in the study design, coordination and collation of laboratory data; performed the statistical analysis; and helped to draft the manuscript. JEML, GAM participated in collation of laboratory data and review of the manuscript. NOA participated in the drafting and review of the manuscript. All authors read and approved the final manuscript.

Author details
[1] Microbiology Department, School of Biomedical and Allied Health Sciences, University of Ghana, P.O. Box 4326, Accra, Ghana, West Africa. [2] Department of Microbiology, Korle-Bu Teaching Hospital, P.O. Box 77, Accra, Ghana, West Africa. [3] Department of Internal Medicine, La General Hospital, P.O.Box PMB La, Accra, Ghana, West Africa.

Acknowledgements
This research/paper has been supported by the University of Ghana—Carnegie Next Generation of Academics in Africa Project with funding from the Carnegie Corporation of New York. We are grateful to the staff of the Microbiology Department of the Korle-Bu Teaching Hospital for their support. We thank Dr. Benjamin Jella Visser and (Department of Tropical Medicine, Infectious Diseases at Academic Medical Center, Tergooi, Netherlands) and Professor George Obeng-Adjei (Center for tropical clinical pharmacology and therapeutics, Ghana) for reviewing the manuscript.

Competing interests
The authors declare that they have no competing interests.

Funding
The study received no specific grant.

References

1. Okeke IN, Klugman KP, Bhutta ZA, Duse AG, Jenkins P, O'Brien TF, Pablos-Mendez A, Laxminarayan R. Antimicrobial resistance in developing countries. Part II: strategies for containment. Lancet Infect Dis. 2005;5:568–80.
2. Reynolds R, Potz N, Colman M, Williams A, Livermore D. Antimicrobial susceptibility of the pathogens of bacteraemia in the UK and Ireland 2001–2002: the BSAC bacteraemia resistance surveillance programme. J Antimicrob Chemother. 2004;53:1018–32.
3. Diekema DJ, Beekmann SE, Chapin KC, Morel KA, Munson E, Doern GV. Epidemiology and outcome of nosocomial and community-onset bloodstream infection. J Clin Microbiol. 2003;41:3655–60.
4. Petti CA, Polage CR, Quinn TC, Ronald AR, Sande MA. Laboratory medicine in Africa: a barrier to effective health care. Clin Infect Dis. 2006;42:377–82.
5. Penno EC, Baird SJ, Crump JA. Cost-effectiveness of surveillance for bloodstream infections for sepsis management in low-resource settings. Am J Trop Med Hyg. 2015;93:850–60.
6. Blomberg B, Manji KP, Urassa WK, Tamim BS, Mwakagile DS, Jureen R, Msangi V, Tellevik MG, Holberg-Petersen M, Harthug S, Maselle SY, Langeland N. Antimicrobial resistance predicts death in Tanzanian children with bloodstream infections: a prospective cohort study. BMC Infect Dis. 2007;7:43.
7. Cosgrove SE. The relationship between antimicrobial resistance and patient outcomes: mortality, length of hospital stay, and health care costs. Clin Infect Dis. 2006;42(Supplement 2):S82–9.
8. Kamga HLF, Njunda AL, Nde PE, Assob JCN, Nsagha DS, Weledji P. Prevalence of septicaemia and antibiotic sensitivity pattern of bacterial isolates at the University Teaching Hospital, Yaoundé, Cameroon. Afr J Clin Exp Microbiol. 2011;12(1):2-8
9. Enweronu-Laryea CC, Newman MJ. Changing pattern of bacterial isolates and antimicrobial susceptibility in neonatal infections in Korle Bu Teaching Hospital, Ghana. East Afr Med J. 2007;84:136–40.
10. Wilkens J, Newman MJ, Commey JO, Seifert H. Salmonella bloodstream infection in Ghanaian children. Clin Microbiol Infect. 1997;3:616–20.
11. Benchimol EI, Smeeth L, Guttmann A, Harron K, Moher D, Petersen I, Sørensen HT, von Elm E, Langan SM. The reporting of studies conducted using observational routinely-collected health data (RECORD) statement. PLoS Med. 2015;12:1–22.
12. Annual Report Korle-Bu Teaching Hospital. 2010.
13. Wayne PA. Clinical and Laboratory Standard Institute (CLSI): performance standards for antimicrobial susceptibility testing. Twenty Second Inf Suppl. 2012;32(3):1–278.
14. Magiorakos A, Srinivasan A, Carey RB, Carmeli Y, Falagas ME, Giske CG, Harbarth S, Hindler JF. bacteria: an international expert proposal for interim standard definitions for acquired resistance. Clin Microbiol Infect. 2012;18:268–81.
15. Ugas MA, Cho H, Trilling GM, Tahir Z, Raja HF, Ramadan S, Jerjes W, Giannoudis PV. Central and peripheral venous lines-associated blood stream infections in the critically ill surgical patients. Ann Surg Innov Res. 2012;6:8.
16. Hojsak I, Strizić H, Mišak Z, Rimac I, Bukovina G, Prlić H, Kolaček S. Central venous catheter related sepsis in children on parenteral nutrition: a 21-year single-center experience. Clin Nutr. 2012;31:672–5.
17. Pronovost PJ, Goeschel CA, Colantuoni E, Watson S, Lubomski LH, Berenholtz SM, Thompson DA, Sinopoli DJ, Cosgrove S, Sexton JB, Marsteller JA, Hyzy RC, Welsh R, Posa P, Schumacher K, Needham D. Sustaining reductions in catheter related bloodstream infections in Michigan intensive care units: observational study. BMJ. 2010;340:c309.
18. Downes KJ, Metlay JP, Bell LM, McGowan KL, Elliott MR, Shah SS. Polymicrobial bloodstream infections among children and adolescents with central venous catheters evaluated in ambulatory care. Clin Infect Dis. 2008;46:387–94.
19. Costello JM, Clapper TC, Wypij D. Minimizing complications associated with percutaneous central venous catheter placement in children: recent advances. Pediatr Crit Care Med. 2013;14:273–83.
20. Acquah S, Quaye L, Sagoe K, Ziem J, Bromberger P, Amponsem AA. Susceptibility of bacterial etiological agents to commonly-used antimicrobial agents in children with sepsis at the Tamale Teaching Hospital. BMC Infect Dis. 2013;13:89.
21. Groß U, Amuzu SK, de Ciman R, Kassimova I, Groß L, Rabsch W, Rosenberg U, Schulze M, Stich A, Zimmermann O. Bacteremia and antimicrobial drug resistance over time, Ghana. Emerg Infect Dis. 2011;17:1879–82.
22. Isendahl J, Manjuba C, Rodrigues A, Xu W, Henriques-normark B, Giske CG, Nauclér P. Prevalence of community-acquired bacteraemia in Guinea-Bissau : an observational study. BMC Infect Dis. 2014;14:1–9.
23. Makoka MH, Miller WC, Hoffman IF, Cholera R, Gilligan PH, Kamwendo D, Malunga G, Joaki G, Martinson F, Hosseinipour MC. Bacterial infections in Lilongwe, Malawi: aetiology and antibiotic resistance. BMC Infect Dis. 2012;12:67.
24. Mckay R, Bamford C, Chb MB, Microbiology M, Town C, Africa S. Community- versus healthcare-acquired bloodstream infections at Groote Schuur Hospital, Cape Town, South Africa. S Afr Med J. 2015;105:363–9.
25. Prasad N, Murdoch DR, Reyburn H, Crump JA. Etiology of severe febrile illness in low- and middle-income countries : a systematic review. PLos One. 2015;10:1–25.
26. Hill PC, Onyeama CO, Ikumapayi UNA, Secka O, Ameyaw S, Simmonds N, Donkor SA, Howie SR, Tapgun M, Corrah T, Adegbola RA. Bacteraemia in patients admitted to an urban hospital in West Africa. BMC Infect Dis. 2007;20:1–8.
27. Laupland KB, Sciences CH, Hospital RI. Incidence of bloodstream infection: a review of population-based studies. Clin Microbiol Infect. 2013;19:492–500.
28. Labi AK, Obeng-Nkrumah N, Addison NO, Donkor ES. Salmonella blood stream infections in a tertiary care setting in Ghana. BMC Infect Dis. 2014;14:3857.
29. MacLennan CA. Out of Africa: links between invasive nontyphoidal Salmonella disease, typhoid fever, and malaria. Clin Infect Dis. 2013;58(5):648–50.
30. Phoba M-F, De Boeck H, Ifeka BB, Dawili J, Lunguya O, Vanhoof R, Muyembe J-J, Van Geet C, Bertrand S, Jacobs J. Epidemic increase in Salmonella bloodstream infection in children, Bwamanda, the Democratic Republic of Congo. Eur J Clin Microbiol Infect Dis. 2014;33:79–87.
31. Obeng-Nkrumah N, Twum-Danso K, Krogfelt KA, Newman MJ. High levels of extended-spectrum beta-lactamases in a major teaching hospital in Ghana: the need for regular monitoring and evaluation of antibiotic resistance. Am J Trop Med Hyg. 2013;89:960–4.
32. Newman MJ, Frimpong E, Donkor ES, Opintan JA, Asamoah-Adu A. Resistance to antimicrobial drugs in Ghana. Infect Drug Resist. 2011;4:215–20.
33. Bush K. Bench-to-bedside review: the role of β-lactamases in antibiotic-resistant gram-negative infections. Crit Care. 2010;14:224.
34. Hackman HK, Brown CA, Twum-Danso K. Antibiotic resistance profile of non-extended spectrum beta-lactamase-producing Escherichia coli and Klebsiella pneumoniae in Accra, Ghana. J Biol Agric Healthc. 2014;4:12–6.
35. Ministry of Health. Republic of Ghana Standard Treatment Guidelines, 6th edn. Accra, Ghana: Ghana National Drugs programme; 2010.
36. Ayisi LA, Adu-Sarkodie Y. Extended-spectrum-beta-lactamase (ESBL) production among Escherichia coli and Klebsiella species in Kumasi, Ghana. J Nat Sci Res. 2015;5:81–6.

12

Genome sequence of *Shigella flexneri* strain SP1, a diarrheal isolate that encodes an extended-spectrum β-lactamase (ESBL)

Ping Shen[1†], Jianzhong Fan[2†], Lihua Guo[1], Jiahua Li[3], Ang Li[1], Jing Zhang[1], Chaoqun Ying[1], Jinru Ji[1], Hao Xu[1], Beiwen Zheng[1*] and Yonghong Xiao[1]

Abstract

Background: Shigellosis is the most common cause of gastrointestinal infections in developing countries. In China, the species most frequently responsible for shigellosis is *Shigella flexneri*. *S. flexneri* remains largely unexplored from a genomic standpoint and is still described using a vocabulary based on biochemical and serological properties. Moreover, increasing numbers of ESBL-producing *Shigella* strains have been isolated from clinical samples. Despite this, only a few cases of ESBL-producing *Shigella* have been described in China. Therefore, a better understanding of ESBL-producing *Shigella* from a genomic standpoint is required. In this study, a *S. flexneri* type 1a isolate SP1 harboring $bla_{CTX-M-14}$, which was recovered from the patient with diarrhea, was subjected to whole genome sequencing.

Results: The draft genome assembly of *S. flexneri* strain SP1 consisted of 4,592,345 bp with a G+C content of 50.46%. RAST analysis revealed the genome contained 4798 coding sequences (CDSs) and 100 RNA-encoding genes. We detected one incomplete prophage and six candidate CRISPR loci in the genome. In vitro antimicrobial susceptibility testing demonstrated that strain SP1 is resistant to ampicillin, amoxicillin/clavulanic acid, cefazolin, ceftriaxone and trimethoprim. In silico analysis detected genes mediating resistance to aminoglycosides, β-lactams, phenicol, tetracycline, sulphonamides, and trimethoprim. The $bla_{CTX-M-14}$ gene was located on an IncFII2 plasmid. A series of virulence factors were identified in the genome.

Conclusions: In this study, we report the whole genome sequence of a $bla_{CTX-M-14}$-encoding *S. flexneri* strain SP1. Dozens of resistance determinants were detected in the genome and may be responsible for the multidrug-resistance of this strain, although further confirmation studies are warranted. Numerous virulence factors identified in the strain suggest that isolate SP1 is potential pathogenic. The availability of the genome sequence and comparative analysis with other *S. flexneri* strains provides the basis to further address the evolution of drug resistance mechanisms and pathogenicity in *S. flexneri*.

Keywords: *Shigella flexneri*, Extended-spectrum β-lactamase, IncFII2, Comparative genomic analysis

Background

Shigella species are a major causative cause of gastrointestinal infections throughout the world, especially

*Correspondence: zhengbw@zju.edu.cn
†Ping Shen and Jianzhong Fan contributed equally to this article
[1] Collaborative Innovation Center for Diagnosis and Treatment of Infectious Diseases, State Key Laboratory for Diagnosis and Treatment of Infectious Diseases, The First Affiliated Hospital, School of Medicine, Zhejiang University, Hangzhou 310003, China
Full list of author information is available at the end of the article

in developing countries [1]. Globally, there are approximately 164.7 million cases per annum, of which 1.1 million people are estimated to die from *Shigella* infections [2]. Based on biochemical and serological properties, the genus *Shigella* comprises four serogroups: *Shigella dysenteriae*, *Shigella flexneri*, *Shigella boydii* and *Shigella sonnei* [2]. *S. flexneri* is endemic in many developing countries and causes more deaths than any other *Shigella* serotypes [3]. In China, shigellosis is the most common gastrointestinal infections [4] and most frequently isolated species responsible for shigellosis in mainland China is *S. flexneri* [5].

Antibiotic treatment is usually recommended for shigellosis as it reduces the duration and severity of symptoms, reduces the excretion of organisms and prevents potentially lethal complications [6]. However, the emergence of extended-spectrum β-lactamase (ESBL)-producing *S. flexneri* is a major public health problem in China, as these strains are associated with critical infections [7]. Most of the CTX-M, SHV, and TEM-type ESBLs genes are located on conjugative plasmids [4]. Moreover, co-existence with other antimicrobial resistance genes is frequently observed in ESBL-producers [8], which makes the choice of effective treatment extremely limited. Increasing instances of ESBL-producing *Shigella* strains isolated from Asia have been reported [1, 2]. So far, only a few cases of ESBL-producing *Shigella* have been described in China [4]. Therefore, a better understanding of ESBL-producing *Shigella* using a genomics approach is required.

The first genome sequence of *S. flexneri* was reported by Jin et al. in 2002 [9]. So far, more than 145 *S. flexneri* strains have been sequenced and analyzed [10]. To extend our understanding of the resistance mechanisms and pathogenesis of ESBL-producing *S. flexneri*, we performed sequencing and genomic analysis of the ESBL-harbouring *S. flexneri* SP1. Comparative genomics analysis of *S. flexneri* SP1 with other *S. flexneri* genomes may improve our understanding of the antibiotic resistance and virulence factors present in *Shigella*.

Methods
Strain information
Shigella flexneri 1a isolate SP1 was isolated from the stool sample of a 76-year-old female diarrhea patient. Standard biochemical tests were performed using the Vitek II system (BioMerieux, France) and species-specific 16S rRNA sequencing was used to confirm the identity of isolate SP1. Serotyping was performed with specific antiserum (Denka-Seiken). Genomic DNA of SP1 was extracted from a single colony of the pure bacterial culture. Possible contamination with other DNA and misassemblies were assessed by performing a BLAST search against the non-redundant database as described previously [11]. The whole genome of SP1 is in the expected size range for a *Shigella* genome and the coverage of the reads was consistent throughout the genome. The assembled draft genome sequence of SP1 was further verified by comparative analysis with the published complete genome sequences of *S. flexneri* strains.

Antimicrobial susceptibility testing
Susceptibility testing for ampicillin, amoxicillin/clavulanic acid, amikacin, aztreonam, piperacillin/tazobactam, cefazolin, cefoxitin, ciprofloxacin, ceftriaxone, cefepime, ertapenem, imipenem, gentamycin, tobramycin, levofloxacin, tigecycline, nitrofurantoin, and trimethoprim were performed by the microbroth dilution method and interpreted according to the CLSI guidelines [12]. *Escherichia coli* strain ATCC 25922 was used as the control strain for susceptibility studies. Late log phase cells were harvested, and genomic DNA was extracted from the pure culture using the DNeasy Blood & Tissue kit (Qiagen, Germany) according to the manufacturer's instructions. For the purpose of bacterial identification, we amplified the 16S rRNA gene with a 16S rRNA universal primer set and the PCR product was sequenced. Ethical approval was granted by the Ethics Committee of the First Affiliated Hospital of Zhejiang University.

Genome sequencing and assembly
The extracted DNA was visualized by agarose gel electrophoresis and quantitated by Qubit 2.0. Whole-genome sequencing was performed on the Illumina HiSeq 4000-PE150 platform. DNA was tailed, ligated to paired-end adaptors and PCR amplified with a 500 bp insert size and a mate-pair libraries with an insert size of 5 kb were used for library construction at the Beijing Novogene Bioinformatics Technology Co., Ltd. Illumina PCR adapter reads and low quality reads from the paired-end and mate-pair library were filtered by the quality control step using Novogene pipeline. All high quality paired reads were assembled using Velvet 1.2.10 [13] into a number of scaffolds. The filtered reads were then passed handled by the next step of the gap-closing.

Genome annotation
Genome annotation included the prediction of coding genes, transfer RNAs, ribosomal RNA, prophage, and clustered regularly interspaced short palindromic repeat sequences (CRISPR). Open reading frames (ORFs) were identified and classified using the Rapid Annotation using Subsystem Technology (RAST) server [14]. Protein classification into functional groups was performed using the Clusters of Orthologous Groups of proteins (COGs) [15]. Transfer RNAs and ribosomal RNA genes rRNAs were detected by tRNAscan-SE [16] and RNAmmer 1.2 software [17], respectively. PHASTER [18] was used to identify prophage and putative phage-like elements and CRISPRFinder [19] was used to identify CRISPR sites. The plasmid replicon was predicted by the PlasmidFinder Tool [20]. ISfinder [21] was employed to search for IS sequences in the genome, with an e-value of 1E−3. plasmidSPAdes was used to produce plasmid sequences from the WGS data [22].

Antibiotic resistance genes prediction and virulence factors analysis
Antibiotic resistance genes were annotated using the comprehensive antibiotic resistance database (CARD)

[23] and Resfinder [24] with default parameters. We further verified all putative antibiotic resistance genes (ARGs) through a BLAST search with cut-off e-value of 1E−0.5. Virulence factors were predicted by using BLAST to search against the VFDB database [25] with an e-value threshold of 1E−5 and also with VirulenceFinder 1.5 [26].

Plasmid characterization

PlasmidFinder 1.3 was used for identify the incompatibility group of the plasmid present in *S. flexneri* SP1 [20]. The plasmid sequence of $bla_{CTX-M-14}$-harboring plasmid from isolate SP1 (named pSP1) was assembled with plasmidSPAdes [22]. Assignment of the plasmid to an incompatibility (Inc) group was performed by multiplex PCR. PCRs were performed as described previously [27].

Phylogenetic analysis and comparative genomic analysis

Comparative genomic analysis was performed by orthology identification method as previously described [11, 28]. Genome sequences of the following representative *S. flexneri* strains were downloaded from the NCBI genome database: *S. flexneri* 2a strain 981 (CP012137), *S. flexneri* S7737 (AMJY00000000), *S. flexneri* 5a strain M90T (CM001474), *S. flexneri* CDC 796.83 (AERO00000000), *S. flexneri* 4343.70 (AFHC00000000), *S. flexneri* NCTC1 (LM651928), *S. flexneri* 2a strain 301 (AE005674), *S. flexneri* G1663 (CP007037), *S. flexneri* Shi06HN006 (CP004057), *S. flexneri* 2003036 (CP004056), *S. flexneri* str 4S BJ10610 (JMRK00000000), *S. flexneri* 4c strain 1205 (CP012140), *S. flexneri* 2002017 (CP001383) and *S. flexneri* 1a strain 0228 (CP012735). Phylogenetic reconstruction and analysis was performed wih the phangorn package, written in the R language [29]. VennDiagram [30] was used to generate the Venn plots of *S. flexneri* SP1, *S. flexneri* str 4S BJ10610, *S. flexneri* 4c strain 1205 (CP012140), *S. flexneri* 2002017, and *S. flexneri* 1a strain 0228.

Results and discussion

General features

We performed whole genome sequencing using the Illumina HiSeq 4000 system with 2×150 bp paired-end reads. After quality control, we assembled the 1095 M bp filtered reads into contigs. The assembled genome of *S. flexneri* SP1 revealed a genome size of 4,592,345 bp with a G+C content of 50.46%. The largest contig consisted of 137,097 bp and the length of N50 contig was 33,394 bp. These scaffolds contain 4798 coding sequences (CDSs), and 100 RNA-encoding genes. The properties and the statistics of the genome are summarized in Additional file 1: Table S1. The resulting genomic size of strain SP1 was similar to previous studies within the range of 4.1–4.8 M bp [31, 32]. Similarly, CDSs numbers were close to the

previous publication [31]. Gene functions were predicted using RAST and COG analysis. RAST server based annotation of the whole genome describes the distribution of subsystems in strain SP1 (Fig. 1a). Proteins responsible for carbohydrates (693 ORFs), amino acids and derivatives (384 ORFs), and cofactors, vitamins, prosthetic groups, pigments (292 ORFs) were abundant among the subsystem categories. The distribution of COGs is illustrated in Fig. 1b. The most abundant COG categories were R (general function prediction only), S (function unknown), E (amino acid transport and metabolism), G (carbohydrate transport and metabolism) and K (transcription). Furthermore, one incomplete prophage region was identified in the genome of SP1. It is a *Salmonella* ST64B-like phage (Acc-No. NC_004313) of 14.1 kb in length and a G+C content of 50.81%. Additionally, six questionable CRISPR loci were detected by CRISPERfinder.

Antimicrobial susceptibility profiles and antibiotic resistance genes

The in vitro antimicrobial susceptibility testing demonstrated that the strain SP1 was resistant to ampicillin, amoxicillin/clavulanic acid, cefazolin, ceftriaxone and trimethoprim, but susceptible to piperacillin/tazobactam, cefoxitin, cefepime, aztreonam, imipenem, amikacin, gentamicin, tobramycin, ciprofloxacin, levofloxacin, tigecycline and nitrofurantoin (Additional file 2: Table S2). We then screened the antibiotic resistance genes (ARGs) in the genome to further explore the genetic basis of multidrug resistance in this strain (Additional file 3: Table S3). In silico analysis revealed the presence of some putative ARGs for different drug classes. We detected genes mediating resistance to aminoglycosides (*aadA24*, *strA* and *strB*), β-lactams ($bla_{CTX-M-14}$ and bla_{OXA-1}), phenicol (*catA1*), tetracycline (*tetD*), sulphonamides (*sul2*), and trimethoprim (*dfrA1*). CTX-M-14 was the most frequent ESBL variant detected in *Shigella* isolates in China, followed by CTX-M-15 [4, 33]. Hitherto, only a few studies have reported the presence of ESBLs in *S. flexneri* [34]. Interestingly, all of the $bla_{CTX-M-14}$-harbouring *S. flexneri* strains were isolated from China [4, 7, 34, 35]. A previous study reported a high prevalence of extended-spectrum cephalosporin resistance *Shigella* mediated mainly by bla_{CTX-M} (mainly $bla_{CTX-M-14}$, 14.1%) in Hangzhou City, Zhejiang Province, China [35]. Our study further indicates the existence of $bla_{CTX-M-14}$-harbouring *S. flexneri* clone may responsible for these *Shigella* infections in this area. In addition, the insertion sequence (IS) elements were frequently detected in upstream of bla_{CTX-M} genes [36]. ISfinder was thus employed to scan the $bla_{CTX-M-14}$ flanking sequences in a range of 6-kb for IS sequences and junction associated proteins. IS*Ecp1* and IS903B were found upstream of $bla_{CTX-M-14}$. IS*Ecp1* belongs to

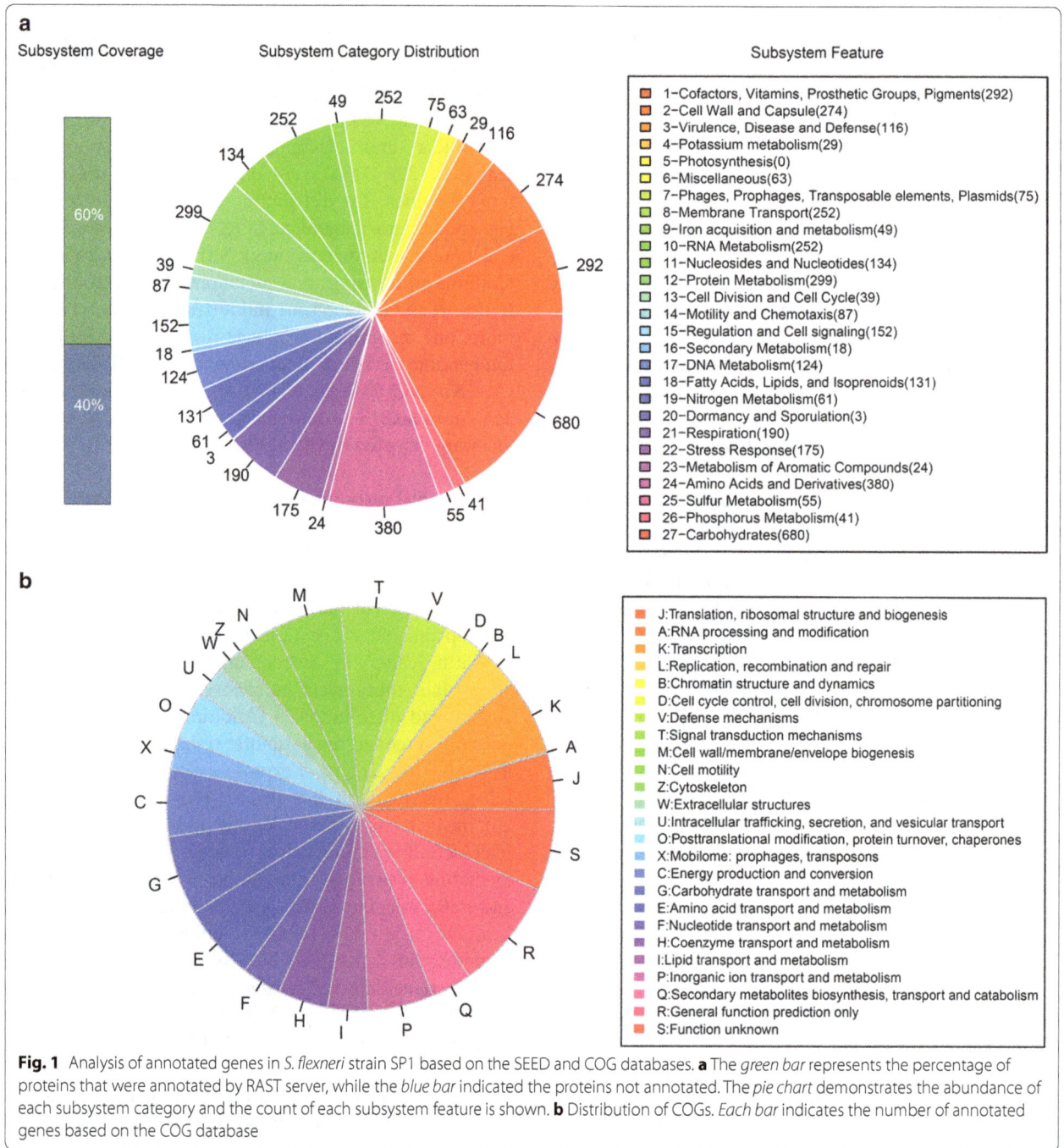

Fig. 1 Analysis of annotated genes in *S. flexneri* strain SP1 based on the SEED and COG databases. **a** The *green bar* represents the percentage of proteins that were annotated by RAST server, while the *blue bar* indicated the proteins not annotated. The *pie chart* demonstrates the abundance of each subsystem category and the count of each subsystem feature is shown. **b** Distribution of COGs. *Each bar* indicates the number of annotated genes based on the COG database

the IS1380 family, which may enhance the expression of $bla_{CTX-M-14/-18}$, $bla_{CTX-M-17}$ and $bla_{CTX-M-19}$ β-lactamase genes [37].

Genetic context of $bla_{CTX-M-14}$ gene

PlasmidFinder and plasmidSPAdes were used to detect the potential plasmids in the whole genome sequence. *In silico* analysis revealed that $bla_{CTX-M-14}$ was located on an IncFII2 plasmid. To further explore the genetic environment of the $bla_{CTX-M-14}$ gene in isolate SP1, using the $bla_{CTX-M-14}$ carrying contig as a query against the nr/nt database revealed sequence homology to the ~74 kb annotated $bla_{CTX-M-14}$-positive IncFII2 plasmid pAC2901 (GenBank: KU987452) from *Citrobacter freundii* strain AC2901 (Fig. 2). Multiple sequence alignments demonstrated that DNA sequences between pSP1 and pAC2901 share >99% identity. Successful dissemination of $bla_{CTX-M-14}$ among *Enterobacteriaceae* isolates from humans, animals and the environment has mainly been associated with IncK, IncF and IncI1 plasmids [38], and there has been only 1 report of a $bla_{CTX-M-14}$ located on an IncFII2 plasmid in the English literature [39]. Here we report for the first time an IncFII2 $bla_{CTX-M-14}$-encoding plasmid in the genus *Shigella*.

Pathogenesis and virulence factors

Shigella flexneri remains a public health concern throughout the world and its pathogenesis should be further investigated. We performed a BLASTP search against the VRDB database and found several known virulence factors. These virulence factors include *Shigella* extracellular protein A (*sepA*), glutamate decarboxylase (*gadA*), invasion plasmid antigen (*ipaH9.8*), long polar fimbriae (*lpfA*), hexosyltransferase homolog (*capU*), invasion protein *Shigella flexneri* (*ipaD*), serine protease autotransporters of *Enterobacteriaceae* (*pic*), VirF transcriptional activator (*virF*), and *Shigella* IgA-like protease homologue (*sigA*). The ability to withstand an acid-challenge of pH 2.5 by *S. flexneri* is a necessary virulence trait, which requires acid-induction of a functional GdaA in the stationary-growth phase [40]. IpaH9.8 is a member of the IpaH family of *Shigella*, which are encoded on the 220 kb virulence plasmid or chromosome and has been shown to be secreted into the host cell where it is targeted to the nucleus [41]. Moreover, LpfA has been linked to virulence in enterohemorrhagic *E. coli* [42]. Earlier reports indicated the SigA is cytopathic for HEp-2 cells and contributes to the intestinal fluid accumulation associated with *S. flexneri* infections [43]. Translocation of effector proteins into host cells and the surrounding space is a common strategy used

by *S. flexneri* to target signaling pathways in the host cell [44], and IpaD and VirF are required to facilitate bacterial invasion of host cells [45]. More importantly, Pic is secreted by pathogenic Gram-negative bacteria through the autotransporter pathway and targets a broad range of human leukocyte adhesion proteins, which represent unique immune-modulating bacterial virulence factors [46]. These data suggest that isolate SP1 is potential pathogenic, which is consistent with the isolation of SP1 from a diarrhea patient.

Comparative analysis with other *S. flexneri* strains

Based on genomes downloaded from the NCBI database, phylogenetic analysis was performed and the resulting tree topology was assessed to identify genetic relatedness between 14 *S. flexneri* isolates and strain SP1 (Fig. 3a). This revealed that SP1 is most closely related to *S. flexneri* str 4S BJ10610, which was also isolated from a severe diarrhea patient and was resistant to multiple drugs [47]. Other *S. flexneri* strains are also has highly similar, except for *S. flexneri* CDC 796.83, suggesting that *S. flexneri* strains show high similarity between different species. A previous study has highlighted that *S. flexneri* has a stable core genome that is equipped with a repertoire of virulence determinants that have enabled it to colonize, and persist, in multiple locations for hundreds of years [48]. A functional genomic comparison was performed between strain SP1 and its four most closely related neighbors: *S. flexneri* str 4S BJ10610 (JMRK00000000), *S. flexneri* 2002017 (CP001383), *S. flexneri* 4c str 1205 (CP012140), and *S. flexneri* 1a str 0228 (CP012735). The Venn diagram indicates the presence of 4449 core conserved genes present in the pan-genome of the analyzed *S. flexneri* isolates (Fig. 3b). Interestingly, a total of 178 strain-specific genes were identified in strain SP1.

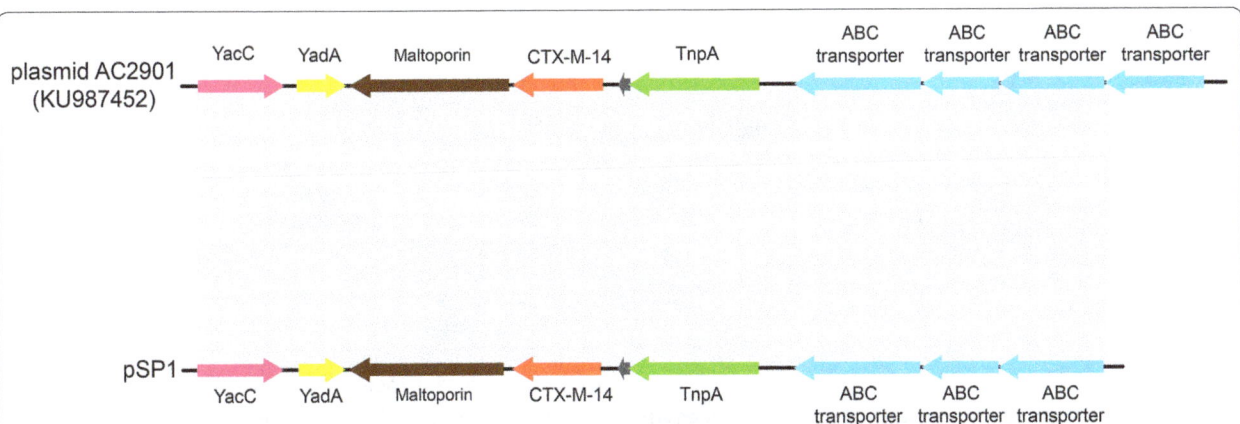

Fig. 2 Genetic organization of scaffolds (portions of genome sequences reconstructed from the whole-genome sequence) containing $bla_{CTX-M-14}$ harbored by plasmid pSP1 and structural comparison with plasmid pAC2901. *Arrows* indicate positions and direction of transcription of genes. Regions with >99% homology are shown in *gray*. Information in parentheses after isolates represents the GenBank accession number

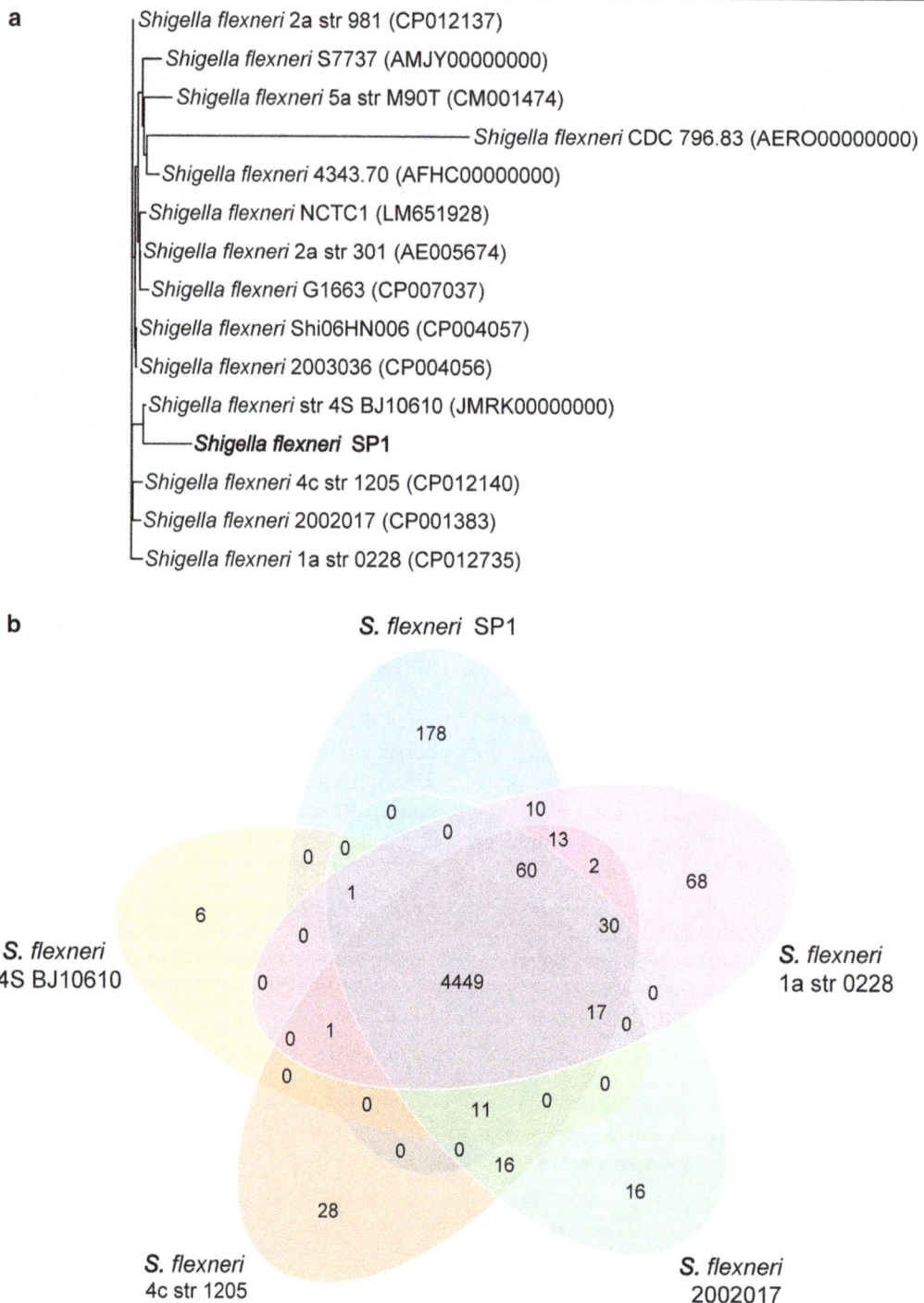

Fig. 3 **a** Phylogenetic tree of *S. flexneri* strain SP1 with 14 other *S. flexneri* isolates. The tree was constructed based on based on alignments of orthologous genes. **b** Venn diagrams showing the orthologous groups in the five most closely related *S. flexneri* genomes. *Numbers* inside the Venn diagrams indicated the number of genes found to be shared among the indicated genomes

Conclusions

As more *S. flexneri* genomes have been sequenced in recent years, comparative genomic studies have progressed rapidly. So far, whole genome studies of *S. flexneri* have exclusively focused on the historical global spread and recent local persistence among these isolates. This work is the first description of the draft genome of a *bla*$_{\text{CTX-M-14}}$-harbouring *S. flexneri* isolate and demonstrates the compares the genome of strain SP1 to other *S. flexneri* isolates. However, the data presented here is a

Genome sequence of Shigella flexneri strain SP1, a diarrheal isolate that encodes...

101

preliminary report on the virulence profile and antibiotic resistance of *S. flexneri* strain SP1. Future studies involving more ESBL-encoding *S. flexneri* isolates from China are urgently needed to study the dynamics of the dissemination of ESBL genes, especially the complete sequence of plasmids carrying these ESBL genes.

Authors' contributions

BZ, PS and JF were involved in the overall experimental design. PS, JF, LG, JL, HX, JJ and CY performed microbiology and molecular biology experiments. BZ, LG and AL generated and analyzed the sequencing data. BZ participated in all discussions of data analysis and wrote the manuscript. All authors read and approved the final manuscript.

Author details

[1] Collaborative Innovation Center for Diagnosis and Treatment of Infectious Diseases, State Key Laboratory for Diagnosis and Treatment of Infectious Diseases, The First Affiliated Hospital, School of Medicine, Zhejiang University, Hangzhou 310003, China. [2] Department of Clinical Laboratory, Hangzhou First People's Hospital, Hangzhou 310006, China. [3] Department of Hospital Infection Control, Zhucheng People's Hospital, Zhucheng 252300, China.

Acknowledgements

Not applicable.

Competing interests

The authors declare that they have no competing interests.

Funding

This work was supported by the National Natural Science Foundation of China (Nos. 81301460 and 81301461); National Key Research and Development Program of China (No. 2016YFD0501105).

References

1. Taneja N, Mewara A, Kumar A, Verma G, Sharma M. Cephalosporin-resistant *Shigella flexneri* over 9 years (2001 2009) in India. J Antimicrob Chemother. 2012;67:1347–53.
2. Tajbakhsh M, Garcia Migura L, Rahbar M, Svendsen CA, Mohammadzadeh M, Zali MR, Aarestrup FM, Hendriksen RS. Antimicrobial-resistant Shigella infections from Iran: an overlooked problem? J Antimicrob Chemother. 2012;67:1128–33.
3. Bennish ML, Wojtyniak BJ. Mortality due to shigellosis: community and hospital data. Rev Infect Dis. 1991;13(Suppl 4):S245–51.
4. Zhang R, Zhou HW, Cai JC, Zhang J, Chen GX, Nasu M, Xie XY. Serotypes and extended-spectrum beta-lactamase types of clinical isolates of *Shigella* spp. from the Zhejiang province of China. Diagn Microbiol Infect Dis. 2011;69:98–104.
5. Yang C, Li P, Zhang X, Ma Q, Cui X, Li H, Liu H, Wang J, Xie J, Wu F, et al. Molecular characterization and analysis of high-level multidrug-resistance of *Shigella flexneri* serotype 4 s strains from China. Sci Rep. 2016;6:29124.
6. Xu Y, Zhuang L, Kang H, Ma P, Xu T, Pan S, Gu B. Prevalence, resistance patterns, and characterization of integrons of *Shigella flexneri* isolated from Jiangsu Province in China, 2001–2011. Eur J Clin Microbiol Infect Dis. 2016;35:1347–53.
7. Zhang W, Luo Y, Li J, Lin L, Ma Y, Hu C, Jin S, Ran L, Cui S. Wide dissemination of multidrug-resistant Shigella isolates in China. J Antimicrob Chemother. 2011;66:2527–35.
8. Zheng B, Dong H, Xu H, Lv J, Zhang J, Jiang X, Du Y, Xiao Y, Li L. Coexistence of MCR-1 and NDM-1 in clinical *Escherichia coli* isolates. Clin Infect Dis. 2016;63:1393–5.
9. Jin Q, Yuan Z, Xu J, Wang Y, Shen Y, Lu W, Wang J, Liu H, Yang J, Yang F, et al. Genome sequence of *Shigella flexneri* 2a: insights into pathogenicity through comparison with genomes of *Escherichia coli* K12 and O157. Nucleic Acids Res. 2002;30:4432–41.
10. Ashton PM, Baker KS, Gentle A, Wooldridge DJ, Thomson NR, Dallman TJ, Jenkins C. Draft genome sequences of the type strains of *Shigella flexneri* held at Public Health England: comparison of classical phenotypic and novel molecular assays with whole genome sequence. Gut Pathog. 2014;6:7.
11. Wang T, Jiang X, Feng C, Li A, Dong H, Wu S, Zheng B. Whole genome sequencing uncovers a novel IND-16 metallo-beta-lactamase from an extensively drug-resistant Chryseobacterium indologenes strain J31. Gut Pathog. 2016;8:47.
12. CLSI. Performance standards for antimicrobial susceptibility testing; 23rd informational supplement. Wayne: M100-S23: Clinical and Laboratory Standards Institute; 2013.
13. Zerbino DR, Birney E. Velvet: algorithms for de novo short read assembly using de Bruijn graphs. Genome Res. 2008;18:821–9.
14. Aziz RK, Bartels D, Best AA, DeJongh M, Disz T, Edwards RA, Formsma K, Gerdes S, Glass EM, Kubal M, et al. The RAST server: rapid annotations using subsystems technology. BMC Genom. 2008;9:75.
15. Natale DA, Shankavaram UT, Galperin MY, Wolf YI, Aravind L, Koonin EV. Towards understanding the first genome sequence of a crenarchaeon by genome annotation using clusters of orthologous groups of proteins (COGs). Genome Biol. 2000;1:RESEARCH0009.
16. Lowe TM, Eddy SR. tRNAscan-SE: a program for improved detection of transfer RNA genes in genomic sequence. Nucleic Acids Res. 1997;25:0955–64.
17. Lagesen K, Hallin P, Rødland EA, Stærfeldt H-H, Rognes T, Ussery DW. RNAmmer: consistent and rapid annotation of ribosomal RNA genes. Nucleic Acids Res. 2007;35:3100–8.
18. Arndt D, Grant JR, Marcu A, Sajed T, Pon A, Liang Y, Wishart DS. PHASTER: a better, faster version of the PHAST phage search tool. Nucleic Acids Res. 2016;44:W16–21.
19. Grissa I, Vergnaud G, Pourcel C. CRISPRfinder: a web tool to identify clustered regularly interspaced short palindromic repeats. Nucleic Acids Res. 2007;35:W52–7.
20. Carattoli A, Zankari E, Garcia-Fernandez A, Voldby Larsen M, Lund O, Villa L, Moller Aarestrup F, Hasman H. In silico detection and typing of plasmids using PlasmidFinder and plasmid multilocus sequence typing. Antimicrob Agents Chemother. 2014;58:3895–903.
21. Siguier P, Varani A, Perochon J, Chandler M. Exploring bacterial insertion sequences with ISfinder: objectives, uses, and future developments. Methods Mol Biol. 2012;859:91–103.
22. Antipov D, Hartwick N, Shen M, Raiko M, Lapidus A, Pevzner PA. plasmidSPAdes: assembling plasmids from whole genome sequencing data. Bioinformatics. 2016;32:3380–7.

23. Jia B, Raphenya AR, Alcock B, Waglechner N, Guo P, Tsang KK, Lago BA, Dave BM, Pereira S, Sharma AN, et al. CARD 2017: expansion and model-centric curation of the comprehensive antibiotic resistance database. Nucleic Acids Res. 2017;45:D566–73.

24. Zankari E, Hasman H, Cosentino S, Vestergaard M, Rasmussen S, Lund O, Aarestrup FM, Larsen MV. Identification of acquired antimicrobial resistance genes. J Antimicrob Chemother. 2012;67:2640–4.

25. Chen L, Zheng D, Liu B, Yang J, Jin Q. VFDB 2016: hierarchical and refined dataset for big data analysis–10 years on. Nucleic Acids Res. 2016;44:D694–7.

26. Kleinheinz KA, Joensen KG, Larsen MV. Applying the ResFinder and VirulenceFinder web-services for easy identification of acquired antibiotic resistance and *E. coli* virulence genes in bacteriophage and prophage nucleotide sequences. Bacteriophage. 2014;4:e27943.

27. Carattoli A, Bertini A, Villa L, Falbo V, Hopkins KL, Threlfall EJ: Identification of plasmids by PCR-based replicon typing. J Microbiol Methods 2005;63:219–28.

28. Zheng B, Li A, Jiang X, Hu X, Yao J, Zhao L, Ji J, Ye M, Xiao Y, Li L. Genome sequencing and genomic characterization of a tigecycline-resistant *Klebsiella pneumoniae* strain isolated from the bile samples of a cholangiocarcinoma patient. Gut Pathog. 2014;6:40.

29. Schliep KP. phangorn: phylogenetic analysis in R. Bioinformatics. 2011;27:592–3.

30. Lam F, Lalansingh CM, Babaran HE, Wang Z, Prokopec SD, Fox NS, Boutros PC. VennDiagramWeb: a web application for the generation of highly customizable Venn and Euler diagrams. BMC Bioinform. 2016;17:401.

31. Rossi O, Baker KS, Phalipon A, Weill FX, Citiulo F, Sansonetti P, Gerke C, Thomson NR. Draft genomes of Shigella strains used by the STOPENTER-ICS consortium. Gut Pathog. 2015;7:14.

32. Zhang N, Lan R, Sun Q, Wang J, Wang Y, Zhang J, Yu D, Hu W, Hu S, Dai H, et al. Genomic portrait of the evolution and epidemic spread of a recently emerged multidrug-resistant *Shigella flexneri* clone in China. J Clin Microbiol. 2014;52:1119–26.

33. Li J, Li B, Ni Y, Sun J. Molecular characterization of the extended-spectrum beta-lactamase (ESBL)-producing *Shigella* spp. in Shanghai. Eur J Clin Microbiol Infect Dis. 2015;34:447–51.

34. Xia S, Xu B, Huang L, Zhao JY, Ran L, Zhang J, Chen H, Pulsrikarn C, Pornruangwong S, Aarestrup FM, Hendriksen RS. Prevalence and characterization of human Shigella infections in Henan Province, China, in 2006. J Clin Microbiol. 2011;49:232–42.

35. Zhang CL, Liu QZ, Wang J, Chu X, Shen LM, Guo YY. Epidemic and virulence characteristic of *Shigella* spp. with extended-spectrum cephalosporin resistance in Xiaoshan District, Hangzhou, China. BMC Infect Dis. 2014;14:260.

36. Wang Y, Song C, Duan G, Zhu J, Yang H, Xi Y, Fan Q. Transposition of ISEcp1 modulates blaCTX-M-55-mediated *Shigella flexneri* resistance to cefalothin. Int J Antimicrob Agents. 2013;42:507–12.

37. Poirel L, Decousser JW, Nordmann P. Insertion sequence ISEcp1B is involved in expression and mobilization of a bla(CTX-M) beta-lactamase gene. Antimicrob Agents Chemother. 2003;47:2938–45.

38. Riccobono E, Di Pilato V, Villagran AL, Bartoloni A, Rossolini GM, Pallecchi L. Complete sequence of pV404, a novel Incl1 plasmid harbouring blaCTX-M-14 in an original genetic context. Int J Antimicrob Agents. 2014;44:374–6.

39. Valat C, Forest K, Billet M, Polizzi C, Saras E, Madec JY, Haenni M. Absence of co-localization between pathovar-associated virulence factors and extended-spectrum beta-lactamase (blaCTX-M) genes on a single plasmid. Vet Microbiol. 2016;192:163–6.

40. Bhagwat AA, Bhagwat M. Comparative analysis of transcriptional regulatory elements of glutamate-dependent acid-resistance systems of *Shigella flexneri* and *Escherichia coli* O157:H7. FEMS Microbiol Lett. 2004;234:139–47.

41. Edwards DJ, Streich FC Jr, Ronchi VP, Todaro DR, Haas AL. Convergent evolution in the assembly of polyubiquitin degradation signals by the *Shigella flexneri* IpaH9.8 ligase. J Biol Chem. 2014;289:34114–28.

42. Dogan B, Suzuki H, Herlekar D, Sartor RB, Campbell BJ, Roberts CL, Stewart K, Scherl EJ, Araz Y, Bitar PP, et al. Inflammation-associated adherent-invasive *Escherichia coli* are enriched in pathways for use of propanediol and iron and M-cell translocation. Inflamm Bowel Dis. 2014;20:1919–32.

43. Al-Hasani K, Navarro-Garcia F, Huerta J, Sakellaris H, Adler B. The immunogenic SigA enterotoxin of *Shigella flexneri* 2a binds to HEp-2 cells and induces fodrin redistribution in intoxicated epithelial cells. PLoS ONE. 2009;4:e8223.

44. Wang F, Jiang Z, Li Y, He X, Zhao J, Yang X, Zhu L, Yin Z, Li X, Wang X, et al. *Shigella flexneri* T3SS effector IpaH4.5 modulates the host inflammatory response via interaction with NF-kappaB p65 protein. Cell Microbiol. 2013;15:474–85.

45. Tobe T, Nagai S, Okada N, Adler B, Yoshikawa M, Sasakawa C. Temperature-regulated expression of invasion genes in *Shigella flexneri* is controlled through the transcriptional activation of the virB gene on the large plasmid. Mol Microbiol. 1991;5:887–93.

46. Ruiz-Perez F, Wahid R, Faherty CS, Kolappaswamy K, Rodriguez L, Santiago A, Murphy E, Cross A, Sztein MB, Nataro JP. Serine protease autotransporters from *Shigella flexneri* and pathogenic *Escherichia coli* target a broad range of leukocyte glycoproteins. Proc Natl Acad Sci USA. 2011;108:12881–6.

47. Li P, Yang C, Wang J, Yi S, Li H, Wang Y, Qiu S, Song H. Draft genome sequence of a new *Shigella flexneri* subserotype, 4S BJ10610. Genome Announc. 2014;2:e00715.

48. Connor TR, Barker CR, Baker KS, Weill FX, Talukder KA, Smith AM, Baker S, Gouali M, Pham Thanh D, Jahan Azmi I, et al. Species-wide whole genome sequencing reveals historical global spread and recent local persistence in *Shigella flexneri*. Elife. 2015;4:e07335.

13

A prospective observational cohort study in primary care practices to identify factors associated with treatment failure in *Staphylococcus aureus* skin and soft tissue infections

Grace C. Lee[1,2*], Ronald G. Hall[3,4], Natalie K. Boyd[1,2], Steven D. Dallas[5], Liem C. Du[6], Lucina B. Treviño[6], Sylvia B. Treviño[6], Chad Retzloff[6], Kenneth A. Lawson[1], James Wilson[1], Randall J. Olsen[7], Yufeng Wang[8] and Christopher R. Frei[1,2]

Abstract

Background: The incidence of outpatient visits for skin and soft tissue infections (SSTIs) has substantially increased over the last decade. The emergence of community-associated methicillin-resistant *Staphylococcus aureus* (CA-MRSA) has made the management of *S. aureus* SSTIs complex and challenging. The objective of this study was to identify risk factors contributing to treatment failures associated with community-associated *S. aureus* skin and soft tissue infections SSTIs.

Methods: This was a prospective, observational study among 14 primary care clinics within the South Texas Ambulatory Research Network. The primary outcome was treatment failure within 90 days of the initial visit. Univariate associations between the explanatory variables and treatment failure were examined. A generalized linear mixed-effect model was developed to identify independent risk factors associated with treatment failure.

Results: Overall, 21% (22/106) patients with *S. aureus* SSTIs experienced treatment failure. The occurrence of treatment failure was similar among patients with methicillin-resistant *S. aureus* and those with methicillin-susceptible *S. aureus* SSTIs (19 vs. 24%; $p = 0.70$). Independent predictors of treatment failure among cases with *S. aureus* SSTIs was a duration of infection of ≥ 7 days prior to initial visit [aOR, 6.02 (95% CI 1.74–19.61)] and a lesion diameter size ≥ 5 cm [5.25 (1.58–17.20)].

Conclusions: Predictors for treatment failure included a duration of infection for ≥ 7 days prior to the initial visit and a wound diameter of ≥ 5 cm. A heightened awareness of these risk factors could help direct targeted interventions in high-risk populations.

Keywords: *Staphylococcus aureus*, Skin and soft tissue infections, Methicillin resistant *Staphylococcus aureus* (MRSA), Epidemiology, Primary care

*Correspondence: leeg3@uthscsa.edu
[2] Pharmacotherapy Education and Research Center, School of Medicine, The University of Texas Health Science Center, 7703 Floyd Curl Dr, MC 6220, San Antonio, TX 78229-3900, USA
Full list of author information is available at the end of the article

Background

The incidence of outpatient and emergency department visits for skin and soft tissue infections (SSTIs) has substantially increased with the emergence of community-associated methicillin-resistant *Staphylococcus aureus* (CA-MRSA) [1]. In the U.S., approximately 80–90% of SSTIs are due to *S. aureus* [2, 3]. Moreover, treatment failure is common after an initial *S. aureus* SSTI episode; recurrence rates have exceeded 50% in some populations [4]. Treatment failure may be multifactorial and can be associated with host factors, disease management, and pathogen features. Two studies set in urgent care and primary care clinics found 35% of patients with CA-MRSA SSTIs experienced treatment failure and 78% reported SSTI recurrence [5, 6]. SSTIs due to CA-MRSA have been implicated to have more serious outcomes compared to community-associated methicillin susceptible *S. aureus* (CA-MSSA) SSTIs; however, there are limited studies evaluating the differences in treatment outcomes in the primary care setting. Furthermore, while there has been a growing body supporting the assessment of early response in treatment failure among hospitalized patients with SSTIs, very little information is available for outpatients [7, 8]. Tools to better identify those who are at higher risk of experiencing treatment failure are needed to better inform treatment decisions in the outpatient setting.

We have recently described the prevalence, treatment characteristics, and costs associated with the management of CA-MRSA SSTIs in South Texas in the primary care setting [9, 10]. The primary objective of this study was to identify risk factors contributing to *S. aureus* SSTI treatment failures.

Methods

Study setting and population

We performed this investigation among a well-described cohort of patients with SSTIs in the primary care setting. Details of this cohort have been described previously [9–11]. Briefly, this study was conducted in collaboration with fourteen clinics within the South Texas Ambulatory Research Network (STARNet), a practice-based research network (PBRN) composed of 108 urban, suburban, and rural primary care clinics distributed throughout the South Texas region, from 2007 to 2014. Patients were eligible for study enrollment if they provided informed consent, were 18 years of age or older, and presented to one of the participating clinics with an SSTI. Healthcare providers collected a wound sample and patient information (e.g., demographics, infection characteristics, clinical information).

Study design

We conducted a prospective observational cohort study to determine predictors of treatment failure. Currently, there is no consensus definition of treatment failure. We have based our definition based on prior studies using a proxy of therapeutic endpoints for SSTIs in the outpatient setting [9–14]. Treatment failure was defined as any of the following events within 90 days of their initial visit: (1) need for a new course or change in antibiotic therapy for SSTI, (2) additional incision and drainage, (3) SSTI at a new site, (4) SSTI at the same site, (5) emergency department visit, or (6) hospital admission. First, we compared the rate of treatment failure for patients with MRSA infections to those with MSSA infections. Next, we identified independent risk factors associated with treatment failure by comparing key characteristics in those patients who did and did not experience treatment failure.

Microbiologic analyses

Samples were plated onto blood agar plates (TSA with 5% sheep blood; Fisher Scientific, Lenexa, KS) and incubated at 35–37 °C for 24 h, then sub-cultured to MRSA selective agar (MRSASelect chromogenic agar plates; Bio-Rad Laboratories, Hercules, CA). Latex agglutination tests (StaphAurex®; Thermo Fisher Scientific, Lenexa, KS), and phenotypic screening tests (cefoxitin) were used for the identification and isolation of MRSA using Vitek 2 AST-GP75 cards (bioMerieux, Durham, NC). Antimicrobial minimum inhibitory concentrations (MICs) were interpreted according to the Clinical and Laboratory Standards Institute document M100-S22 (2012). Multidrug resistance (MDR) was defined as resistant to >2 antimicrobial classes. For molecular analysis, multilocus sequence types (MLST) were assigned for 98 isolates using whole genome sequence data according to designated MLST (http://www.mlst.net) as described previously [11].

Data collection and variables

Clinical information included patient gender, race (Black, White, Other), ethnicity (Hispanic, Non-Hispanic), past medical history (e.g., diabetes, peripheral vascular disease, chronic non-infectious skin disorder, HIV/AIDS, cancer, actively receiving chemotherapy, immunosuppression), health care-related work history, skin infection history, height, infection characteristics (e.g., location, duration, size, deepest tunnel depth, erythema, smell, ulceration, drainage, abscess, satellites), incision and drainage procedures, and antibiotics prescribed. A BMI ≥ 30 kg/m^2 was used to indicate obesity status. A 110 kg weight cutoff was used to indicate 'high body weight'.

This is consistent with previous literature associating high body weight with antimicrobial dosing outcomes [15–17]. In addition, this cut-off was internally derived using a Classification and Regression Tree (CART) analysis which found a significant node at 110 kg that partitioned the data associated with treatment failure.

Statistical analyses

First, a bivariable analysis was conducted comparing variables between the 'treatment failure' and 'no treatment failure' groups. The Breslow-Day test was used to identify possible effect modification; any $p \leq 0.05$ was considered an effect modifier. A generalized linear mixed-effect model was developed to identify independent risk factors; clinic site was set as the random effect. Covariates included MRSA phenotype, largest diameter size of the wound ≥ 5 cm, and duration of skin infection prior to visit of ≥ 7 days. Adjusted odds ratios (ORs) and 95% confidence intervals (CIs) were reported. A $p \leq 0.05$ was used to determine statistical significance. SPSS 22.0® (IBM Corp, Armonk, NY) was used for all statistical comparisons.

Results

Among cases with positive *S. aureus* SSTIs, 106 cases (61%) had 90-days follow-up information. Overall, 22 (21%) cases experienced treatment failure. Treatment failure occurred in 19% (13) of cases with initial MRSA SSTIs and 24% (9) with MSSA SSTIs ($p = 0.70$). In bivariable analysis, factors associated with treatment failure included Black race, weight ≥ 110 kg, MDR, duration of skin infection prior to visit ≥ 7 days, lesion diameter ≥ 5 cm, lesion size ≥ 25 cm^2, and abscess formation (Table 1). Multivariable analysis showed no significant difference in the likelihood of treatment failure between MRSA and MSSA (aOR, 0.42 (0.12–1.42); $p = 0.16$). Independent predictors of treatment failure among cases with *S. aureus* SSTIs were duration of skin infection prior to visit ≥ 7 days [aOR, 6.02 (95% CI 1.74–19.61)], and a lesion diameter size ≥ 5 cm [aOR, 5.25 (95% CI 1.58–17.20)].

Infection location, specific treatment strategies, or prescribed antimicrobial agents were not significantly associated with treatment failure. The proportion of discordant antimicrobial agents prescribed was higher in the treatment failure group than in the no-failure group, but did not reach statistical significance (11 vs. 4%, $p = 0.20$) which may be an artifact of the small sample size. MRSA isolates had significantly lower susceptibility to ciprofloxacin ($p < 0.01$) and erythromycin ($p < 0.01$). Two isolates (1 MRSA and 1 MSSA) were D-test positive.

Molecular analysis (Fig. 1) was conducted on 98 isolates: 56% (65/116) of CA-MRSA and 43% (32/75) of CA-MSSA. All MRSA isolates and 68% of MSSA isolates were MLST strain type (ST) 8. Other MSSA strain types included: ST5, ST12, ST-15, ST-20, ST-45, and ST-59. Four isolates had undefined MLST designation. Furthermore, 95% of *S. aureus* SSTI treatment failures were ST-8 compared to 84% of cases with no treatment failure ($p = 0.32$).

Discussion

Over the past 10 years, ambulatory care visits for SSTIs have increased exponentially. The worldwide emergence of CA-MRSA strains has made the management of *S. aureus* SSTIs extremely complicated and challenging [2, 3]. A clinical approach to the management of *S. aureus* SSTIs is to identify risk factors to predict those who are more likely to experience treatment failure.

Although it has been postulated that CA-MRSA related SSTIs may be associated with worse outcomes, SSTIs caused by MRSA did not have worse outcomes than those caused by MSSA in the South Texas community. Miller et al. found similar 30-day response rates among patients with CA-MRSA and CA-MSSA infection (23 [33%] of 70 vs. 13 [28%] of 47 patients; $p = 0.55$). In addition, patients with CA-MSSA infections were more likely to be re-hospitalized and to subjectively believe that they had not been cured [18]. Moreover, a previous randomized clinical trial of children with suspected *S. aureus* SSTIs found that the incidence of recurrence did not differ between children with MRSA vs. MSSA baseline infections [14]. Our findings further support the notion that the methicillin resistance phenotype is not a reliable predictor for clinical outcomes of community associated *S. aureus* infections. Rather, community associated *S. aureus* should be considered a single entity when evaluating virulence risks.

Identifying predictors for clinical failure can help target more aggressive treatment, monitoring, and decolonization procedures. This study identified that duration of infection 7 days and longer prior to the initial visit was the strongest predictor of treatment failure. This may be related to the natural course of infection that patients were presenting at a time of maximum intensity of inflammation and infection. Moreover, it may be that longer duration of an active *S. aureus* infection without proper treatment may have increased the likelihood for household or fomite transmission, both which have been shown to be important factors for infection recurrence [19–21]. This finding is in contrast to a recent study that found longer duration of symptoms was among the factors related to early response (at day 3). However, the investigation evaluated antibiotic response at day 3 among hospitalized SSTI patients; therefore, may not necessarily be associated with long-term outcomes

Table 1 Risk factors associated with treatment failure among patients with community-associated *S. aureus* skin and soft tissue infections

Characteristic	Overall, n = 106	No failure, n = 84	Treatment failure, n = 22	OR (95% CI)	p	aOR (95% CI)	p
Mean age, years (±SD)	41 (±14)	40 (±13)	45 (±13)		0.15		
Gender							
Male	53 (50%)	44 (52%)	9 (41%)	0.63 (0.24–1.63)	0.34		
Race/ethnicity							
Black	8 (8%)	4 (5%)	4 (18%)	4.44 (1.02–19.47)	0.03		
Hispanic	78 (74%)	64 (76%)	14 (64%)	0.547 (0.20–1.49)	0.23		
Diabetes	28 (26%)	21 (25%)	7 (32%)	1.40 (0.50–3.89)	0.52		
Obese (BMI ≥ 30)[b]	50 (54%)	38 (50%)	12 (71%)	2.40 (0.77–7.48)	0.12		
Weight ≥110 kg	19 (20%)	12 (15%)	7 (37%)	3.21 (1.05–9.80)	0.04		
Chronic non-infectious skin disorder	1 (1%)	1 (1%)	0	0.99 (0.97–1.01)	1.00		
Immunosuppressed at time of visit	2 (2%)	2 (2%)	0	0.98 (0.94–1.01)	1.00		
Provides healthcare to others	2 (2%)	1 (1%)	0	0.99 (0.97–1.01)	1.00		
MRSA phenotype	68 (65%)	55 (66%)	13 (59%)	0.87 (0.49–1.56)	0.65	0.42 (0.12–1.42)	0.16
MDR	29 (27%)	10 (12%)	19 (86%)	2.85 (1.07–7.62)	0.03		
Prior SSTI	35 (33%)	27 (32%)	8 (36%)	1.21 (0.45–3.20)	0.71		
Prior antibiotic history	16 (15%)	11 (13%)	5 (23%)	1.95 (0.60–6.36)	0.32		
Duration of infection prior to visit ≥7 days	48 (48%)	32 (40%)	16 (76%)	4.80 (1.59–14.41)	<0.01	6.02 (1.74–20.87)	<0.01
Severity							
Largest diameter ≥5 cm	49 (48%)	34 (42%)	15 (71%)	3.53 (1.24–10.02)	0.01	5.25 (1.58–17.42)	<0.01
Lesion area ≥25 cm^2	37 (35%)	24 (29%)	13 (59%)	3.55 (1.34–9.39)	0.01		
Infection characteristics							
Erythema	78 (74%)	61 (74%)	17 (77%)	1.23 (0.40–3.72)	0.72		
Drainage	56 (53%)	45 (54%)	11 (50%)	0.84 (0.33–2.16)	0.72		
Ulceration	30 (29%)	22 (27%)	8 (36%)	1.58 (0.59–4.29)	0.43		
Abscess	76 (72%)	56 (67%)	20 (91%)	4.82 (1.05–22.14)	0.03		
Location							
Lower extremity	35 (33%)	26 (31%)	9 (41%)	1.54 (0.59–4.06)	0.38		
Head/neck/face	11 (10%)	10 (12%)	1 (5%)	0.35 (0.40–2.91)	0.45*		
Trunk	24 (23%)	17 (20%)	7 (32%)	1.84 (0.65–5.22)	0.26*		
Axilla	13 (12%)	11 (13%)	2 (9%)	0.66 (0.14–3.24)	0.61*		
Upper extremity	6 (6%)	5 (6%)	1 (5%)	0.75 (0.08–6.79)	1.00*		
Groin/buttock	17 (16%)	14 (17%)	3 (14%)	0.79 (0.21–3.03)	1.00*		
Treatment							
I&D only	4 (4%)	3 (4%)	1 (5%)	1.01 (0.91–1.12)	1.00		
I&D + antibiotics	57 (59%)	43 (51%)	14 (64%)	1.30 (0.68–2.51)	0.41		
Antibiotics only	32 (33%)	27 (36%)	5 (24%)	0.84 (0.63–1.13)	0.29		
Antibiotics							
Trimethoprim–sulfamethoxazole	81 (76%)	65 (77%)	16 (73%)	0.78 (0.27–2.27)	0.65		

including post-treatment failure and recurrence that were evaluated in the current study [7]. Importantly, this finding further supports the proposition that time to effective treatment is essential in the management of SSTIs, and possibly, that patients presenting with longer duration (≥7 days) of infections may require more aggressive measures and/or follow-up monitoring.

In addition, a lesion diameter of greater than 5 cm was associated with treatment failure. Lesion size has been used as a proxy for severity in several syndromes of

A prospective observational cohort study in primary care practices to identify factors...

107

Table 1 continued

Characteristic	Overall, n = 106	No failure, n = 84	Treatment failure, n = 22	OR (95% CI)	p	aOR (95% CI)	p
Doxycycline	12 (11%)	9 (11%)	3 (14%)	1.32 (0.32–5.34)	0.71		
Clindamycin	7 (7%)	5 (6%)	2 (9%)	1.58 (0.26–8.75)	0.63		
Cephalexin	9 (9%)	7 (8%)	2 (9%)	1.10 (0.21–5.71)	1.00		
Discordant therapy	5 (5%)	3 (4%)	2 (11%)	2.82 (0.44–18.24)	0.26		

Note there were no cases of patients with the peripheral vascular disease, human immunodeficiency virus, cancer, and receipt of chemotherapy

MRSA methicillin resistant *S. aureus*, *MSSA* methicillin susceptible *S. aureus*, *SD* standard deviation, *OR* odds ratio, *CI* confidence interval, *aOR* adjusted odds ratio, *SSTI* skin and soft tissue infection, *BMI* body mass index, *I&D* incision and drainage

* Fishers exact test was used

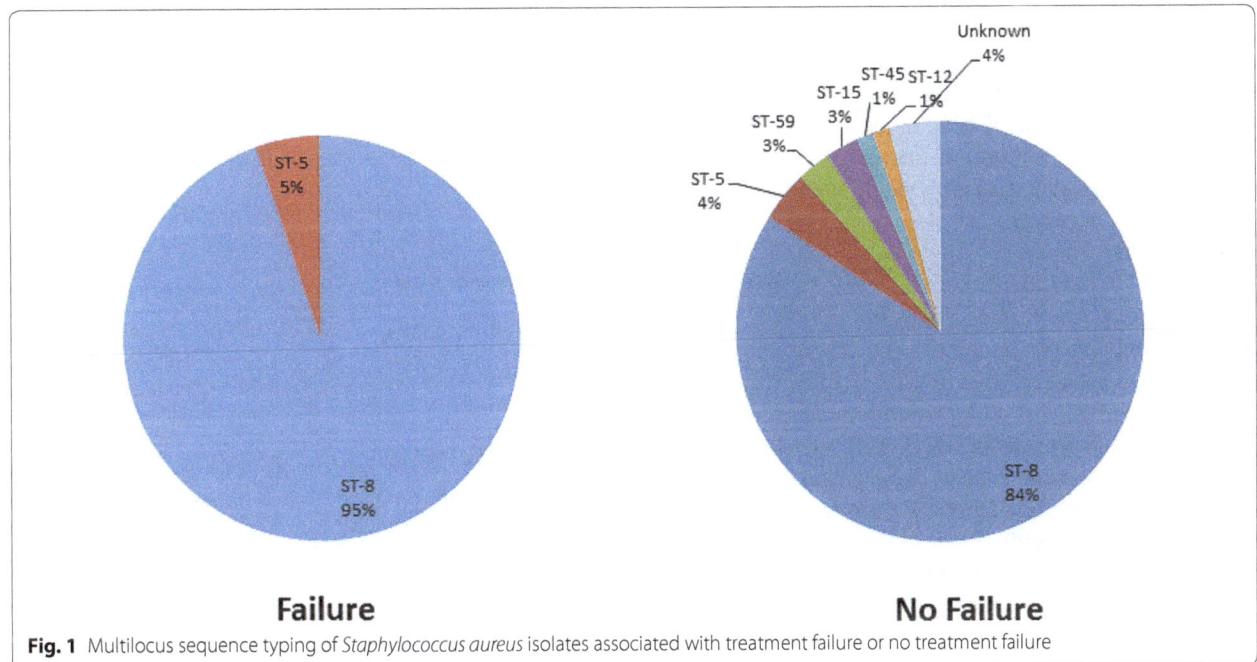

Fig. 1 Multilocus sequence typing of *Staphylococcus aureus* isolates associated with treatment failure or no treatment failure

skin infections, including necrotizing fasciitis and surgical site infections [22]. The 5 cm threshold used in this study was based on data from an observational study, in which abscesses larger than 5 cm were associated with treatment failure [23]. This investigation found a significant predictor of hospitalization on the first follow-up was having an infected area >5 cm in diameter at the initial evaluation (33% of patients with diameter >5 cm were later hospitalized vs. none with diameter ≤5 cm; $p = 0.004$). Other studies have also identified lesion size as an important indicator for severity and suggest treatment stratification approaches [24–26]. In the most recent guidelines for acute bacterial skin and skin structure infection (ABSSSI) clinical trials, the FDA recommends an evaluation of lesion size as a more quantitative assessment of infection severity and the change in lesion size at 48 to 72 h as the new primary endpoint [27].

Our findings provide further support to assess initial lesion sizes to predict infection severity and treatment outcomes.

Specific treatment strategies or type of prescribed antimicrobial agents were not found to be independent factors associated with treatment failure. It should be noted that because of the limited sample size, this study was not designed to perform direct comparisons of treatment approaches and antibiotic therapies. Larger investigations are needed to compare the role of treatment strategies and antibiotic regimens.

In our molecular analyses, ST-8 was the predominant strain type and was more likely to be found in patients whose treatment failed. However, this 11% absolute difference did not reach statistical significance due to the size of our cohort. This might suggest that the pathogenicity of community associated *S. aureus* may be based on the genetic background or lineage rather than the methicillin susceptibility phenotype. A more thorough investigation on the genomic characteristics of these strains is currently underway.

There are limitations to this study. First, we did not account for social and behavioral risk factors that may be associated with *S. aureus* SSTIs and/or clinical outcomes. Second, we used laboratory diagnosis to identify *S. aureus* cases. Patients presenting with SSTIs with no culture or were culture-negative may have different characteristics. The small sample size limited the ability to identify risks associated with lower exposures. Compliance of antimicrobials prescribed was not assessed. Finally, there may be limited generalizability to other regions outside of South Texas. To our knowledge, this is the first prospective study evaluating the clinical and epidemiological factors of *S. aureus* SSTI treatment failure in the primary care setting, adding important findings to the sparse literature in this growing population.

Conclusions

The rates of treatment failure were similar among patients with CA-MRSA SSTIs to those with CA-MSSA SSTIs. Independent predictors for treatment failure included a duration of infection for greater than 7 days prior to the initial visit and a wound diameter of ≥ 5 cm. A heightened awareness of these risk factors could help direct clinical management and public health interventions in high-risk populations. Future large prospective investigations are required to validate these findings and to assess optimal treatment approaches.

Abbreviations

SSTIs: skin and soft tissue infections; CA-MRSA: community-associated methicillin resistant *S. aureus*; CA-MSSA: community-associated methicillin susceptible *S. aureus*; STARNet: South Texas Ambulatory Research Network; PBRN: practice-based research network; MICs: minimum inhibitory concentrations; MDR: multidrug resistance; MLST: multilocus sequence type; CART: classification and regression tree; ORs: odds ratios; CIs: confidence intervals; aOR: adjusted odd ratio; SD: standard deviation; BMI: body mass index; I&D: incision and drainage; ST: strain type.

Authors' contributions

Conception and design of work: GCL and CRF; Data collection: GCL, SDD, LCD, LBT, SBT, CRF; Data analysis and interpretation: GCL, RGH, CRF; Drafting of manuscript: GCL; Critical revision of manuscript: RGH, NKB, KAL, JAW, RJO, YW, CRF. All authors read and approved the final manuscript.

Author details

[1] College of Pharmacy, University of Texas at Austin, Austin, TX, USA. [2] Pharmacotherapy Education and Research Center, School of Medicine, The University of Texas Health Science Center, 7703 Floyd Curl Dr, MC 6220, San Antonio, TX 78229-3900, USA. [3] School of Pharmacy, Texas Tech University Health Sciences Center, Dallas, TX, USA. [4] Dose Optimization and Outcomes Research (DOOR) Program, Dallas, TX, USA. [5] Department of Clinical Laboratory Sciences, School of Health Professions, University of Texas Health Science Center, San Antonio, TX, USA. [6] South Texas Ambulatory Research Network, The University of Texas Health Science Center, San Antonio, TX, USA. [7] Department of Pathology and Genomic Medicine, Houston Methodist Hospital and Research Institute, Houston, TX, USA. [8] Department of Biology, The University of Texas San Antonio, San Antonio, TX, USA.

Acknowledgements

The authors would like to thank their South Texas Ambulatory Research Network (STARNet) and Area Health Education Center (AHEC) colleagues, including Paula Winkler, who assisted with the administrative aspects of the study. We also thank Khine Tun for editing and formatting the manuscript.

Competing interests

The authors declare that they have no competing interests.

Declaration

The University of Texas Health Science Center Institutional Review Board granted approval for this study.

Funding statement

This study was funded by an investigator-initiated research grant from Pfizer to Dr. Frei. Dr. Frei was also supported by the U.S. National Institutes of Health in the form of a KL2 Career Development Award (NIH/NCRR 5KL2 RR025766, PI-Robert Clark).

References

1. Pallin DJ, Egan DJ, Pelletier AJ, Espinola JA, Hooper DC, Camargo CA Jr. Increased US emergency department visits for skin and soft tissue infections, and changes in antibiotic choices, during the emergence of community-associated methicillin-resistant *Staphylococcus aureus*. Ann Emerg Med. 2008;51:291–8.
2. Ray GT, Suaya JA, Baxter R. Incidence, microbiology, and patient characteristics of skin and soft-tissue infections in a U.S. population: a retrospective population-based study. BMC Infect Dis. 2013;13:252.
3. Ray GT, Suaya JA, Baxter R. Microbiology of skin and soft tissue infections in the age of community-acquired methicillin-resistant *Staphylococcus aureus*. Diagn Microbiol Infect Dis. 2013;76:24–30.
4. Creech CB, Al-Zubeidi DN, Fritz SA. Prevention of recurrent *Staphylococcal* skin infections. Infect Dis Clin North Am. 2015;29:429–64.
5. Frei CR, Miller ML, Lewis JS 2nd, et al. Trimethoprim–sulfamethoxazole or clindamycin for community-associated MRSA (CA-MRSA) skin infections. J Am Board Fam Med. 2010;23:714–9.
6. Parchman ML, Munoz A. Risk factors for methicillin-resistant Staphylococcal aureus skin and soft tissue infections presenting in primary care: a South Texas Ambulatory Research Network (STARNet) study. J Am Board Fam Med. 2009;22:375–9.
7. Bruun T, Oppegaard O, Hufthammer KO, et al. Early response in cellulitis: a prospective study of dynamics and predictors. Clin Infect Dis. 2016;15:1034–41.
8. Amara S, Adamson RT, Lew I, et al. Clinical response at Day 3 of therapy and economic outcomes in hospitalized patients with acute bacterial skin and skin structure infection (ABSSSI). Curr Med Res Opin. 2013;29:869–77.
9. Forcade NA, Parchman ML, Jorgensen JH, et al. Prevalence, severity, and treatment of community-acquired methicillin-resistant *Staphylococcus aureus* (CA-MRSA) skin and soft tissue infections in ten medical clinics in Texas: a South Texas Ambulatory Research Network (STARNet) study. J Am Board Fam Med. 2011;24:543–50.

10. Labreche MJ, Lee GC, Attridge RT, et al. Treatment failure and costs in patients with methicillin-resistant *Staphylococcus aureus* (MRSA) skin and soft tissue infections: a South Texas Ambulatory Research Network (STARNet) study. J Am Board Fam Med. 2013;26:508–17.

11. Lee GC, Long SW, Musser JM, et al. Comparative whole genome sequencing of community-associated methicillin-resistant *Staphylococcus aureus* sequence type 8 from primary care clinics in a Texas community. Pharmacotherapy. 2015;35:220–8.

12. Bocchini CE, Mason EO, Hulten KG, et al. Recurrent community-associated *Staphylococcus aureus* infections in children presenting to Texas Children's Hospital in Houston Texas. Pediatr Infect Dis J. 2013;32:1189–93.

13. Fritz SA, Hogan PG, Hayek G, et al. Household versus individual approaches to eradication of community-associated *Staphylococcus aureus* in children: a randomized trial. Clin Infect Dis. 2012;54:743–51.

14. Kaplan SL, Forbes A, Hammerman WA, et al. Randomized trial of "bleach baths" plus routine hygienic measures vs. routine hygienic measures alone for prevention of recurrent infections. Clin Infect Dis. 2014;58:679–82.

15. Rubino CM, Van Wart SA, Bhavnani SM, Ambrose PG, McCollam JS, Forrest A. Oritavancin population pharmacokinetics in healthy subjects and patients with complicated skin and skin structure infections or bacteremia. Antimicrob Agents Chemother. 2009;53:4422–8.

16. Falagas ME, Karageorgopoulos DE. Adjustment of dosing of antimicrobial agents for bodyweight in adults. Lancet. 2010;375:248–51.

17. Gillon JE, Cassat JE, Di Pentima MC. Validation of two vancomycin nomograms in patients 10 years of age and older. J Clin Pharmacol. 2014;54:35–8.

18. Miller LG, Quan C, Shay A, et al. A prospective investigation of outcomes after hospital discharge for endemic, community-acquired methicillin-resistant and -susceptible *Staphylococcus aureus* skin infection. Clin Infect Dis. 2007;44:483–92.

19. Miller LG, Diep BA. Clinical practice: colonization, fomites, and virulence: rethinking the pathogenesis of community-associated methicillin-resistant *Staphylococcus aureus* infection. Clin Infect Dis. 2008;46:752–60.

20. Uhlemann AC, Dordel J, Knox JR, et al. Molecular tracing of the emergence, diversification, and transmission of *S. aureus* sequence type 8 in a New York community. Proc Natl Acad Sci USA. 2014;111:6738–43.

21. Uhlemann AC, Kennedy AD, Martens C, Porcella SF, Deleo FR, Lowy FD. Toward an understanding of the evolution of *Staphylococcus aureus* strain USA300 during colonization in community households. Genome Biol Evol. 2012;4:1275–85.

22. Stevens DL, Bisno AL, Chambers HF, et al. Practice guidelines for the diagnosis and management of skin and soft tissue infections: 2014 update by the infectious diseases society of America. Clin Infect Dis. 2014;59:147–59.

23. Lee MC, Rios AM, Aten MF, Mejias A, Cavuoti D, McCracken GH Jr, Hardy RD. Management and outcome of children with skin and soft tissue abscesses caused by community-acquired methicillin-resistant *Staphylococcus aureus*. Pediatr Infect Dis J. 2004;23:123–7.

24. Miller LG, Daum RS, Chambers HF. Antibacterial treatment for uncomplicated skin infections. N Engl J Med. 2015;372:2460.

25. Miller LG, Daum RS, Creech CB, et al. Clindamycin versus trimethoprim-sulfamethoxazole for uncomplicated skin infections. N Engl J Med. 2015;372:1093–103.

26. Eron LJ, Lipsky BA, Low DE, et al. Managing skin and soft tissue infections: expert panel recommendation. J Antimicrob Chemother. 2003;52(Suppl 1):i3–17.

27. Itani KM, Shorr AF. FDA guidance for ABSSSI trials: implications for conducting and interpreting clinical trials. Clin Infect Dis. 2014;58(1):S4–9.

14

Rapid screening for antibiotic resistance elements on the RNA transcript, protein and enzymatic activity level

Alexander Rohde[1,2*], Jens Andre Hammerl[1] and Sascha Al Dahouk[1]

Abstract

Background: The emerging threat posed by antibiotic resistance has affected public health systems all over the world. Surveillance of resistant bacteria in clinical settings and identifying them in mixed cultures is of paramount importance and can contribute to the control of their spreading. Culture-independent monitoring approaches are highly desirable, since they yield results much faster than traditional susceptibility testing. However, many rapid molecular methods like PCR only detect the sole presence of a potential resistance gene, do not provide information regarding efficient transcription, expression and functionality and, in addition, cannot assign resistance genes to species level in mixed cultures.

Methods: By using plasmid-encoded TEM β-lactamase mediated ampicillin resistances as a proof of principle system, we (1) developed a fluorescence in situ hybridization-test (FISH) capable to detect the respective mRNAs, (2) implemented an immunofluorescence test to identify the corresponding proteins and (3) compared these two microscopic tests with an established colorimetric nitrocefin assay to assess the enzymatic activity.

Results: All three methods proved to be suitable for the testing of antibiotic resistance, but only FISH and immunofluorescence were able to differentiate between susceptible and resistant bacteria on the single cell level and can be combined with simultaneous species identification.

Conclusions: Fluorescence in situ hybridization and immunofluorescence tests are promising techniques in susceptibility testing since they bridge the gap between the slow, but accurate and sound cultural methods and molecular detection methods like PCR with much less functional relevance.

Keywords: Antibiotic resistance, Fluorescence in situ hybridization, β-Lactamases, Plasmids

Background

The emergence of antibiotic resistance is threatening the public health in industrialized as well as developing countries, resulting in therapy failure and increased health-care expenditures [1, 2]. Monitoring the occurrence of antibiotic resistance is one important component to control its spreading and, consequently, numerous surveillance programs have been implemented [3–6]. The susceptibility of bacterial isolates towards certain antimicrobials is mainly assessed by slow cultural methods, which require the availability of pure isolates. However, in clinical settings rapid susceptibility testing is extremely crucial to initiate appropriate therapeutic measures because any delay might increase morbidity, mortality and long-term sequelae; therefore, alternative testing methods are gaining importance in hospital care [7]. Screening ubiquitous biofilms in hospitals consisting of multiple different bacterial species or blood samples containing mixed cultures for resistance genes can be carried out by PCR-testing; however, detected resistance genes can neither be attributed to a specific species, nor can it prove a functional resistance. Therefore, culture-independent assays on the single cell level, preferably coupled with the simultaneous species identification, are

*Correspondence: alexander.rohde@bfr.bund.de
[1] Department of Biological Safety, Federal Institute for Risk Assessment, Diedersdorfer Weg 1, 12277 Berlin, Germany
Full list of author information is available at the end of the article

highly desirable, not only for academic purposes, but also in clinical or environmental microbiology. β-lactamases are one of the most frequently encountered mediators of antimicrobial resistance. Among them, TEM β-lactamases encoded on plasmids represent especially interesting targets because mobile elements like plasmids can easily spread antibiotic resistance. To detect the presence of these resistance elements, three culture-independent methods appear to be capable of fulfilling this task. Firstly, the detection of TEM β-lactamase mRNA transcripts can be performed by a modified version of fluorescence in situ hybridization (FISH), which was initially developed for eukaryotes and has recently also been successfully used for prokaryotes [8–10]. Previous attempts using FISH were mainly restricted to detect single mutations in the highly abundant rRNAs conferring resistance to antibiotics targeting ribosomes, e.g. macrolides [11, 12]; however, by applying dozens of probes simultaneously (instead of only one) mRNAs with much lower concentrations can be detected as well. In parallel with mRNA detection, FISH can be used to simultaneously identify the bacterial species based on their ribosomal RNA [7, 11]. Secondly, immunofluorescence stainings of the proteins with specific antibodies represent a further alternative and can also be used for concurrent species identification [13]. Thirdly, chromogenic substrates like nitrocefin offer a way to test the enzymatic activity of TEM β-lactamases [14, 15]. Apart from these methods, reverse transcription PCR assays (RT-PCR) are an additional possibility enabling the detection of efficient transcription [16–18]. However, in contrast to FISH and immunofluorescence stainings, RT-PCR cannot detect resistance elements on the single cell level. In this work, we established a FISH assay to detect TEM mRNAs encoded on different kind of plasmids and, additionally, an immunofluorescent staining to detect the corresponding proteins and compared these methods with the traditional nitrocefin assay to screen for functional β-lactamases.

Methods

Strains and cultivation

Escherichia coli strain DH5α carrying either the high copy number plasmids pLitmus38 (AMP^r) and pUC18 (AMP^r) or the medium copy number vector pBR328 (AMP^r, TET^r, CHL^r) with a low plasmid stability were used as well as the *E. coli* reference strain ATCC 35218, a reference strain producing TEM-1 β-lactamases [19–21]. On the plasmids pLitmus38, pUC18 and pBR328 a TEM-1 gene confers resistance towards ampicillin. Susceptibility of these bacterial strains was tested by Etest® (bioMerieux, France) according to manufacturer specifications and all AMP^r *E. coli* strains

possessed MICs >256 µg/ml. As negative controls, DH5α (MIC <1.5 µg/ml) and GeneHogs (MIC <2 µg/ml; Thermo Fisher Scientific, USA) without plasmids were used as susceptible *E. coli* strains as well as *Y. pseudotuberculosis* ATCC 29833 (MIC <0.125 µg/ml). Two clinical *Klebsiella pneumoniae* isolates, K2 with an intermediate resistance (MIC <24 µg/ml) and the highly resistant strain My6107 (MIC >256 µg/ml), and *Yersinia enterocolitica* DSM 13030 (MIC >256 µg/ml) were used as ampicillin-resistant strains expressing non-TEM β-lactamases. *E. coli* and *K. pneumoniae* were grown in LB medium at 37 °C, *Y. enterocolitica* and *Y. pseudotuberculosis* at 28 °C. To exhibit antibiotic stress, bacterial cultures were grown in LB medium containing ampicillin in a concentration of 100 µg/ml.

In addition, 25 *E. coli* isolates from different environmental samples and with different TEM-variants (Additional file 1: Figure S1) were used to verify the inclusivity and sensitivity of the established FISH and immunofluorescence assays. To test whether the newly developed assays are applicable for mixed bacterial cultures, samples containing different species (*Salmonella enterica*, thermophilic *Campylobacter* spp., *Listeria* spp., *Y. enterocolitica*, *E. coli* O157) were prepared as described earlier [22].

Fish

Bacterial cultures were fixed by adding three volumes of 4 % (vol/vol) PBS/formaldehyde mixture (Carl Roth, Germany). Samples were incubated for 2 h at 4 °C and then washed three times by centrifugation and resuspension in PBS. Cells were resuspended in a 50 % Ethanol/PBS (vol/vol) mixture and either used directly or stored at −20 °C. 10 µl of each sample were pipetted on glass slides (miacom® diagnostics, Germany), dried shortly on a 52 °C hot plate (miacom® diagnostics) and dehydrated in 50, 80 and 96 % ethanol for 3 min each. The slides were coated with 10 µl hybridization buffer (1 M NaCl, 20 mM Tris–HCl (pH 7.2), 0.01 % SDS, 15 % formamide) containing FISH probes in an accumulated concentration of 800 nM (or approximately 20 nM for each FISH probe). FISH probes hybridized in a light-protected humidity chamber at 30 °C for at least 1.5 h. Slides were rinsed in distilled cold water for a few seconds, followed by washing for 10 min (310 mM NaCl, 20 mM Tris–HCl (pH 7.2), 0.01 % SDS) at 30 °C. Slides were again rinsed twice in distilled water, immediately air-dried and embedded in Roti®-Mount FluorCare DAPI (Carl Roth). FISH probes were designed with the Stellaris Probe Designer and synthesized and labelled with CalFluor Red 610 by Biosearch Technologies (Petaluma, USA). The *bla*-gene of pBR328 (GenBank accession #: L08858.1) was used to construct the FISH probes as listed in Table 1. A conventional

Table 1 Oligonucleotides used to detect TEM mRNA and Enterobacteriaceae (as a positive hybridization control)

Probe name	Sequence (5′→3′)	Target	Detection purpose
Enterobac-Alexa488	TCGTGTTTGCACAGTGCTGTGTTT	23S rRNA	Enterobacteriaceae (adapted with minor modifications from Bohnert et al. [23])
Enterobac-Komp	TCGTGTTTGCAGAGTGCTGTGTTT	23S rRNA	Competitor for Enterobacteriaceae detection (adapted with minor modifications from Bohnert et al. [23])
Bla-TEM-CalFluor610	GGAAATGTTGAATACTCAT AAAAGGGAATAAGGGCGAC CAGGAAGGCAAAATGCCGC GCGTTTCTGGGTGAGCAAA CAGCATCTTTTACTTTCAC CTCGTGCACCCAACTGATC GATCCAGTTCGATGTAACC CAAGGATCTTACCGCTGTT GTTCTTCGGGGCGAAAACT AAGTGCTCATCATTGGAAA CGCCACATAGCAGAACTTT CGTCAACACGGGATAATAC GACCGAGTTGCTCTTGCCC TCTGAGAATAGTGTATGCG GTGAGTACTCAACCAAGTC TAAGATGCTTTTCTGTGAC CTCTTACTGTCATGCCATC TTATGGCAGCACTGCATAA CCGCAGTGTTATCACTCAT TCGTTGTCAGAAGTAAGTT TTAGCTCCTTCGGTCCTCC CCATGTTGTGCAAAAAAGC CAAGGCGAGTTACATGATC TCAGCTCCGGTTCCCAACG CGTCGTTTGGTATGGCTTC CAGGCATCGTGGTGTCACG GCAACGTTGTTGCCATTGC GTTCGCCAGTTAATAGTTT GCCGGGAAGCTAGAGTAAG CCATCCAGTCTATTAATTG GTCCTGCAACTTTATCCGC GAAGGGCCGAGCGCAGAAG CAGCAATAAACCAGCCAGC GCTCACCGGCTCCAGATTT CAATGATACCGCGAGACCC TACCATCTGGCCCCAGTGC TAACTACGATACGGGAGGG CCTGACTCCCGTCGTGTA TATTTCGTTCATCCATAGT CACCTATCTCAGCGATCTG ACCAATGCTTAATCAGTGA	mRNA	TEM β-lactamase mRNA

FISH probe developed by Bohnert et al. targeting the ribosomes of Enterobacteriaceae (Enterobac and the unlabeled competitor Enterobac-Komp) was used as a positive hybridization control (Table 1; [23]). FISH probe lyophilisates were diluted in distilled water and stored at −20 °C until usage. Each bacterial strain was tested in three independent hybridization experiments.

Immunofluorescence

Bacterial cultures were prepared as described for FISH. After drying on a glass slide, the bacteria were permeabilized with lysozyme (Carl Roth, 10 mg/ml) for 7 min and afterwards rinsed shortly with water. Samples were then blocked with blocking buffer [2 % of bovine serum albumin in PBS (Sigma-Aldrich, USA)] for 1 h at room temperature. Subsequently, the primary antibody [anti-(TEM) β-lactamase ab12251 (mouse); abcam, United Kingdom], diluted 1:200 in blocking buffer, was added and incubated either overnight at 6 °C (for sequential stainings) or 1 h at room temperature. Slides were rinsed shortly with water and washed three times with PBS and, finally, with blocking buffer for 3 min each. Slides were then incubated with the secondary antibody (goat anti-mouse IgG-Alexa Fluor® 488 ab150117, abcam), diluted

1:300 in blocking buffer, for 1 h at room temperature. Slides were again rinsed shortly with water and washed three times with PBS for 3 min each, once more rinsed with water, air-dried and embedded in Roti®-Mount FluorCare DAPI. Each bacterial strain was stained in three independent immunofluorescence assays.

Fluorescence microscopy

Microscopy was carried out with an AxioScope fluorescence microscope using a 100× N-achroplan Ph3 M27 oil objective (Zeiss, Germany). Images were acquired by the AxioCam MRm and further processed for overlay of different fluorophore channels by using the imaging software ZEN 2012 (Zeiss).

Nitrocefin assay

Nitrocefin (Merck Millipore, Germany) was dissolved in DMSO (PanReac Applichem, Germany) in a concentration of 5 mg/ml. 50 µl of this stock solution was added to 950 µl PBS. 50 µl of this nitrocefin working solution was added to 150 µl of a bacterial culture. Alternatively, a colony was picked from an agar plate and suspended in 50 µl nitrocefin working solution on a glass slide. A colour change from yellow to red was considered as proof for functional β-lactamases. Each bacterial strain was tested three times.

Results and discussion

The FISH assay proved to be sensitive enough to detect signals in all TEM β-lactamase producing strains. FISH signals were highly specific and showed no hybridization with susceptible *E. coli* strains without plasmids conferring resistance or with species which possess other types of β-lactamases (Additional file 2: Figure S2). Interestingly, the transcription pattern varied among individual cells of a pure culture (Fig. 1a) and depended on the tested plasmids as well as on the growth phase: *E. coli* strains harbouring pLitmus38 and pUC18 showed significantly stronger signals than *E. coli* ATCC 35218 or strains with pBR328. In addition, stationary cultures exhibited stronger FISH signals than exponentially growing cultures, which might be a result of a slower metabolism or prolonged mRNA half-lives. The FISH assay could be easily combined with conventional rRNA-FISH for bacterial identification, as exemplified by the simultaneous use of the FISH probe Enterobac. Notably, not all cells which were stained via conventional ribosome FISH staining showed detectable transcription rates of the TEM β-lactamase (Fig. 1a), which can be explained with a natural variation in the transcription rates on the single cell level, a phenomenon which has been observed for other mRNAs before [9, 10]. In contrast to the ribosome staining by the conventional FISH probe Enterobac,

the mRNA signal was not evenly distributed throughout the bacterial cell. Instead, several distinct foci can be observed (Fig. 1a), which is in accordance with previously published reports about mRNA distribution in prokaryotes [9, 10].

Immunofluorescence staining of the TEM β-lactamase protein showed a more even signal distribution among the bacterial cells than the RNA-signals determined by mRNA FISH (compare Fig. 1a, b). Stationary cultures also showed stronger signals compared to exponentially growing bacteria. As expected for a protein which is secreted in the periplasm, ring-shaped halo-like structures around the cells were observed, especially for pUC18 *E. coli* strains (Fig. 1b, right), whereas strains harbouring pLitmus38 and pBR328 as well as *E. coli* ATCC 35218 showed protein accumulations mainly in the cell poles (Fig. 1b, left). In accordance with FISH, antibody staining produced stronger signals for pLitmus38 and pUC18 than for pBR328 and *E. coli* ATCC 35218. Bacteria without a TEM gene were not stained by immunofluorescence (Additional file 3: Table S1).

To elucidate the correlation between transcription and protein level, a sequential FISH and immunofluorescence staining was performed (Fig. 2). However, a clear association between both signals could not be inferred. Some cells showed a pronounced immunofluorescence signal, thus detectable amounts of protein, but a negative FISH signal (thus no detectable mRNAs) or vice versa.

To verify that both assays can be applied to environmental samples, 25 *E. coli* strains with different TEM-variants (TEM-1, TEM-30, TEM-52) were tested. All 25 isolates were detected by immunofluorescence and showed protein accumulations mainly in the cell poles. However, four strains exhibited a rather weak antibody staining. Likewise, the FISH signals of two strains were too weak to be reliably detected (Additional file 1: Figure S1). However, a combination of both methods enabled clear results. This combined testing might be useful to avoid false-negative results and is especially advisable if samples with strong background fluorescence are examined like food matrices or filtrates [22, 24].

To demonstrate that the detection of antibiotic resistance in samples with many different species is possible, mixed microbial cultures were prepared containing a resistant *E. coli* strain as well as *Listeria* spp., *Campylobacter* spp. and Enterobacteriaceae like *Y. enterocolitica*, *S. enterica* and susceptible *E. coli* (all without TEM-elements). Both methods, FISH and immunofluorescence, reliably identified resistant bacteria within this mixture (Fig. 3).

The nitrocefin assay is an established general assay to identify the presence of most types of β-lactamase producing strains. All *E. coli* strains with the high copy

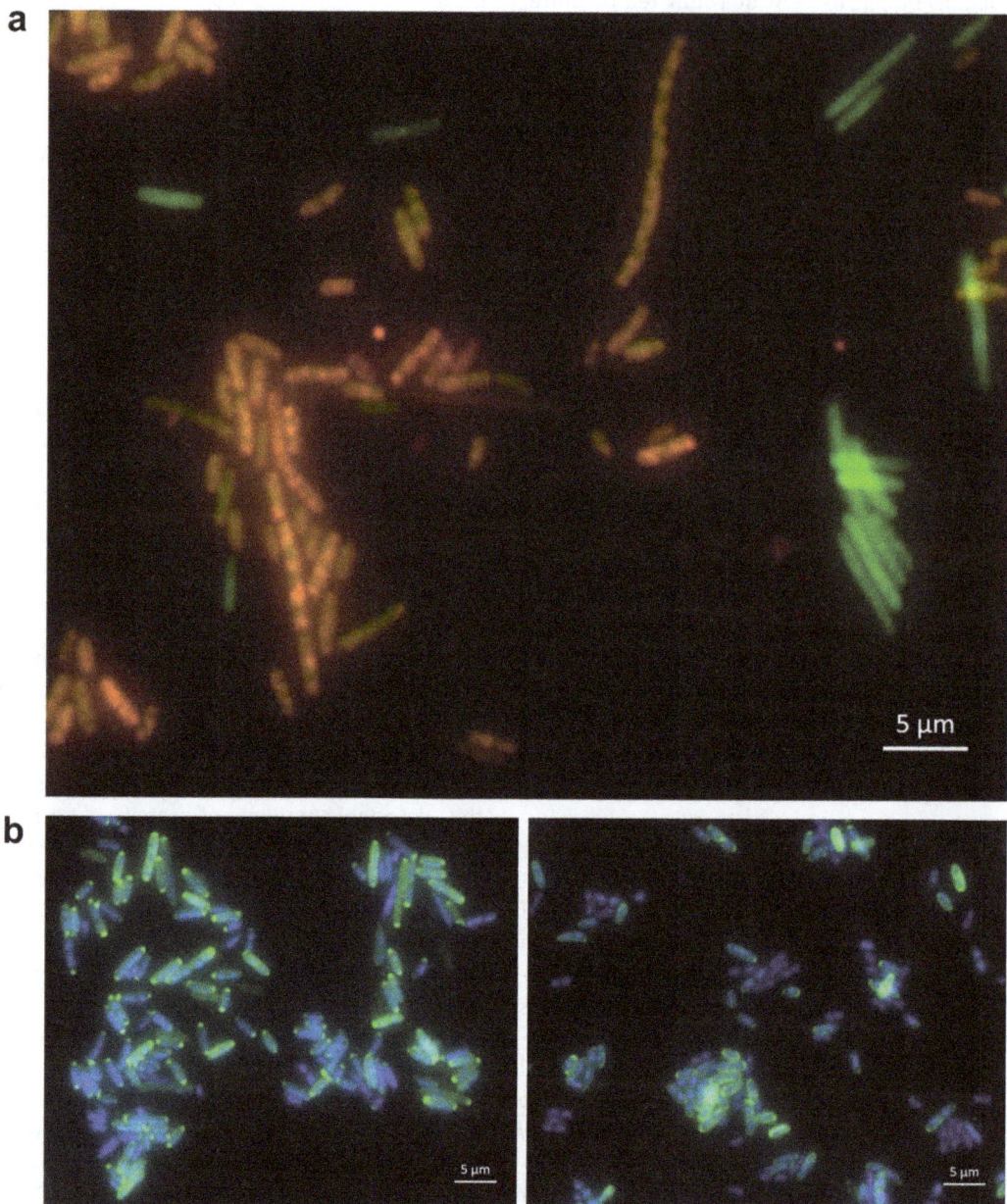

Fig. 1 Detection of TEM β-lactamase mRNAs and the respective protein in *E. coli*. **a** FISH staining of TEM β-lactamase mRNA in *E. coli* harboring pLitmus38 (*red*) and the ribosomal RNAs by Enterobac (*green*). **b** Antibody (*green*) and DNA/DAPI (*blue*) staining of the TEM β-lactamases in *E. coli* harboring pLitmus38 (*left*) or pUC18 plasmids (*right*)

number plasmids pUC18 and pLitmus38 as well as *K. pneumoniae* My6107 were rapidly tested positive for β-lactamase in a few minutes, both by colony smear as well as in liquid cultures, whereas all susceptible strains produced negative results (Additional file 4: Figure S3). Interestingly, the colour change for *Y. enterocolitica*, *K. pneumoniae* K2, *E. coli* ATCC 35218 and strains harbouring the plasmid pBR328 with a low stability and a relatively weak β-lactamase production [20] was less pronounced, especially in liquid cultures without selection pressure, and took significantly longer than for the resistant *E. coli* strains with high copy plasmids, which showed a much more rapid substrate turnover (Additional file 4: Figure S3). We also tried to use nitrocefin to visualize β-lactamase activity on the single cell level. However, nitrocefin was not retained within the periplasm and was, thus, unable to distinguish resistant from susceptible cells using microscopy. It has to be noted that

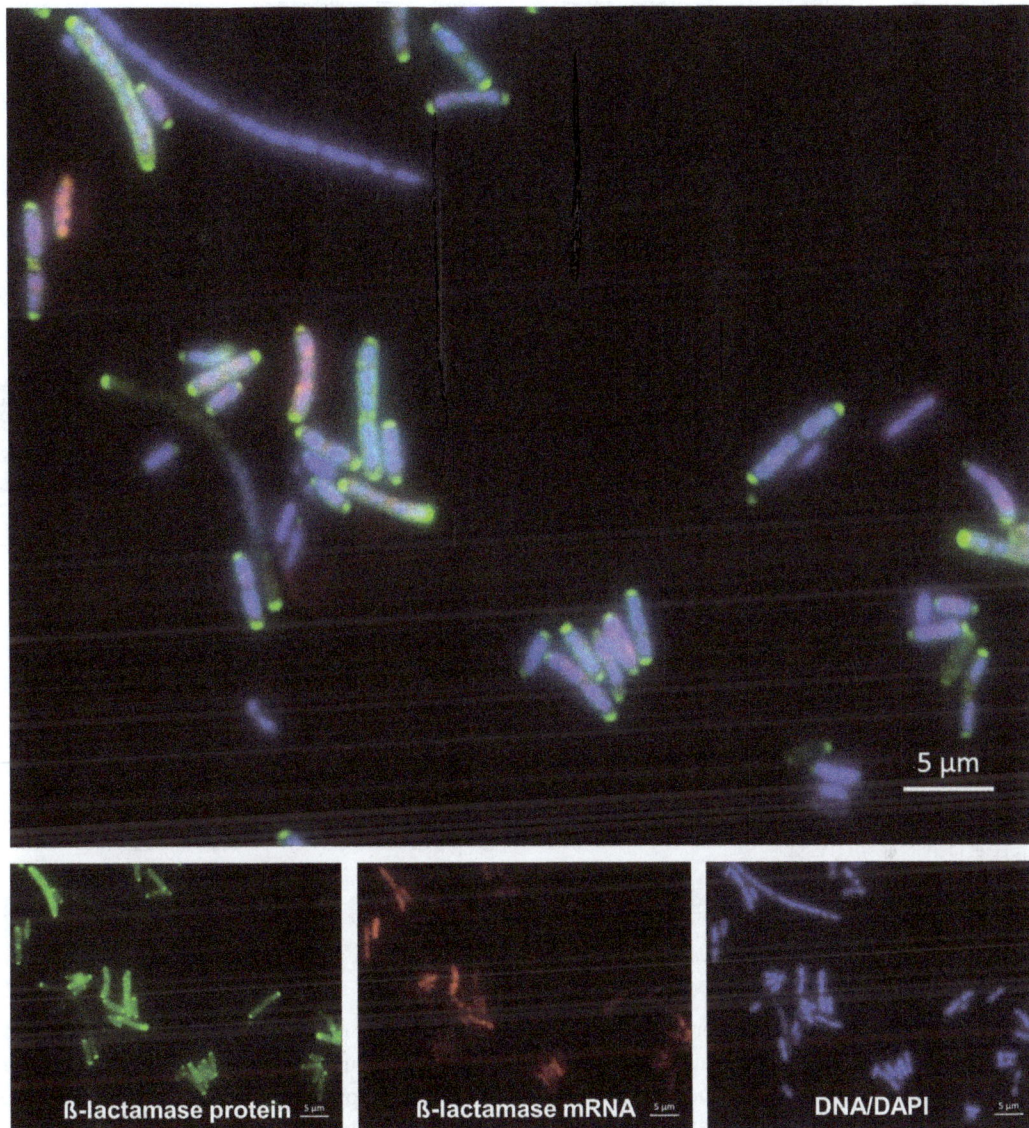

Fig. 2 Simultaneous staining of TEM mRNA and TEM protein in *E. coli* harboring pLitmus38. The upper image shows the merge of the mRNA signal (*red*), the protein level (*green*) and the DNA/DAPI staining (*blue*). The three images below show each fluorescence channel separately

also fluorogenic β-lactamase substrates like CCF2-AM are available, but these substrates are much more expensive and their application is mainly limited to eukaryotic reporter gene assays.

In summary, all three methods are able to detect antibiotic resistance, in particular in case of constitutive moderate transcription and expression rates, and produce congruent results with regard to signal strength. However, there are intrinsic strength and weaknesses of each technique (Table 2). The fast, affordable and easy nitrocefin activity assay can sense the presence of a broad range of β-lactamases and is not confined to TEM-like proteins. In addition, detecting biological activity is probably the most meaningful way to search culture-independently for antibiotic resistance. However, nitrocefin is hardly suitable for single cell microscopy, is not very sensitive in the presence of only low numbers of resistant bacteria and, in contrast to FISH and immunofluorescence, cannot be used for the simultaneous species identification on the single cell level. The β-lactamase antibody staining proved to be a highly convenient and robust system, yielding strong and specific signals. However, it is the slowest of all three methods and depends on the availability of suitable (and rather costly) antibodies. Mutations, which are frequent events in the evolution of antibiotic resistance genes, might easily compromise antibody binding. Finally, multi-probe mRNA

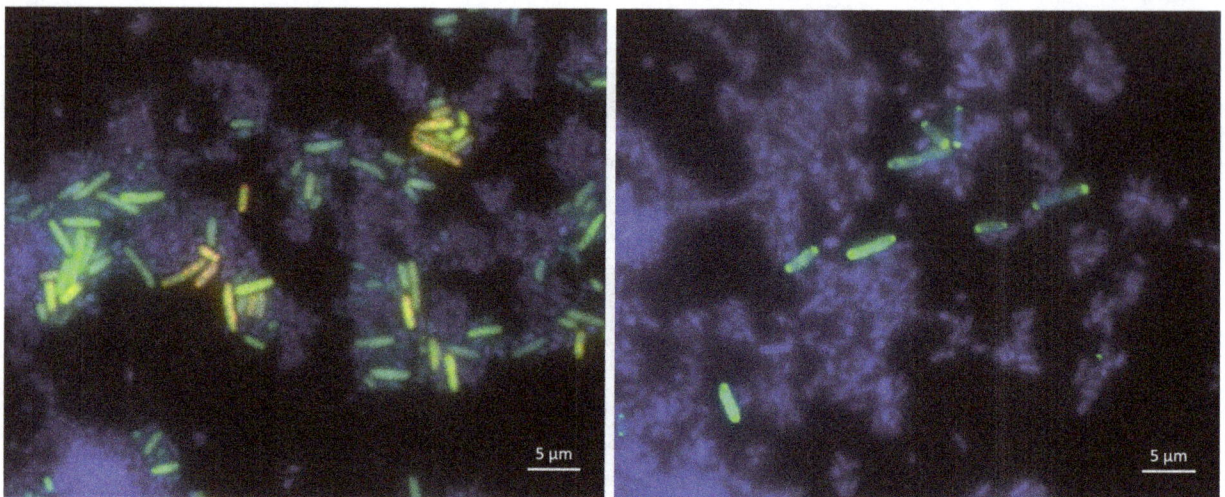

Fig. 3 Detection of resistance in mixed microbial samples. *Left* FISH staining of TEM β-lactamase mRNA in resistant *E. coli* (*red*), ribosomal RNA staining of all Enterobacteriaceae (*green*) and DNA/DAPI staining of all bacteria in the sample. *Right* Antibody staining of TEM β-lactamases expressing *E. coli* (*green*) and DNA/DAPI staining of all bacteria in the sample

Table 2 Comparison of culture-independent techniques applied for the screening of antibiotic resistance

Detection method	FISH	Immunofluorescence	Nitrocefin assay
Target	mRNA	Protein	Enzymatic activity
Speed (h)	5	7	<1
Costs	Moderate	Moderate/high	Low
Simultaneous species identification	Possible	Possible	Not possible
Specificity	Narrow, type-specific (e.g. TEM)	Narrow, type-specific (e.g. TEM)	Broad
Drawbacks	Transcription is no correlate for efficient expression	Specific antibodies required	Not suitable on the single cell level

FISH assays employing up to 50 probes per target mRNA are able to effectively detect groups of related gene products. Efficient detection of mRNAs has been previously performed by RT-PCR; the additional advantage of FISH, however, lies in the detection of resistance on the single cell level, enabling refined insights in multi-species mixed communities and samples. Recently, we developed an extensive set of free-combinable FISH probes targeting the rRNA of various pathogenic bacteria [22]. The assay presented here is a valuable enhancement of these tests. Convenient mRNA FISH assays are not only conceivable to screen for antibiotic resistance elements but are also promising tools to identify the transcription of toxins and other virulence factors. In contrast to the detection by antibodies, mutations are unlikely to affect the detection via FISH, since the use of 50 probes or more tolerates hybridization failure of a few probes. However, monitoring the transcription has the least biological relevance and does neither prove efficient translation nor sufficient biological effectivity.

Conclusions

Fluorescence in situ hybridization and immunofluorescence tests represent promising and affordable tools for susceptibility testing on the single cell level. They combine the speed of other rapid and culture-independent methods with the ability of the cultural methods to obtain functional information and, furthermore, have the potential for simultaneous species identification.

Abbreviations

FISH: fluorescence in situ hybridization; PCR: polymerase chain reaction; RNA: ribonucleic acid; mRNA: messenger RNA; rRNA: ribosomal RNA; RT-PCR: reverse transcription PCR; AMP^r: ampicillin resistance; TET^r: tetracycline resistance; CHL^r: chloramphenicol resistance; MIC: minimal inhibitory concentration; *Y. pseudotuberculosis*: *Yersinia pseudotuberculosis*; *E. coli*: *Escherichia coli*; *K. pneumoniae*: *Klebsiella pneumoniae*; *Y. enterocolitica*: *Yersinia enterocolitica*; LB: lysogeny broth; PBS: phosphate-buffered saline; DAPI: 4′,6-diamidino-2-phenylindole; DMSO: dimethyl sulfoxide; ATCC: American Type Culture Collection.

Authors' contributions
AR, JAH and SAD designed the study. AR carried out the experiments and analyzed the data. AR, JAH and SAD drafted the manuscript. All authors read and approved the final manuscript.

Author details
[1] Department of Biological Safety, Federal Institute for Risk Assessment, Diedersdorfer Weg 1, 12277 Berlin, Germany. [2] Department of Biology, Chemistry and Pharmacy, Free University Berlin, Takustr. 3, 14195 Berlin, Germany.

Acknowledgements
Not applicable.

Competing interests
The authors declare that they have no competing interests.

Funding
This work was supported by a grant of the German Federal Ministry of Education and Research and was executed within the framework of the project ZooGloW (FKZ 13N12697). The funders had no role in study design, data collection and interpretation, or the decision to submit the work for publication.

References

1. Paphitou NI. Antimicrobial resistance: action to combat the rising microbial challenges. Int J Antimicrob Agents. 2013;42(Suppl):S25–8.
2. Arias CA, Murray BE. Antibiotic-resistant bugs in the 21st century–a clinical super-challenge. N Engl J Med. 2009;360:439–43.
3. Acar JF, Moulin G. Integrating animal health surveillance and food safety: the issue of antimicrobial resistance. Rev Sci Tech. 2013;32:383–92.
4. Johnson AP. Surveillance of antibiotic resistance. Philos Trans R Soc Lond B Biol Sci. 2015;370:1–12.
5. Moyaert H, de Jong A, Simjee S, Thomas V. Antimicrobial resistance monitoring projects for zoonotic and indicator bacteria of animal origin: common aspects and differences between EASSA and EFSA. Vet Microbiol. 2014;171:279–83.
6. Fluit AC, van der Bruggen JT, Aarestrup FM, Verhoef J, Jansen WT. Priorities for antibiotic resistance surveillance in Europe. Clin Microbiol Infect. 2006;12:410–7.
7. Frickmann H, Masanta WO, Zautner AE. Emerging rapid resistance testing methods for clinical microbiology laboratories and their potential impact on patient management. Biomed Res Int. 2014;2014:1–18.
8. Raj A, van den Bogaard P, Rifkin SA, van Oudenaarden A, Tyagi S. Imaging individual mRNA molecules using multiple singly labeled probes. Nat Methods. 2008;5:877–9.
9. Skinner SO, Sepúlveda LA, Xu H, Golding I. Measuring mRNA copy number in individual Escherichia coli cells using single-molecule fluorescent in situ hybridization. Nat Protoc. 2013;8:1100–3.
10. So LH, Ghosh A, Zong C, Sepúlveda LA, Segev R, Golding I. General properties of transcriptional time series in Escherichia coli. Nat Genet. 2011;43:554–60.
11. Trebesius K, Panthel K, Strobel S, Vogt K, Faller G, Kirchner T, Kist M, Heeseman J, Haas R. Rapid and specific detection of Helicobacter pylori macrolide resistance in gastric tissue by fluorescent in situ hybridisation. Gut. 2000;46:608–14.
12. Haas M, Essig A, Bartelt E, Poppert S. Detection of resistance to macrolides in thermotolerant Campylobacter species by fluorescence in situ hybridization. J Clin Microbiol. 2008;46:3842–4.
13. Hujer AM, Keslar KS, Dietenberger NJ, Bethel CR, Endimiani A, Bonoma RA. Detection of SHV beta-lactamases in Gram-negative bacilli using fluorescein-labeled antibodies. BMC Microbiol. 2009;9:1–4.
14. Kaase M, Lenga S, Friedrich S, Szabos F, Sakinc T, Kleine B, Gatermann SG. Comparison of phenotypic methods for penicillinase detection in Staphylococcus aureus. Clin Microbiol Infect. 2008;14:614–6.
15. Papanicolaou GA, Medeiros AA. Discrimination of extended-spectrum beta-lactamases by a novel nitrocefin competition assay. Antimicrob Agents Chemother. 1990;34:2184–92.
16. Corvec S, Caroff N, Espaze E, Marraillac J, Drugeon H, Reynaud A. Comparison of two RT-PCR methods for quantifying ampC specific transcripts in Escherichia coli strains. FEMS Microbiol Lett. 2003;228:187–91.
17. Dumas JL, van Delden C, Perron K, Köhler T. Analysis of antibiotic resistance gene expression in Pseudomonas aeruginosa by quantitative real-time-PCR. FEMS Microbiol Lett. 2006;254:217–25.
18. Fu Y, Zhang F, Zhang W, Chen X, Zhao Y, Ma J, Bao L, Song W, Ohsugi T, Urano T, Liu S. Differential expression of bla (SHV) related to susceptibility to ampicillin in Klebsiella pneumoniae. Int J Antimicrob Agents. 2007;29:344–7.
19. Evans PD, Cook SN, Riggs PD, Noren CJ. LITMUS: multipurpose cloning vectors with a novel system for bidirectional in vitro transcription. Biotechniques. 1995;19:130–5.
20. Covarrubias L, Cervantes L, Covarrubias A, Soberon X, Vichido I, Blanco A, Kupersztoch-Portnoy YM, Bolivar F. Construction and characterization of new cloning vehicles. V. mobilization and coding properties of pBR322 and several deletion derivatives including pBR327 and pBR328. Gene. 1981;13:25–35.
21. Vieira J, Messing J. The pUC plasmids, an M13mp7-derived system for insertion mutagenesis and sequencing with synthetic universal primers. Gene. 1982;19:259–68.
22. Rohde A, Hammerl JA, Al Dahouk S. Detection of foodborne bacterial zoonoses by fluorescence in situ hybridization. Food Control. 2016;69:297–305.
23. Bohnert J, Hübner B, Botzenhart K. Rapid identification of Enterobacteriaceae using a novel 23S rRNA-targeted oligonucleotide probe. Int J Hyg Environ Health. 2000;203:77–82.
24. Rohde A, Hammerl JA, Appel B, Dieckmann R, Al Dahouk S. FISHing for bacteria in food–a promising tool for the reliable detection of pathogenic bacteria? Food Microbiol. 2015;46:395–407.

15

Antibiotic resistant airborne bacteria and their multidrug resistance pattern at University teaching referral Hospital in South Ethiopia

Fithamlak Bisetegen Solomon*, Fiseha Wada Wadilo, Amsalu Amache Arota and Yishak Leka Abraham

Abstract

Background: Hospitals provide a reservoir of microorganisms, many of which are multi-resistant to antibiotics. Emergence of multi-drug resistant strains in a hospital environment, particularly in developing countries is an increasing problem to infection treatment. This study aims at assessing antibiotic resistant airborne bacterial isolates.

Methods: A cross-sectional study was conducted at Wolaita Sodo university teaching and referral Hospital. Indoor air samples were collected by using passive air sampling method. Sample processing and antimicrobial susceptibility testing were done following standard bacteriological techniques. The data was analyzed using SPSS version 20.

Results: Medically important bacterial pathogens, Coagulase negative *staphylococci* (29.6%), *Staphylococcus aureus* (26.3%), *Enterococci* species, *Enterococcus faecalis* and *Enterococcus faecium* (16.5%), *Acinetobacter* species (9.5%), *Escherichia coli* (5.8%) and *Pseudomonas aeruginosa* (5.3%) were isolated. Antibiotic resistance rate ranging from 7.5 to 87.5% was detected for all isolates. *Acinetobacter* species showed a high rate of resistance for trimethoprim-sulfamethoxazole, gentamicin (78.2%) and ciprofloxacin (82.6%), 28 (38.9%) of *S. aureus* isolates were meticillin resistant, and 7.5% *Enterococci* isolates of were vancomycin resistant. 75.3% of all bacterial pathogen were multi-drug resistant. Among them, 74.6% were gram positive and 84% were gram negative. Multi-drug resistance were observed among 84.6% of *P. aeruginosa*, of 82.5% *Enterococcii*, *E. coli* 78.6%, *S. aureus* 76.6%, and Coagulase negative *staphylococci* of 73.6%.

Conclusions: Indoor environment of the hospital was contaminated with airborne microbiotas, which are common cause of post-surgical site infection in the study area. Bacterial isolates were highly resistant to commonly used antibiotics with high multi-drug resistance percentage. So air quality of hospital environment, in restricted settings deserves attention, and requires long-term surveillance to protect both patients and healthcare workers.

Keywords: Airborne, Bacteria, Antibiotic, Resistance, Multi-drug resistance

Background

Hospital environment plays a significant role in the occurrence of nosocomial infection since it harbors a diverse population of microorganisms [1]. Bacterial pathogens of medical importance like *Pseudomonas aeruginosa, Staphylococcus aureus, Escherichia coli,* *Enterococci, Acinetobacter* spp. and Coagulase-negative *staphylococci* are a common cause of healthcare-associated infection which could able to survive and persist for long period of time in the hospital environment and have resistant disinfectants potential. The persistence ability of bacterial pathogens in hospital environment associated with a background rise in various types of nosocomial infections and could reach the sick patients through sources like air [2–5].

*Correspondence: fitha2007@yahoo.com
School of Medicine, College of Health Sciences, Wolaita Sodo University,
PO Box: 138, Wolaita Sodo, Ethiopia

Operation theatre, delivery room, and intensive care unit are settings where patients are at a greater risk than the outside environment and could be polluted with bacterial pathogens released into it from various sources [6]. Environmental surface reservoirs like floors, the number of visitors, extent of indoor traffic, time of day and the number of materials brought in from outside and antibiotic resistance aggravate the extent of air bacterial microbiota [7, 8]. The uncontrolled movement of air in and out of the hospital environment makes the bacterial persistence worse since these infectious microorganisms may spread easily into the environment through sneezing, coughing, talking and contact with hospital materials. It can affect not only patients admitted to rooms in which the prior occupants tested positive for a pathogen but also other patients in the facility and even patients in other facilities in a network [9].

Hospitals provide a reservoir of microorganisms, many of which are multi-resistant to antibiotics. The emergence of resistance to antimicrobial agents is a global public health problem particularly in pathogens causing nosocomial infections which contributed to the morbidity, mortality, increased health care costs resulting from treatment failures, and longer hospital stays [1, 10].

The emergence of multi-drug resistant (MDR) strains in a hospital environment, particularly in developing countries is an increasing infection control problem presented a challenge in the provision of good quality patient care associated with high frequency of hospital acquired infections of which emergence, and reemergence of difficult-to-treat nosocomial infections in patients with increased antibiotic resistance rate [11, 12].

Frequently encountered MDR bacteria, methicillin-resistant *S. aureus*, cephalosporins, and extended spectrum beta-lactamase producing *Enterobacteriaceae*, ceftazidime-resistant *P.* aeruginosa, Imipenem-resistant *A. baumannii* and vancomycin-resistant *Enterococci* are commonly encountered in the hospital environment [13–15].

Post surgical site infection, urinary tract infection and respiratory infection are the common hospital acquired infection in this study area of which air could be the potential source. The susceptibility pattern of the isolates to commonly used antibiotics in this area will also provide enormous options for clinicians to select appropriate antibiotics for empirical therapy. So this study aims at the isolation and antibiotic susceptibility pattern of potentially pathogenic airborne bacteria in restricted settings of the hospital setup.

Study area

The study was conducted at Wolaita Sodo University teaching and referral Hospital (WSUTRH), Sodo, located South Central Ethiopia. It's serving people in catchment's area of 2 million people. The hospital has 320 beds for inpatient service which are on medical, pediatrics, surgical, gynecology and obstetrics ward.

Study design

The Hospital-based cross-sectional study design was conducted in WSUTRH from November 2015–March 2015.

Sample size

Sample number were determined in convenience in which 72 settle plate samples were collected in each ward (Delivery room, operation theater, and intensive care unit) for continuous 3 months which gives a total sample size of 216 airborne samples.

Sampling techniques

The air samples were collected from November 1–March 30, 2015 (1st week of the months) once a week during Monday's since the patient load is higher in the study area. The air samples were collected in a day considering the most representative hours (at 8–9 AM, at 11 AM–12 PM, 4–5 PM) after a preliminary survey by considering the fact that a higher patient, staff and attendee load could become the highest burden for acquiring infection through air way. Indoor air samples were collected from delivery room, intensive care unit and operation theatre. Settle plate or passive air sampling method was used. A nine cm diameter sterile Petri dish with 20 ml tryptic soy agar (TSA) was left open to the air for an hour, a meter above the floor and a meter from the wall [16]. Self-contamination was prevented by wearing sterile surgical gloves, mouth masks, and protective gown. Petri-plates were labeled with sample number, hospital ward, date and time of sample collection. Two agar plates were placed at each of the selected wards with 5 m apart. Soon after collection; samples were transported to the microbiology laboratory in sealed plastic bags.

Processing of specimens and preliminary identification

Following collection, 3–5 colonies on TSA were inoculated into MacConkey agar, blood agar plates 5% (BAP), brain heart infusion agar, Mannitol salt agar (Oxoid, LTD), and Bile-aesculin-azide agar (BEAA) (Biomerieux, France) selective medium. The inoculated agar plate was incubated at 35 °C for 24–48 h. Then the growth was inspected to identify the bacteria. Microbial growth on the agar media was identified by colonial morphology, Gram staining, and biochemical tests, oxidase, catalase, coagulase, citrate, indole test, growth in 6.5% NaCl and turbidity, voges-prosquaer, hippurate hydrolysis, pigment production and mannitol fermentation. Isolates were determined and characterized based on Bergy manual of determinative bacteriology [17].

Antibiotic susceptibility testing

Susceptibility testing was performed on isolates based on the Kirby–Bauer diffusion technique [18]. The grades of susceptibility pattern were recognized as sensitive, intermediate and resistant by comparison of the zone of inhibition as indicated in Clinical lab science institute [19] standard 2014. The antibiotics tested for both gram negative and gram positive bacteria (Oxoid, Basingtone, UK) were amikacin (30 µg), ampicillin (10 µg), amoxicillin (25 µg), amoxicillin-clavulanic acid (30 µg), cefoxitin (30 µg), ceftazidime (30 µg), ceftriaxone (30 µg), chloramphenicol (30 µg), ciprofloxacin (5 µg), clindamycin (2 µg), doxycycline (30 µg), erythromycin (15 µg), gentamicin (10 µg), imipenem (10 µg), norfloxacin (10 µg), penicillin G (10 units), tetracycline (30 µg), trimethoprim-sulphamethoxazole (25 µg), and vancomycin (30 µg). Antibiotics were selected based on local availability, literature, effectiveness and CLSI Guidelines.

MDR was defined as acquired non-susceptibility to at least one agent in three or more antimicrobial categories [20].

Pan resistance-Resistance for all antibiotics tested.

Quality controls

Standard operating procedures were prepared and followed from sample collection to reporting. Culture medias was prepared based on the manufactures instruction then the sterility of culture media was checked by incubating 5% of the batch at 35–37 °C overnight and observing bacterial growth. Those culture medias which showed growth were discarded. Antibiotic discs potency was checked by using *S. aureus* ATCC25923, *E. coli* ATCC 25922 and *P. aeruginosa* ATCC 27853 strains as control organisms.

Data analysis

Statistical analysis was performed by using SPSS version 20 software program and descriptive statistics were used.

Ethical considerations

The proposal was approved by the ethical review committee of Wolaita Sodo University. An official letter was written from the university to WSUTRH administrator. The result of the study was communicated to the responsible bodies for any beneficiary or corrective measures.

Results

Total numbers of 216 air samples were collected from delivery room (DR), intensive care unit (ICU), and operation theatre (OT). 195 (90.2%) settle plates were showed a positive bacterial growth for any one of the bacteria. Significant proportions of bacterial pathogens of nosocomial importance like Coagulase negative *staphylococci, S. aureus, Enterococci* spp., *E. fecalis*, 72.5% and *E. faecium*, 27.5%, *Acinetobacter* spp., *E. coli*, and *P. aeruginosa* were also detected. CoNS (72/243) were the highest prevalent bacteria in three wards followed by *S. aureus* 45.8% (64/243). Coagulase negative *staphylococci* 37.8% were the most accountable bacteria in the delivery room followed by *S. aureus* 42.2% (27/64). On the other hand, *S. aureus* was the most abundant bacteria identified in the OR 27/59 (45.85). CoNS and *S. aureus* was the most isolated bacteria in the ICU Fig. 1.

Antibiotic resistance rate of air-borne bacterial pathogens

Antibiotic resistance range of 7.5 up to 87.5% was detected among gram-positive isolates of which CoNS showed a high level of resistance for chloramphenicol 68.1% and trimethoprim-sulfamethoxazole 66.7%. *S. aureus* isolates depicted 87.5% resistance to chloramphenicol and 28 (38.9%) were MRSA isolates. *Enterococci* spp. showed resistant for trimethoprim-sulfamethoxazole 77.5% and ampicillin, 70%. Eight isolates in this study were vancomycin-resistant *Enterococci* (VRE).

Gram-negative bacterial isolates showed resistance ranging from 15.4–87% of which *Acinetobacter* spp. showed a high rate of resistance (>65%) for all antibiotics tested. Ampicillin and doxycycline resistant *E. coli* isolates 71.4 and 78.6% respectively were identified. Imipenem, ceftazidime, and ciprofloxacin resistance *P. aeruginosa* isolates with the rate of resistance, 38.5, 23.1, and 76.9% were also isolated respectively (Table 1).

MDR pattern of gram-positive airborne bacterial pathogens

Seventy-five percent of all bacterial pathogens were multi-drug resistant (MDR) of which 74.6% were gram positive and 84% were gram negative. *Enterococci* spp. accounts 82.5% MDR prevalence of which three isolates were pan-resistant and seven isolates were resistant for three antibiotics (chloramphenicol + gentamicin + trimethoprim-sulfamethoxazole. Seventy-three (73.6%) CoNS became MDR of which two isolates depicted pan-resistance. *S. aureus* isolates showed the very high level of MDR rate, 76.6% (Table 2).

MDR pattern of gram-negative airborne bacterial pathogens

Overall MDR rate of gram negative bacteria were 84%. The vast majorities (91.3%) of *Acinetobacter* spp. were MDR with two pan-resistant isolates and 84.6% of the isolates, four pan-resistances, were MDR. Eighty percent of *E. coli* isolates were having multi-drug resistance

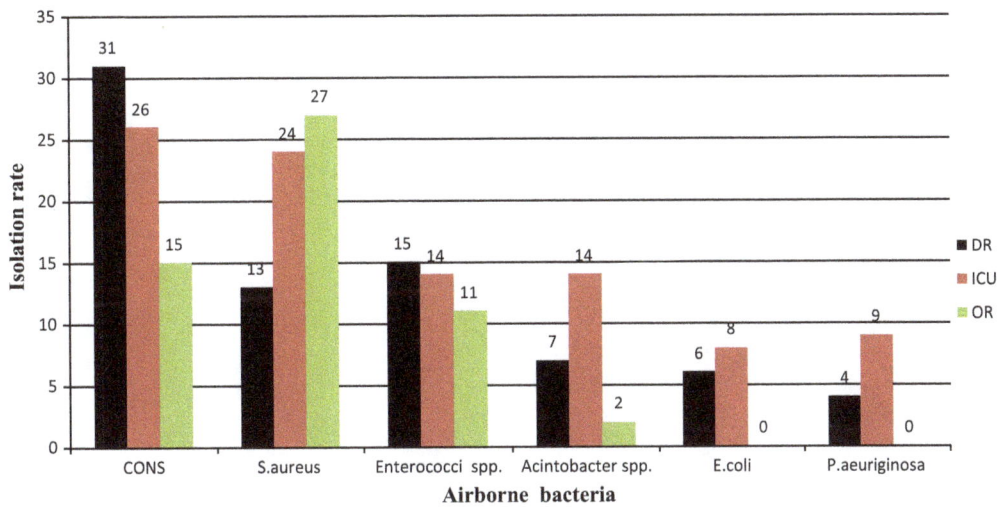

Fig. 1 Distribution of airborne bacterial pathogens in wards of WSUTRH, November–March 2015. *DR* delivery room, *ICU* intensive care unit, *OR* operation theater

Table 1 Antimicrobial resistance pattern of airborne bacterial pathogens of nosocomial importance in WSUTRH, November–March 2015

Resistance

Antibiotics	Gram positive			Gram negative		
	CoNS (72)	*S. aureus* (64)	*Entrococci* spp. (40)	*Acinetobacter* spp. (23)	*E. coli* (14)	*P. aeruginosa* (13)
AMP	ND	ND	28 (70)	ND	10 (71.4)	ND
AMK	ND	ND	11 (27.5)	16 (69.6)	2 (15.4)	6 (46.2)
AMX-CLA	ND	ND	ND	ND	5 (35.7)	ND
AZT	20 (27.8)	17 (26.6)	13 (32.5)	ND	ND	ND
CAF	49 (68.1)	56 (87.5)	25 (62.5)	ND	ND	ND
CF	24 (32.8)	28 (38.9)	ND	ND	ND	ND
CFZ	ND	ND	ND	15 (65.2)	ND	3 (23.1)
CIP	23 (31.9)	25(39.1)	23 (57.5)	19 (82.6)	7 (50)	8 (61.5)
CN	35 (48.6)	21 (32.8)	12 (30)	18 (78.2)	2 (15.4)	8 (61.5)
CRO	ND	ND	14 (35)	18 (78.2)	5 (35.6)	8 (61.5)
CPH	ND	ND	27 (67.5)	ND	ND	ND
DA	12 (16.7)	16 (25)	16 (40)	ND	ND	ND
DOX	ND	ND	ND	20 (87)	10 (71.4)	ND
ERT	ND	ND	ND	ND	ND	ND
IMP	ND	ND	ND	ND	7 (50)	5 (38.5)
NOR	ND	ND	ND	ND	ND	9 (69.2)
PEN	ND	ND	30 (75)	ND	ND	ND
TMP-SXT	48 (66.7)	35 (54.7)	31 (77.5)	19 (82.6)	5 (35.7)	9 (69.2)
VAN	ND	ND	3 (7.5)	ND	ND	ND

Amk amikacin, *Amp* ampicillin, *Amx* amoxicillin, *Amo-cla* amoxicillin-clavulinic acid, *CF* cefoxitin, *Cro* ceftriaxone, *CFZ* ceftazidime, *Cph* cephalothin, *Caf* chloramphenicol, *Cip* ciprofloxacin, *DA* clindamycin, *DOX* doxycycline, *Ert* erythromycin, *Cn* gentamicine, *IMP* imipenem, *Nor* norfloxacin, *PEN* penicillin, *Tmp-Sxt* trimethoprim-sulfamethoxazole, *VAN* vancomycin, *ND* not done

of which 11.1% of the isolates depicted MDR pattern of ampicillin + amoxicillin-clavulanic acid + cephalothin + ciprofloxacin + trimethoprim-sulfamethoxazole) (Table 3).

Discussion

CoNS, and *S. aureus*, identified in this study is in line with previous findings conducted in, Ethiopia [21, 22], Nigeria [23], Kashmir [24], Nepal [25], and Iran [26]. CoNS and

Table 2 Multi drug resistant pattern of airborne gram positive bacterial isolates in WSUTRH November–March 2015

Bacteria	Quantity	Antibiotics pattern	Frequency	Class
Enterococci spp.	Max	AMK, AMP, AZT, CAF, CIP, CN, CPH, CRO, DA, PEN, TMP-SXT, VAN	3	9
	Min	AMK, TMP-SXT, PEN	2	3
		CAF, CN, TMP-SXT	7	3
		DA, PEN, TMP-SXT	2	3
CoNS	Max	AZT, CAF, CF, CIP, CN, DA, DOX, TMP-SXT	2	8
	Min	CAF, DOX, TMP-SXT	8	3
		AZT, CAF, TMP-SXT	2	3
		CF, CN, TMP-SXT	6	3
		DOX, CIP, TMP-SXT	8	3
S. aureus	Max	AZT, CAF, CF, CIP, CN, DA, DOX, TMP-SXT	4	8
	Min	CF, DA, TMP-SXT	7	3
		AZT, CAF, DOX	8	3
		CN, CIP, TMP-SXT	8	3

Max maximum number of resistance pattern, *Min* minimum number of resistance pattern

Table 3 Multi-drug resistance pattern of airborne gram negative bacterial pathogens in WSUTRH from November–March 2015

Bacteria	Quantity	Antibiotic pattern	No	Class
P. aeruginosa	Max	AMK, CFZ, CIP, CN, CRO, IMP, NOR, TMP-SXT	2	5
		AZT, CFZ, CIP, CN, IMP, NOR	1	
		AMK, CIP, CN, NOR, TMP-SXT	2	
	Min	AMK, CIP, CN, CRO	2	3
Acinetobacter spp.	Max	AMK, CFZ, CIP, CN, CRO, DOX, TMP-SXT	4	5
		AMK, CFZ, CIP, CN, DOX, TMP-SXT	3	
		AMK, CFZ, CIP, CRO, DOX, TMP-SXT	4	
		CIP, CN, CRO, DOX, TMP-SXT	3	
	Min	CFZ, CN, CRO, DOX	4	3
E. coli	Max	AMK, AMP, AM-CLA, CN, CRO, DOX, TMP-SXT	2	6
	Min	AMP, CIP, DOX, IMP	3	4
		AMP, DOX, IMP, TMP-SXT	3	

S. aureus were the predominant bacterial isolates in all setups in this study which could be associated with their ability to persist and resist the harsh environmental condition and to suspend in the air particles [9]. *S. aureus*, was the most prevalent bacteria in the air of operation theatre. This finding is corroborated with findings done previously which has the same [21–23, 26]. This might be because of its survival ability on the environmental surface, ability to resist disinfection and could also have an association with the fact that *S. aureus* was the main cause of post-surgical site infection in this hospital.

Enterococci spp. (*E. fecalis* and *E. faecium*) reported in this study were also identified in previous studies isolated elsewhere in Nigeria [23] and Iran [27]. Whereas *Acinetobacter* spp. 9.3% was the most common gram-negative bacteria in this study which could be supported by its higher survival ability (3 days to 11 months) in the environment. Our finding couldn't be compared with other airborne studies in Ethiopia since it is not reported even though these bacteria were reported elsewhere, Taiwan 13.4% [28] and Iran 42% [26] in restrict settings like ICU and OT. *Enterococci* and *Acinetobacter* spp. did not reported previously from air studies in Ethiopia. This could possibly be due to many reasons, the investigator's attention to these pathogens, requirement of high sterility aseptic techniques with enriched bacterial media (selective) and reporting of these bacteria in family name (*streptococci*) rather than species name.

The isolation percentage of *E. coli* (7.5%) in this study is lower as compared with the 13.5% detected in Khartoum [29] hospital and 15.2% reported in Taiwan hospital [28]. This could be due to the use of active air sampling in Taiwan hospital and difference in ward and number of patients attended in reference to Khartoum hospital as compared and *E. coli* is one of the commonest causes of urinary tract infections, 35% prevalence in the study setting where *E. coli* accounts 31.4%, and is commonly present in appendix abscess, peritonitis, cholecystitis, septic wounds and bedsores, bacteraemia and endotoxic shock, particularly in surgical or otherwise debilitated patients [30].

Pseudomonas aeruginosa prevalence (5.3%) in this study is relatively comparable with other similar study in North Ethiopia [22] but much less than 28% [31] and 52% [10] reported previously which could be due to the difference in methodology, sampling place or magnitude of nosocomial infection in specific localities. *P. aeruginosa* associated infection is a recognized public health threat often acquired from the hospital environment and contaminated medical devices. It is not only an important cause of morbidity but also increases the stay of the patient in the hospital and increases the cost of treatment [32].

Indoor air quality in a hospital environment is of great concern to patients, attendants, and clinical staff which could be a cause for nosocomial infections and outbreak. High level of airborne bacteria in the hospital is an alarming call since these settings are places where actual surgical procedures, severely sick, and post-surgical rehabilitated patients are admitted and delivery services are handled.

Antibiotic resistant infections add considerable and avoidable costs to the health care system of which it adds 20 billion USD in excess direct health care cost with additional costs to low society of productivity as high as 35 billion USD [33].

Thirty-nine percent of MRSA prevalence in the current study is higher than 26.6% [34], 18.1% [35] and 7.7% [22] reported in Ethiopia which could be explained by difference in sampling site where most of the resistant isolates in the current study were identified in the intensive care unit where repeated exposure to antibiotics is administered. The frequency of antibiotic administration and magnitude of nosocomial infection in each locality also may differ. Emergence of drug resistant strains especially methicillin-resistant *S. aureus* is a serious problem in hospital environments and infections caused by MRSA strains, 51% prevalence (hospital lab record for 8 years) are associated with longer hospital stay, prolonged antibiotic administration, and higher cost than infections caused by methicillin-susceptible *S. aureus* strains [36]. high prevalence of MRSA strains from the environment, 39% could become the main factors for 51% resistance rate from clinical isolates.

Seventy 70 and 75% resistance prevalence for ampicillin and penicillin G *Enterococci* spp. in this study has a great implication since these antibiotics are preferable in the treatment of enterococcal infections [37] and the growing incidence of infections is a great concern due to multidrug resistance. Vancomycin-resistant *Enterococci* (VRE) 9.1% prevalence in the current study make the scenario worse since vancomycin is the preferred choice in the case where this bacteria became resistant to other antibiotics. CoNS and *S. aureus* also showed a high level of resistance for chloramphenicol and trimethoprim-sulfamethoxazole.

Gram-negative bacteria showed a high level of MDR rate than gram-positive bacteria in the current study

that *Acinetobacter* spp. and *P. aeruginosa* showed high resistance rate for most of the antibiotics. *Acinetobacter* spp. showed the highest rate of resistance with a minimum resistance of 61.5%, this could possibly be due to the bacterial ability to resist many antibiotics or could possibly be due to selective pressure or abusing of the drugs in the hospital where 86.6% prevalence were recorded for commonest antibiotics like ciprofloxacin, and gentamicin. A higher number of resistances to effective antibiotics like ceftazidime 23.1% and imipenem 38.5% to *Acinetobacter* are a major public health problem since their disclosure could possibly lead to a therapeutic impasse in the hospital.

Higher levels of *P. aeruginosa* resistance were noticed for TMP-SXT 69.2%, gentamicin 61.5% and ceftriaxone 61.5% which is comparable with the study conducted in Ethiopia [31] of which 95, 62.5, and 58.2% resistance were detected on TMP-SXT, gentamicin and ceftriaxone antibiotics respectively.

Conclusions and recommendation

Higher prevalence airborne bacteria of clinical concern, CoNS, *S. aureus*, *Enterococci* spp., *Acinetobacter* spp., *P. aeruginosa* and *E. coli* were found in WSUTRH. This could be significant factors for the high prevalence of post-surgical site infection and respiratory tract infection in the study area. High MDR resistance rate (>70%) of the isolates on the hospital air is a clinical concern since antibiotic resistant rate increased in alarming rate. Effective and new antibiotics, like ceftazidime and imipenem resistance, for the study area in the hospital air could be projected to the patients and could pose major problem for antibiotic stewardship programs. So this findings deserves attention, and requires effective infection control measures like proper disinfection and regular cleaning, restriction of patient relatives' movement in and out of the wards/units to protect both patients and healthcare workers. Though isolates were not identified from patients in this study, the role of contaminated indoor air could be pathogenic if contact is established with patients; it is pertinent that their presence should be controlled.

Abbreviations

DR: delivery room; ICU: intensive care unit; MDR: multi drug resistant; OT: operation theatre; TMP-SXT: trimethoprim-sulfamethoxazole; WSUTRH: Wolaita Sodo University teaching referral Hospital.

Authors' contributions

FS: Conceived the study, FS, AR YA, and FW: Participated in the design of the study and performed the statistical analysis, FS, FW: Interpreted the data: FS:

Obtained ethical clearance and permission for study: FW: Supervised data collectors: FS, FW: Drafting the article or revisiting it critically for important intellectual content. All authors read and approved the final manuscript.

Acknowledgements
We would like to thank Wolaita Sodo University for funding this research and teaching referral Hospital nurses and medical laboratory staffs for data collection and processing.

Competing interests
The authors declare that they have no competing interests.

Ethics approval
The study proposal got ethical approval from Wolaita Sodo University ethical review Board.

Funding
The funding for this study was granted by Wolaita Sodo University. The funding body had no influence on study design, data collection, analysis and interpretation of data, writing of the manuscript and in the decision to submit the manuscript for publication.

References

1. Muhammad UK, Isa MA, Aliyu ZM. Distribution of potential nosocomial pathogens isolated from environments of four selected hospital in Sokoto, North Western Nigeria. J Microbiol Biotechnol Res. 2013;3:139–43.
2. Osaro EF, Ufuoma IO, Dorcas AO. Hospital indoor airborne microflora in private and government owned hospitals in Benin City, Nigeria. WJMS. 2008;3:34–8.
3. Tayh G. Risk factors and antimicrobial resistance of pathogens isolated from Burn Units at Local Hospitals in Gaza Strip, Palestine. 2011. http://library.iugaza.edu.ps/thesis/96729.pdf.
4. Anguzu J, Olil D. Drug sensitivity patterns of bacterial isolates from septic post-operative wounds in a regional referral hospital in Uganda. Afr Health Sci. 2007;7:148–54.
5. Hidron AI, Edwards JR, Patel J, Horan TC, Sievert DM, Pollock DA. Antimicrobial-resistant pathogens associated with healthcare-associated infections: annual summary of data reported to the national healthcare safety network at the Centers for Disease Control and Prevention, 2006–2007. Infect Control Hosp Epidemiol. 2008;29:996–1011.
6. Nunes GZ, Martins SA, Altoe FL, Nishikawa MM. Indoor air microbiological evaluation of offices, hospitals, industries, and shopping centers. Mem Inst Oswaldo Cruz. 2005;100:351–7.
7. Suzuki A, Namba Y, Matsuura M, Horisawa A. Bacterial contamination of floors and other surfaces in operating rooms: a 5-year survey. J Hyg. 1984;9393:559–66.
8. CDC. Antibiotic resistance threats in the United States. http://www.cdc.gov/drugresistance/pdf/ar-threats-2013-508.pdf.
9. Roy FC, Sarah S, Charles D. The role of the healthcare environment in the spread of multidrug-resistant organisms: update on current best practices for containment. Ther Adv Infect Dis. 2014;2:79–90.
10. Davane M, Suryawanshi N, Pichare A, Nagoba B. *Pseudomonas aeruginosa* from hospital environment. J Microbiol Infect Dis. 2014;4:42–3.
11. Asghar AH, Faidah HS. Frequency and antimicrobial susceptibility of gram-negative bacteria isolated from 2 hospitals in Makkah, Saudi Arabia. Saudi Med J. 2009;30:1017–23.
12. WHO. The evolving threats of antimicrobial resistance, option for action.2012; ISSN 9789241503181.
13. Centers for Disease Control and Prevention. Healthcare infection control advisory committee. Guidelines for environmental infection control in healthcare facilities. Atlanta; 2003.
14. Guidelines for the prevention and control of multi-drug resistant organisms (MDRO) excluding MRSA in the healthcare setting. Royal College of Physicians clinical advisory group on healthcare associated infections in association with HSE quality and patient safety; 2012.
15. Lee TB, Baker OG, Lee JT, Scheckler WE. Recommended practices for surveillance. Am J Infect Control. 1998;26:277–88.
16. Pasquarella C, Pitzurra O, Savino A. The index of microbial air contamination (review). J Hosp Infect. 2000;46:241–56.
17. Bergey. Manual of systematic bacteriology volume 1 to 5; 2014.
18. Bauer AW, Kirby WM, Sherris JC, Turck M. Antibiotic susceptibility testing by a standardized single disk method. Am J Clin Pathol. 1996;45:493–6.
19. CLSI performance standards for antimicrobial susceptibility testing; twenty-fourth informational supplement, M100-S24; 2014.
20. Magiorakos AP. Multidrug-resistant, extensive drug resistant and pandrug-resistant bacteria, an international expert proposal for interim standard definitions for acquired. Clin Microbiol Infect. 2012;18:268–81.
21. Chalachew G, Gebre K, Wondewosen T. Indoor air bacterial load and antibiotic susceptibility pattern of isolates in operating rooms and surgical wards at Jimma University specialized hospital, Southwest Ethiopia. Ethiop J Health Sci. 2011;21:9–17.
22. Tewelde T, Yibrah B, Kibrom G. Microbial contamination of operating theatre at Ayder Referral Hospital, Northern Ethiopia. Int J Pharm Sci Res. 2015;6:1264–8.
23. Ekhaise FO, Isitor EE, Idehen O, Emoghene AO. Airborne microflora in the atmosphere of an hospital environment of University of Benin Teaching Hospital (UBTH), Benin City, Nigeria. World J Agric Sci. 2010;6:166–70.
24. Singh K, Dar FA, Kishor K. Bacterial contamination in operating theaters of district hospital Budgam in Kashmir division. Innov J Med Health Sci. 2013;3:62–5.
25. Pradhan SB, Shrestha CD. Microbiological surveillance of hospital environment in a Medical College Hospital in Kathmandu, Nepal. Int J Infect Microbiol. 2012;1:76–9.
26. Alireza A, Sanam M. Microbial profile of air contamination in hospital ward. Iran J Pathol. 2012;7:168–74.
27. Awosika SA, Olajubu FA, Amusa NA. Microbiological assessment of indoor air of a teaching hospital in Nigeria. Asian Pac J Trop Biomed. 2012;2:465–8.
28. Ping YH, Zhi YS, Chi HC, Walter D. Airborne and surface-bound microbial contamination in two intensive care units of a medical center in central Taiwan. Aerosol Air Qual Res. 2013;13:1060–9.
29. Sanaa OY, Amani E. Isolation of potential pathogenic bacteria from the air of hospital-delivery and nursing rooms. J Appl Sci. 2010;10:1011–4.
30. Collee JG, Duguid JP, Fraser AG, Marmion BP. Mackie and MaCartney. Practical medical microbiology. 13th ed. London: Churchill Livingstone; 1989. p. 432–44.
31. Mitiku M, Ali S, Kibru G. Antimicrobial drug resistance and disinfectants susceptibility of *Pseudomonas aeruginosa* isolates from clinical and environmental samples in Jimma University Specialized Hospital, Southwest Ethiopia. Am J Biomed Life Sci. 2015;2:40–5.
32. Awoke D. Longitudinal bacteriology of burn patients at Yekatit 12 hospital burn center, Addis-Ababa, Ethiopia AAU electronic library 1–51; 2011.
33. Frieden T. Centers for Disease Control and Prevention. Antibiotic resistance threats in the United States.CDC; 2013.
34. Teklu S, Getenet B, Tesfaye K, Tsegaye S. Bacterial contamination, bacterial profile and antimicrobial susceptibility pattern of isolates from stethoscopes at Jimma University Specialized Hospital. Ann Clin Microbiol Antimicrob. 2013;12:39.
35. Edosa, K. Bacterial profile and antibiotic sensitivity pattern of the isolates from operating room environments in government hospitals in Addis Ababa, Ethiopia.AAU electronic library:1–53; 2015.
36. Kirecci E, Miraloglu M. A research of nasal methicillin-resistant/sensitive staphylococcus aureus and pharyngeal beta-hemolytic Streptococcus carriage in midwifery students in Kahramanaras, Turkey. Ethiop J Health Dev. 2010;24:57–60.
37. Murray BE. Vancomycin-resistant enterococcal infections. N Engl J Med. 2000;342:710.

16

Ethnomedicines and anti-parasitic activities of Pakistani medicinal plants against *Plasmodia* and *Leishmania* parasites

Akash Tariq[1,2]*, Muhammad Adnan[2], Rahila Amber[3], Kaiwen Pan[1], Sakina Mussarat[2] and Zabta Khan Shinwari[4]

Abstract

Background: Leishmaniasis and malaria are the two most common parasitic diseases and responsible for large number of deaths per year particularly in developing countries like Pakistan. Majority of Pakistan population rely on medicinal plants due to their low socio-economic status. The present review was designed to gather utmost fragmented published data on traditionally used medicinal plants against leishmaniasis and malaria in Pakistan and their scientific validation.

Methods: Pub Med, Google Scholar, Web of Science, ISI Web of knowledge and Flora of Pakistan were searched for the collection of data on ethnomedicinal plants. Total 89 articles were reviewed for present study which was mostly published in English. We selected only those articles in which complete information was given regarding traditional uses of medicinal plants in Pakistan.

Results: Total of 56 plants (malaria 33, leishmaniasis 23) was found to be used traditionally against reported parasites. Leaves were the most focused plant part both in traditional use and in in vitro screening against both parasites. Most extensively used plant families against Leishmaniasis and Malaria were *Lamiaceae* and *Asteraceae* respectively. Out of 56 documented plants only 15 plants (*Plasmodia* 4, *Leishmania* 11) were assessed in vitro against these parasites. Mostly crude and ethanolic plant extracts were checked against *Leishmania* and *Plasmodia* respectively and showed good inhibition zone. Four pure compounds like artemisinin, physalins and sitosterol extracted from different plants proved their efficacy against these parasites.

Conclusions: Present review provides the efficacy and reliability of ethnomedicinal practices and also invites the attention of chemists, pharmacologist and pharmacist to scientifically validate unexplored plants that could lead toward the development of novel anti-malarial and anti-leishmanial drugs.

Keywords: Ethnomedicines, Malaria, Leishmaniasis, Phytochemicals, In vitro activities

Background

Leishmaniasis and malaria are two most common parasitic diseases and infects a large number of human populations worldwide. Leishmaniasis is endemic disease of almost 88 countries in which about 350 million peoples are at risk of infection [1]. Malaria is a major public health problem throughout the world and causes one million deaths per year particularly in developing countries [2].

Leishmaniasis is caused by an obligate intracellular protozoan parasite of genus *Leishmania* while transmitted to humans and other animals by many species of phlebotomus sand flies [3, 4]. The main causative agents for leishmaniasis are *Leishmania tropica*, *Leishmania major*, *Leishmania aethiopica*, *Leishmania donovani* and *Leishmania infantum*. The four main clinical types of leishmaniasis are cutaneous leishmaniasis, mucocutaneous leishmaniasis, diffuse cutaneous leishmaniasis and visceral leishmaniasis. Among these visceral

*Correspondence: atm_bot@hotmail.com
[2] Department of Botany, Kohat University of Science and Technology, Kohat 26000, Pakistan
Full list of author information is available at the end of the article

leishmaniasis is very fatal if left untreated. About 90 % cases of visceral leishmaniasis are reported from many countries like Brazil, Bangladesh, Sudan, India and Nepal [5, 6]. Leishmaniasis is a complex group of diseases produces various symptoms in host depending upon parasite's type [7]. Commonly used allopathic drugs against leishmaniasis are pentavalent antimonials like sodium stibogluconate and meglumine antimoniate etc. These allopathic drugs are mostly unaffordable to the local people and are also not safe due to their toxicity on living system. Many drugs need long term administration to recover from the disease and show side effects depending on the patient's reaction to medicine [8].

Malaria is caused by an intra-erhytrocytic protozoan parasite of the genus *Plasmodium* and transmitted by female anopheles mosquito [9]. The four main species of *Plasmodia* which infects humans are *Plasmodium falciparum, Plasmodium vivax, Plasmodium knowlesi, Plasmodium malariae*, and *Plasmodium ovale*. Globally the most important species is *P. falciparum* causing severe and potentially fatal malaria [2, 10]. For the treatment of malaria many drugs like chloroquine, halofantrine, pyrimethamine, mefloquine, quinine and artemisinin are used [2, 4]. Many problems like resistance of the parasites to drugs, lack of effective vaccines, resistance of mosquito vectors to insecticides and socioeconomic problems rendering treatment of malaria through chemotherapy ineffective [11, 12].

Leishmaniasis and malaria has become a particular problem in the rural areas of Pakistan of all the provinces [13]. Approximately 66 % people of Pakistan live in rural areas [14] and majority of the rural population in Pakistan is poor and cannot afford such expensive drugs for the treatment of leishmaniasis and malaria [15, 16]. Mostly in rural areas peoples depend on medicinal plants for the treatment of various diseases particularly leishmaniasis and malaria [17]. Traditional medicines are extensively using in Pakistan due to easily affordability and efficacy against various diseases [18, 19].

The present review was designed to gather utmost fragmented published literature on anti-malarial and anti-leishmanial plants used by local people in Pakistan. This review will also provide information on in vitro screening and phytochemical investigation of documented plants against these parasites. Future outcomes of this review are to provide evidences regarding the efficacy and reliability of ethnomedicines against *Leishmania* and *Plasmodia* parasites, identify scientific gaps present in current knowledge and to recommend future research areas for the development of effective anti-malarial and anti-leishmanial drugs with fewer side effects.

Methods

This review paper was designed by collecting and consulting large number of mostly published literature on medicinal plants used to treat leishmaniasis and malaria in Pakistan. Pub Med, Google Scholar, Web of Science, ISI Web of Knowledge and Flora of Pakistan were searched for the collection of data on ethnomedicinal plants. Plant list and Tropicos were searched for the corrections of plant scientific names, publication authors, synonyms and families. Different search indicators like ethnomedicinal plants used against leishmaniasis and malaria, in vitro activity of different medicinal flora of Pakistan, epidemiology of leishmaniasis and malaria in world, prevalence of leishmaniasis and malaria in Pakistan, drug resistance potential of *Leishmania* and *Plasmodia* parasites were used for the collection of data from the database. Total 89 articles were reviewed for present study which was mostly published in English. We selected only those articles in which complete information was given regarding traditional use of medicinal plants in Pakistan. In-vitro activity of those plants has been mentioned which were checked against *Leishmania and plasmodia* parasites. On the bases of selected data from literature, three tables were formulated using Microsoft Excel 2007 and Microsoft Word 2007. Tables 1 and 2 were formulated on medicinal plants used to treat leishmaniasis and malaria in Pakistan. These tables contains plant name, family, local name, part used, study area and phytochemistry. Table 3 was formulated on anti-parasitic activity of medicinal plants against *L. tropica, L. major* and *P. falciparum*. Concentration of plant's extract (µg/ml) and their inhibition (%) against parasites were also mentioned. Pure compounds isolated from ethnomedicinal plants and assessed against these parasites have also been mentioned in this review article. Chemical structures of compounds were drawn using ChemDraw software and shown in (Figs. 1, 2 and 3) (CambridgeSoft\ChemOffice2004\ChemDraw).

Medicinal plants used to treat leishmaniasis in Pakistan

Leishmaniasis is a neglected tropical disease. Visceral leishmaniasis and cutaneous leishmaniasis are the two main clinical types of leishmaniasis widespread in Pakistan. The incidence of visceral leishmaniasis has been reported from Dera Ismail Khan, Quetta, Tank, Hazara Division, Northern areas and Azad Jammu Kashmir [20]. About 90 % cases of cutaneous leishmaniasis have been reported from all the provinces of Pakistan [21]. The reported endemic areas of cutaneous leishmaniasis are Dir, Chitral, Swat, Mansehra, Dera Ghazi khan, Gilgat, Skardu, Abbotabad, Azad Kashmir, Chilas, Rawalpindi,

Table 1 Medicinal plants used to treat leishmaniasis in Pakistan

S. no	Botanical name/family name	Common and or local/name (s)	Part used	Area	Phytochemistry	Citation
1	Aloe vera (L.) Burm.f./Xanthorrhoeaceae (= Aloe barbadense Mill./Liliaceae)	Kuwargandal, Aloe vera	Leaves	Dera Ismail Khan, Kohat	Sitosterol	[61], [25, 57]
2	Asparagus gracilis L./Asparagaceae	Shagandal	Aerial parts	Islamabad	Glycosides, tannins, saponins	[22]
3	Asparagus asiaticus L./Berberidaceae (= Berberis baluchistanica Ahrendt.)	Zarch	Roots	Kalat	Alkaloids, flavonoids, saponins, diterpenes, phenols	[62]
4	Trachyspermum ammi (L.) Sprague/Apiaceae (= Carumcopticum L./Umbelliferae)	Ajwain	Whole plant	Quetta	NA	[48]
5	Citrullus colocynthis L. Schrad/Cucurbitaceae	Bitter apple, Kortuma	Fruits	Nushki	Ursolic acid, cucurbitacin E 2-0-β-D-glucopyranoside and cucurbitacin I 2-0-β-D-glucopyranoside, alkaloids, flavonoids, saponins, tannins, terpenoids, diterpenes, coumarins	[35]
6	Juniperus M.Bieb./Cupressaceae	Juniper	Fresh berries	Ziarat	Alkaloids, flavonoids, saponins, diterpenes, phenols	[37]
7	Jurinea dolomiaea Boiss./Compositae	Nazar zela	Roots	Kohistan	Alkaloids, flavonoids, saponins, terpenoids, phenols	[22]
8	Melia azedarach L./Meliaceae	Neem, Chinaberry tree, Persian lilac	Green fruits	Islamabad	Phenols	[21]
9	Nepeta praetervisa Rech.f./Lamiaceae	Simsok	Leaves	Kalat	Carbohydrate, tannins, phenols, alkaloids, flavonoids, diterpenes, quinones, cardiac glycosides, terpenoids, triterpenoids, coumarins	[63]
10	Onosma griffithii Vatke/Boraginaceae	Golden drop	Whole Plant	Malakand	NA	[64]
11	Perotis hordeiformisNees ex Hook. &Arn./Poaceae	Kikuyu grass	Leaves	Soorab	Alkaloids, flavonoids, saponins, diterpenes, phenols	[65]
12	Physalis minima L./Solanaceae	Pygmy Ground cherry, Gooseberry	Whole plant	Karachi	Physalins	[66]
13	Rhazya stricta Decne./Apocynaceae	Aizwarg	Leaves	Nushki	Alkaloids, flavonoids, saponins, diterpenes, phenols	[34]
14	Salvia bucharica Popov/Lamiaceae	Sage, Gul-e-Kakar	Leaves	Quetta	NA	[67]
15	Sarcococca wallichii Stapf/Buxaceae (= Sarcococca coriacea Mull. Arg.)	NA	Roots	Karachi	Steroidal alkaloids	[68]
16	Sarcococca hookeriana Baill./Buxaceae	Sweet box	Whole plant	Karachi	Steroidal alkaloids	[66]
17	Sida cordata L. (Burm.f.) Borss. Waalk./Malvaceae	Simak	Whole plant	Islamabad	Phenols, saponins, flavonoids	[22]
18	Stellaria media L. Vill./Caryophyllaceae	Gander	Whole plant	Islamabad	Glycosides, flavonoids, phenols, saponins, terpenoids	[22]
19	Swertia chirata Roxb ex./Gentianaceae	Chirata	Seeds	D. I. Khan	Amarogentin, amaroswerin, sweroside	[69]
20	Tamarix aphylla (L.) H.Karst./Tamaricaceae	Ghaz, Tamarisk, Salt cedar	Barks	Kohat	NA	[25]
21	Thuspeinanta brahuica (Boiss.) Briq./Lamiaceae	NA	Leaves	Kalat	Alkaloids, flavonoids, saponins, phenols, diterpenes	[70]
22	Tylophora hirsute Wight/Apocynaceae (= Asclepiadaceae)	Damvel	Aerial parts	Malakand	NA	[71]

NA indicates data not available

Table 2 Medicinal plants used to treat malaria in Pakistan

S. no	Botanical name/family name	Common and or local name (s)	Area	Part used	Phytochemistry	Citation
1	*Acacia nilotica* L. (Delile)/Leguminosae (= Fabaceae)	Kikar	Mardan	Leaves	Terpenoids	[72]
2	*Ajuga integrifolia* Buch.-Ham./Lamiaceae (= *Ajugabracteosa* Wall ex Benth./Labiatae)	Rati buti	Maradori valley	Leaves	NA	[73]
3	*Allium cepa* L./Amaryllidaceae (= Liliaceae)	Piaz	Bannu	Bulb	NA	[74]
4	*Artemisia annua* L./Compositae (= Asteraceae)	Afsantin jari, Sweet Wormwood	Northern areas Maradori valley	Whole plant Root	Artemisinin	[75] [75]
5	*Artemisia japonica* Thunb./Compositae (= Asteraceae)	Barmar, Basna Tashang	Northern areas	Whole plant	Artemisinin	[75]
6	*Artemisia maritime* L./Compositae (= Asteraceae)	Tarkh, Zoon, Rooner	Northern areas	Whole plant	Artemisinin	[75]
7	*Artemisia scoparia* Waldst. and Kitam./Compositae (= Asteraceae)	Lungi booti	Bhimber	Flowering shoots	Artemisinin	[76]
8	*Azadirachta indica* A.Juss./Meliaceae	Neem	D. I. Khan	Seeds, Leaves	Limonoid (gedunin)	[73]
9	*Bupleurum longicaule* Wall. ex DC./Apiaceae	Proshi	Maradori valley	Root	NA	[73]
10	*Calotropis procera* (Aiton) Dryand./Apocynaceae (= Asclepiadaceae)	Sodom apple, Mudar, Milk weed	Cholistan desert Karachi	Root	Alkaloids, Flavonoids, Nitrogen, Crude protein, Crude fiber, Soluble phosphates	[77] [16]
11	*Capparis spinosa* L./Capparidaceae	Kaveer	Chitral	Flowers	NA	[78]
12	*Trachyspermum ammi* (L.) Sprague/Apiaceae (= *Carumcopticum* L./Umbelliferae)	Ajwain	Quetta	Whole plant	NA	[48]
13	*Datura stramonium* L./Solanaceae	Jimson weed	Faisalabad	Leaves	Alkaloids, flavonoids, saponins, glycosides, tannic acid, vitamin C, steroids	[79]
14	*Dodonaea viscosa* (L.) Jacq./Sapindaceae	Ghwarasky	Allai valley	Seeds	NA	[80]
15	*Enicostemma hyssopifolium* Willd./Gentianaceae	Chhota Chirayata, Nagajihva	Karachi	Whole plant	NA	[16]
16	*Eucalyptus camaldulensis* Dehnh./Myrtaceae	River red gum	Karachi	Leaves, stem	NA	[16]
17	*Fagonia cretica* L./Zygophyllaceae	Azghakey	Mardan	Leaves	Terpenoids	[72]
18	*Helianthus annuus* L./Compositae (= Asteraceae)	Maera stargay gul, Sunflower	Bannu	Leaves	NA	[74]
19	*Melia azedarach* L./Meliaceae	Neem, Chinaberry Tree	Islamabad	Green fruits	Phenols	[19]
20	*Moringa oleifera* Lam./Moringaceae	Sajna, Marango, Moonja	Faisalabad	Whole plant	NA	[81]
21	*Nerium oleander* L./Apocynaceae	Adelfa, Rose bay	Faisalabad	Leaves	Alkaloids	[79]
22	*Origanum majorana* L./Lamiaceae	Sweet marjoram	Faisalabad	Aerial parts	NA	[36]
23	*Origanum vulgare* L./Lamiaceae	Satar, Pot marjoram	Faisalabad	Aerial parts	NA	[36]

Table 2 continued

S. no	Botanical name/family name	Common and or local name (s)	Area	Part used	Phytochemistry	Citation
24	*Peganum harmala* L./ Nitrariaceae (= Zygo-phyllaceae)	Harmal	Northern areas	Seeds	β-carboline alkaloid (isoharmine), harmaline, harmine	[82]
25	*Polygonatum verticillatum* (L.) All./Asparagaceae	Worlds Solomon's seal	Swat	Aerial parts	α-Bulnesene, Linalyl, acetate, eicosadienoic, docosane, pentacosane, piperitone	[83]
26	*Psidium guajava* L./Myrtaceae	Amrood	Mardan	Leaves	Terpenoids	[72]
27	*Swertia chirata* Roxb ex./ Gentianaceae	Chirata	D. I. Khan	Seeds	Glycosides: Amarogentin, amaroswerin, sweroside	[69]
28	*Swertia paniculata*Wall./ Gentianaceae	Momera	Allaivalley	Whole plant	NA	[80]
29	*Tagete sminuta* L./Compositae(= Asteraceae)	Marigold	Northern areas, Abbotabad	Seeds	Terpenoids, saponins, tannins, flavonoids, alkaloids	[45, 84]
30	*Viburnum nervosum*D. Don/Caprifoliaceae (= Adoxaceae)	NA	Azad Jammu Kashmir	Whole plant	Butilinol, oleanolic acid, butilinic acid, urosolic acid,α-amyrin, β-sitosterol	[85]
31	*Vincetoxicum stocksii* Ali &Khatoon/Apocynaceae (= Asclepiadaceae)	NA	Quetta	Whole plant	NA	[48]
32	*Viola odorata* L./Violaceae	Banafsha	Maradori valley	Whole plant	NA	[73]
33	*Xanthium strumarium* L./ Compositae (= Asteraceae)	Desi Arinad	Allai valley	Leaves	NA	[80]

NA indicates data not available

Khuzdar, Jacobabad, Lasbela, Derabughti, Rajanpur, Quetta, Qila Saifullah, Qila Abdullah, Pishan, Dera Ismail Khan, Larkana and Dadu [22]. These areas are foot hills of mountainous range and situated in North, South and South-Western Pakistan covering about all the provinces including Azad Kashmir. Growth and development of vector sandfly is promoted by the environmental conditions of these endemic areas [23].

Most of the above mentioned regions of Pakistan are rural in nature lacking modern health and education facilities and inhabitants of these regions have low economic status due to least income sources. Moreover, rural people rely on their rich traditional knowledge for their primary health care due to high cost of allopathic drugs [19]. Present review showed that traditional people use 23 medicinal plants belonging to 19 families for the treatment of leishmaniasis (Table 1). Other areas of Pakistan are also known for containing variety of medicinal plants and classic traditional healing practices but scientific documentation has not been yet done. The most widely used plant families for the treatment of leishmaniasis in Pakistan are *Lamiaceae* (four plants), *Liliaceae* (two plants) and *Asclepiadaceae* (two plants). The family

Lamiaceae and *Liliaceae* usually ranks high in ethnomedicinal studies not only in Pakistan but throughout the world [24–26]. Perez et al. [27] also reported high number of plants belonging to *Lamiaceae* family having anti-parasitic activity including leishmaniasis. Present findings indicate that *Lamiaceae* family contains variety of anti-parasitic secondary metabolites and should be given focus in future studies. Other reasons of its wide use might be due to higher abundance of these plants in different regions and strong traditional beliefs [28–30]. Almost all plant parts are found to have anti-leishmanial activity but most preferred parts in Pakistan are leaves, fruits, roots and aerial parts. Leaves are also the most focused part of plant in in vitro screening against leishmaniasis not only in Pakistan but other countries of world [31, 32]. Most of the metabolic processes take place in leaves result in production of different secondary metabolites; therefore, it might be attributed with its wider utilization for in vitro screening and traditional medicines [33]. In some areas like Quetta, Islamabad and Malakand whole plant is used to treat leishmaniasis which is major threat to the conservation status of these medicinal plants. People should be educated regarding

Table 3 In-vitro screening of traditionally used anti-leishmanial and anti-malarial plants against *Leishmania* and *Plasmodia* parasites

Plant name	Part used	Parasite type	Extract	Concentration (µg/ml)	Inhibition (%)	Citation
Aloe vera	Leaves	*Leishmania tropica*	Crude methanol	25	15	[25]
				50	27	
				75	43	
				100	66	
Artemisia annua	Leaves	*Plasmodium falciparum*	Aqueous	0.095	50	[86]
Azadiracha indica	Leaves	*Plasmodium falciparum*	Ethanol	2.4	50	[36]
				2.5	50	
Asparagus asiaticus	Roots	*Leishmania major*	Crude methanol	25	22	[63]
				50	34	
				250	42	
				500	51	
			Amphotericin B (Reference drug as a control)	25	50	
				50	75	
				250	88	
				500	100	
Citrullus colocynthis	Fruits	*Leishmania major*	Crude methanol	25	67	[35]
				50	71	
				250	88	
				500	100	
Juniperus excels	Fresh berries	*Leishmania major*	Crude methanol	25	49	[37]
				50	58	
				250	88	
				500	97	
Melia azedarach	Fruit	*Leishmania tropica*	Aqueous	1500	55.9	[86]
				2500	67.4	
				5000	80.4	
Moringa oleifera	Leaves	*Plasmodium falciparum*	Acetone	400	59.8	[31]
Nepeta praetervisa	Leaves	*Leishmania major*	Methanol	25	39	[62]
				50	54	
				250	68	
				500	78	
Peganum harmala	Seeds	*Plasmodium falciparum*	Ethanol	12.5	91	[58]
				25	97.4	
				50	98.5	
				100	99.8	
			Chloroquine	NA	99.6	
Perotis hordeiformis	Leaves	*Leishmania major*	Methanol	25	47	[65]
				50	58	
				250	70	
				500	80	
			Amphotericin B (Reference drug as a control)	25	50	
				50	75	
				250	88	
				500	100	

Table 3　continued

Plant name	Part used	Parasite type	Extract	Concentration (µg/ml)	Inhibition (%)	Citation
Rhazya stricta	Leaves	*Leishmania major*	Crude methanol	25	65	[34]
				50	70	
				250	92	
				500	100	
Salvia bucharica	Leaves	*Leishmania major*	Crude methanol	25	44	[67]
				50	40	
				250	59	
				500	75	
Tamarix aphylla	Barks	*Leishmania tropica*	Crude methanol	25	20	[25]
				50	28	
				75	54	
				100	84	
Thuspeinanta brahuica	Leaves	*Leishmania major*	Crude methanol	25	40	[87]
				50	58	
				75	70	
				100	82	
			Amphotericin B (Reference drug as a control)	25	50	
				50	75	
				75	88	
				100	100	

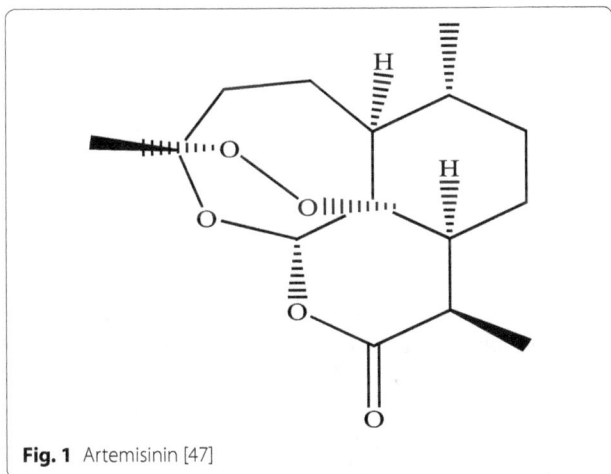

Fig. 1　Artemisinin [47]

proper harvesting of these valuable anti-leishmanial plants for sustainable utilization.

In-vitro activities of anti-leishmanial plants

Majority of the modern allopathic drugs of the world have developed on the basis of traditional knowledge of the people regarding medicinal plants. Among 23 medicinal plants used against leishmaniasis in Pakistan only 11 plants have been studied worldwide for their in vitro activity against *L. major* and *L. tropica* parasites and documented in the present review. Anti-leishmanial activity of medicinal plants has shown excellent activity against *Leishmania* parasite (Table 3). Different plant parts have been used for extract formation experimentally among which leaves, fruits and roots are most widely used parts. This result gives an indication about the reliability of traditional ethnomedicinal knowledge and efficacy of these practices. Different plant extracts like crude methanol and methanol have been used at different concentrations (µg/ml) for their efficacy against *L. major* and *L. tropica* but crude methanol extract is most commonly used [34]. Crude methanol extraction of plant parts is also practiced in other parts of the world. Crude methanolic extract of different plants have shown strong inhibition zone ranges from 65 to 100 % at different concentrations ranging from 25 to 500 µg/ml against *L. major* parasite [34, 35], while methanolic extract of different plant parts having concentration of about 25–500 µg/ml shown optimum inhibition zone ranging from 39 to 80 %. Aqueous extract of a plant have shown inhibition zone ranging from 55.9 to 80.4 % at concentration of about 25–5000 µg/ml [35, 36]. Plant extracts have been proved more effective against leishmaniasis as compared to allopathic drugs due to less toxicity [36]. Therefore it is imperative to investigate and explore medicinal plants scientifically for the development of novel anti-leishmanial drugs of strong efficacy. Experimental investigation of different plants have shown presence of phytochemical constituents such as alkaloids,

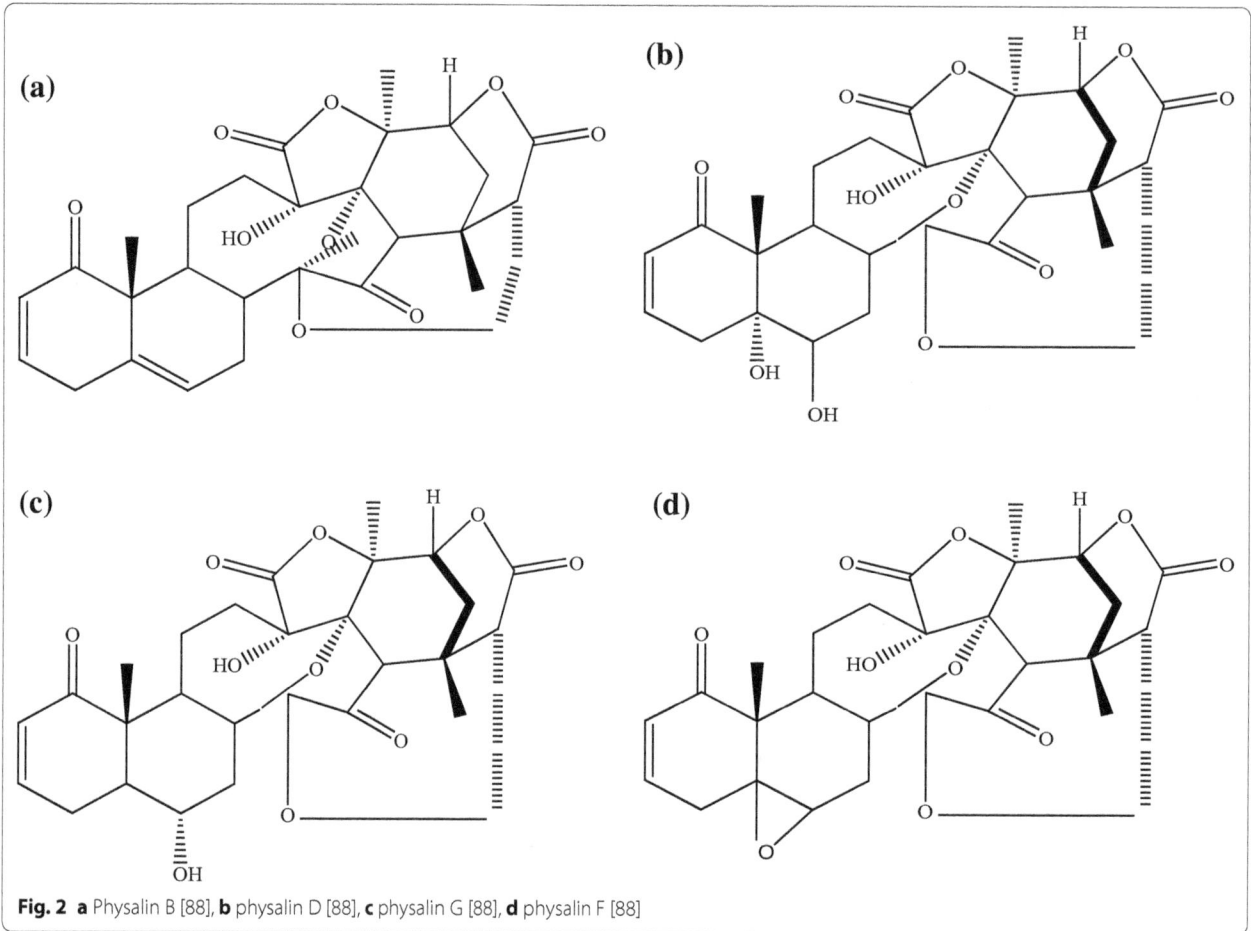

Fig. 2 a Physalin B [88], **b** physalin D [88], **c** physalin G [88], **d** physalin F [88]

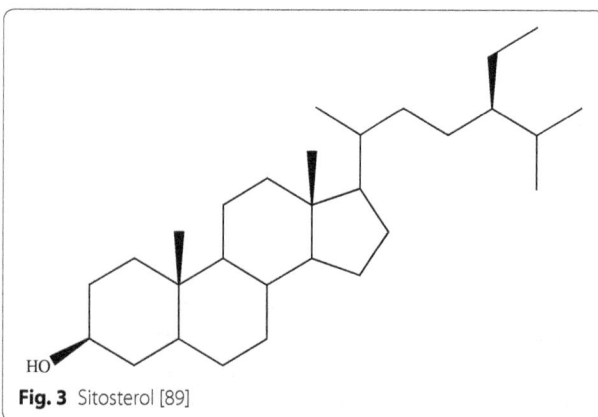

Fig. 3 Sitosterol [89]

flavonoids, carbohydrates, diterpenes, saponins, phenols and tannins that might be responsible for their inhibitory activities against *Leishmania* parasites [36, 37]. Very few studies conducted on the purification of pure compounds from above mentioned plants and should be given focus in future.

Medicinal plants used to treat malaria in Pakistan

In modern medical terms, malaria can be defined as infection caused by red blood cells parasite belonging to genus *Plasmodium*. Malaria is a major serious public health problem caused by *P. falciparum* and *P. vivax*, the two most prevalent *Plasmodium* species throughout the world. Approximately 64 % cases of malaria caused by *P. vivax* and about 36 % cases by *P. falciparum* in Pakistan [38]. According to WHO report about 1.6 million cases of malaria were reported in endemic areas per year [39]. The cases of malaria infection are reported from Sindh, Punjab, Khyber Pakhtunkhwa, Baluchistan and FATA areas. In these regions malaria often occurs in poor people because majority of population in these regions are rural with very low socioeconomic status. The environment of these areas promotes optimum growth of female Anopheles vector [40]. Reason behind high prevalence of malaria in poor people of Pakistan might be due to that malaria strike in the season when economic conditions are more difficult for the people. In Brazil 99 % malarial cases are reported and transmitted in Amazon region, where population consists of tribal people and immigrants from other regions [40]. History has proven traditional medicines to be the best source of effective anti-malarial e.g. *Cinchona* spp. and *Artemisia annua* L. [41].

Chloroquine is the most commonly used antibiotic for the treatment of malaria not only in Pakistan but throughout the world [38]. Low income status of poor people and emergence of antibiotic resistance of parasite encourage the use of traditional medicines for the treatment of malaria. Ethnomedicinal used of plants are common throughout the world including Pakistan [42]. Present review documented 33 anti-malarial plants traditional being use in Pakistan (Table 2). The most widely used plant families for the treatment of malaria in Pakistan are *Asteraceae* (9 plants), *Gentianaceae*, *Lamiaceae* and *Asclepiadaceae* (3 plants each). The medicinal plants belonging to these families are extremely used for medicinal purposes including anti-malarial purposes not only in Pakistan but throughout the world [43–45] that might be due to greater availability or high traditional values of these plants in different regions. Traditional healers mostly used leaves for the preparation of ethnomedicinal recipes against malaria and these findings are not surprising because leaves are the most focused plant part throughout the world [44, 46]. In different regions of Pakistan mostly whole plant is used for the treatment of malaria due to the presence of important compounds. It is considered to be one of the major causes of extinction of highly valuable medicinal plants in many areas of Pakistan.

In-vitro activities of anti-malarial plants

In present review, among 33 medicinal plants used to treat malaria in Pakistan, only 4 plants have been investigated experimentally throughout the world for their in vitro activity against *P. falciparum* (Table 3). Only two plant parts, seeds and leaves have been used for extract preparation. Different plant extracts like acetone, aqueous and ethanol have been used scientifically at different concentrations (μg/ml) for their efficacy against *P. falciparum* [32, 37, 47]. Ethanol extraction of plants is also followed throughout the world due to its polar nature [42]. Ethanolic extracts of two different plants like *Azadiracha indica* and *Peganum harmala* have shown strong inhibition zone ranging from 50 to 99.8 % at concentration of about 2.4–100 μg/ml against *P. falciparum*. Acetone extract of *Artemisia annua* show 50 % inhibition zone at concentration of about 0.095 μg/ml and aqueous extracts of *Moringa oleifera* show optimum inhibition zone 59.8 % at concentration of 400 μg/ml. These results show the strong efficacy of plants extracts against *P. falciparum* in comparison with standard drug. Phytochemical

screening of different plant extracts have not been studied in detail but experimentally studied plant parts mostly contain alkaloids, flavonoids, saponins, tannins and terpenoids that might be responsible for anti-parasitic activities of these plants. Other plants needs in vitro exploration and phytochemical screening that could lead toward extraction of some novel compounds/drugs against *Plasmodium* parasite.

Medicinal plants with both anti-leishmanial and anti-malarial potential

Three plants *Melia azedarach* L. (*Meliaceae*), *Vincetoxicum stocksii* L. (*Asclepiadaceae*) and *Carum copticum* L. (*Umbelliferae*) have been used for the treatment of both leishmaniasis and malaria which show their high potential for anti-parasitic activity [19, 48]. But in vitro activity of only one plant *M. azedarach* has been investigated experimentally against *Leishmania* parasite. Aqueous extract of fruit of *M. azedarach* showed strong inhibition zone of about 55.9, 67.4 and 80.4 % against *L. tropica* at three different concentrations 1500, 2500 and 5000 μg/ml, respectively (Table 3). Present finding is very interesting because it gives an indication about strong efficacy of these candidate medicinal plants for future research against malaria.

Active phyto-compounds against *Leishmania* and *Plasmodia* parasites

Only three compounds isolated from traditionally used anti-leishmanial and anti-malarial plants of Pakistan were investigated for their anti-parasitic activity.

Artemisinin

In present review four plant species of *Artemisia* used in Pakistan to treat malaria (Table 2). The genus *Artemisia* has great importance in pharmaceutics as it is used in traditional medicines to treat various diseases especially malaria not only in Pakistan but throughout the world [49–51]. In-vitro study of *Artemisia* plants shows that they contain an important chemical compound Artemisinin, Sesquiterpenoid lactone. Artemisinin (Fig. 1) is extracted from the leaves of *Artemisia* and known to have best antimalarial activity. WHO recommended the Artemisinin combination therapy for the treatment of malaria caused by *P. falciparum* [2, 52]. *Artemisia annua*, a good source of Artemisinin is endemic plant of China and used as folk medicine to treat malaria for about 2000 years [52]. Artemisinin have also been reported for good antiviral, anti-cancer and anti-leishmanial activity [53].

Physalins

Several physalins (Steroidal lactone) were isolated from various species of genus *Physalis* belonging to the family

Solanaceae. Physalins (Fig. 2) have both anti-leishmanial and anti-malarial potential [54, 55]. Four types of physalins B, D, G and F (Fig. 2a–d) were isolated from *Physalis angulata*. The in vitro and in vivo activity of physalins B and F showed potent anti-leishmanial activity against various *Leishmania* parasites like *L. brazillenesis, L. amazonensis, L. major* and *L. chagasi* [55, 56]. Physalins B, D, G and F have also been reported for their anti-malarial activity against *P. falciparum* [54].

Sitosterol

Aloe barbadense is an important medicinal plant having bioactive compounds reported for their anti-leishmanial activity. Sitosterol (Fig. 3) is an important compound extracted from the leaves of *Aloe vera*. It inhibits the growth of promastigotes of *L. donovani*, a causative agent for life threatening visceral leishmaniasis disease. The active components of *Aloe vera* target the CDC42 protein in comparison with a natural inhibitor Sacramine B [57].

Antibiotic resistance of *Leishmania* and *Plasmodia* parasites

Literature review showed that both *Leishmania* and *Plasmodium* parasites have shown resistance to various antibiotics that are being used for the treatment of leishmaniasis and malaria. Various antibiotics have been used for the treatment of malaria worldwide like chloroquine, halofantrine, pyrimethamine, mefloquine, quinine and artemisinin [2, 4]. The in vitro investigation of chloroquine showed resistance range from 69.8 to 99.6 % against *P. falciparum* [58, 59].

The most commonly used drugs for the treatment of leishmaniasis are pentavalent antimonials like sodium stibogluconate and meglumine antimoniate. Beside these many other drugs like amphotericin, ambisome (lipid formulation of amphotericin), miltefosine (impavido), pentamidine and paromomycin were discovered to treat leishmaniasis [60]. All types of *Leishmania* parasites show resistance against one drug or other [19, 60]. Due to emerging potential of drug resistance of parasites, high cost of allopathic drugs and their side effects encourages the use of traditional medicines among local population worldwide.

Conclusions and future recommendations

Pakistan has tremendous potential regarding the use of ethnomedicines for the treatment of multiple diseases including malaria and leishmaniasis. This review provides a scientific rationale for the traditional uses of medicinal plants against these diseases. Traditional healers of different regions have strong knowledge to utilize medicinal plants. In-vitro screening of traditionally used anti-parasitic plants have proven the efficacy of such plants. Crude

plant extracts, methanolic and other extracts were effective in antimalarial and anti-leishmanial activities. Mostly, leaves of documented plants are traditionally used and also for in vitro screening. Different classes of compounds exist in the documented plants including alkaloids, flavonoids and terpenoids. Very few compounds have so far been isolated from the documented plants and tested in vitro against studied leishmanial and malarial parasites. In pure compounds, ursolic acid and cucurbitacin in *C. colocynthis* while glycosides and alkaloids isolated from *R. stricta* possess anti-leishmanial activities. On the other side, compounds such as limonoids (gedunin) from *A. indica* while β-carboline alkaloids, Harmaline and Harmine isolated from *P. harmala* have proven in vitro and in vivo anti-plasmodial activities. Hence, these plant species must be explored for the identification of more such compounds to be used against *Leishmania* and *Plasmodium* parasites. Moreover in the present era, parasites are showing resistance to common allopathic drugs, while on the other side medicinal plants have proven their effectiveness as anti-parasitic drugs. It is therefore imperative to conduct future studies on the unexplored documented plants both in vitro and in vivo for the development of novel drugs. On the basis of findings in this review, following recommendations are suggested:

- Ethnomedicinal studies provide baseline information for future scientific research, therefore it is recommended to expedite exploration of anti-parasitic plants not only in Pakistan but throughout the world.
- Traditional healers mostly use *Lamiaceae* and *Asteraceae* families for the treatment of leishmaniasis and malaria, respectively. It invites the attention of worldwide researchers to explore species belonging to these families both phytochemically and pharmacologically.
- Among all plant parts, leaves have taken more focus both in traditional medicines as well as in in vitro studies. Other plant parts should also be brought under the spotlight for the potential discovery of different compounds.
- Different extracts of documented plants have been used worldwide against leishmaniasis and *Plasmodia*. Crude extracts have been given more preference against leishmaniasis while only very few plants have been tested in vitro against *Plasmodia*. Extracts like methanolic, ethanolic, n-hexane should also be valued against both parasites that could be helpful in extraction of some novel compounds.
- More attention should be given towards the isolation of pure compounds from these plants, and their in vitro investigations against leishmanial and malarial parasites.

- In-vivo studies should also be brought under the focus in order to pharmacologically validate these traditional plants.
- Action mechanism of different extracts and pure compounds on the studied parasites should also be studied in future research.
- Toxicity of these plants should also be tested on living system that would be helpful in proving the reliability of traditional medicines.

Abbreviations
WHO: World health organization; FATA: Federally Administered Tribal Areas.

Authors' contributions
All authors contributed to this work. All authors have read and approved the final manuscript.

Author details
[1] Key Laboratory of Mountain Ecological Restoration and Bioresource Utilization & Ecological Restoration Biodiversity Conservation Key Laboratory of Sichuan Province, Chengdu Institute of Biology, Chinese Academy of Sciences, Chengdu 610041, China. [2] Department of Botany, Kohat University of Science and Technology, Kohat 26000, Pakistan. [3] Department of Zoology, Kohat University of Science and Technology, Kohat 26000, Pakistan. [4] Department of Biotechnology, Quaid-i-Azam University Islamabad, Islamabad 44000, Pakistan.

Acknowledgements
The authors are indebted to all those who worked and are currently working on various aspects related to the prevention of Malaria and Leishmaniasis.

Competing interests
The authors declare that they have no competing interests.

References
1. Ngurea PK, Kimutaib A, Zipporah W, Rukungad G, Tonui WK. A review of Leishmaniasis in Eastern Africa. J Nanjing Med U. 2009;23:79–86.
2. Shahinas D, Folefoc A, Pillai DR. Targeting *Plasmodium falciparum* Hsp90: towards reversing antimalarial resistance. Pathogens. 2013;2:33–54.
3. Pradeep D, Steven S, Philippe D, Atul M, Roshan T, Niyamat AS, Dipika S, Arvind P, Rhonda S. Annual incidence of visceral leishmaniasis in an endemic area of Bihar, India. Trop Med Int Health. 2010;10:1365.
4. Nahrevanian H, Milan BS, Kazemi M, Hajhosseini R, Mashhadi SS, Nahrevanian S. Antimalarial Effects of Iranian Flora *Artemisia sieberi* on *Plasmodium berghei* In vivo in mice and phytochemistry analysis of its herbal extracts. Malar Res Treat. 2012. doi:10.1155/2012/727032.
5. Uzun S, Uslular C, Yucel A, Acar MA, Ozpoyraz M, Memisoglu HR. Cutaneous leishmaniasis evaluation of 3074 cases in Cukurova region of Turkey. Br J Dermatol. 1999;140:347–50.
6. Alavi-Naini R, Fazaeli A, Dempsey OT. Topical treatment modalities for old world cutaneous leishmaniasis: a review. Prague Med Rep. 2012;113:105–18.
7. Zand M, Narasu ML. Vaccination against leishmaniasis. Ann Biol Res. 2013;4:170–4.
8. Croft SL, Coombs GH. Leishmaniasis-current chemotherapy and recent advances in the search for novel drugs. Trends Parasitol. 2003;19:502–8.
9. Hardman JG, Limbird LE. Drugs used in the chemotherapy of malaria in The Goodman and Gilman's Pharmacologicalbases of Therapeutics. 10th ed. New York: McGraw-Hill; 2001.
10. Leslie T, Mikhail A, Mayan I, Cundill B, Anwar M, Bakhtash SH, Mohammed N, Rahman H, Zekria R, Christopher JMW. Mark Rowland Rapid diagnostic tests to improve treatment of malaria and other febrile illnesses: patient randomised effectiveness trial in primary care clinics in Afghanistan. Br Med J. 2014;348:1–13.
11. Fidock DA, Rosenthal PJ, Croft SL, Brun R, Nwaka S. Antimalarial drug discovery: efficacy models for compound screening. Nat Rev Drug Discov. 2004;3:509–20.
12. Douradinha B, Doolan DL. Harnessing immune responses against *Plasmodium* for rational vaccine design. Trends Parasitol. 2011;27:274–83.
13. Bhutto AM, Soomro RA, Nonaka S, Hashiguchi Y. Detection of new endemic areas of cutaneous leishmaniasis in Pakistan: a 6-year study. Int J Dermatol. 2003;42:543–8.
14. Ikram AU, Zahra NB, Shinwari ZK, Qaiser M. Ethnomedicinal review of folklore medicinal plants belonging to family Apiaceae of Pakistan. Pak J Bot. 2015;47:1007–14.
15. Tiuman TS, Santos AO, Nakamura TU, Filho BPD, Nakamura CV. Recent advances in Leishmaniasis treatment. Int J of Infect Dis. 2011;15:525–32.
16. Qasim M, Abideen Z, Adnan MY, Ansari R, Gul B, Khan MA. Traditional ethno-botanical uses of medicinal plants from coastal areas of Pakistan. J Coastal Life Med. 2014;2:22–30.
17. Jeruto P, Lukhoba C, Ouma G, Otieno D, Mutai C. An ethnobotanical study of medicinal plants used by the Nandi people in Kenya. J Ethnopharmacol. 2008;116:370–6.
18. Shah SMH, Shah SMM, Nisar M, Khan FA, Ali M. Khanl. Antimicrobial activities of medicinal plants used in folk remedies in Pakistan. J Pharm Res. 2012;5:2057–60.
19. Khan I, Yasinzai MM, Mehmood Z, Ilahi I, Khan J, Khalil AT, Saqib MS, Rahman WU. Comparative study of green fruit extract of *Melia azedarach* Linn. with its ripe fruit extract for antileishmanial, larvicidal, antioxidant and cytotoxic activity. Am J Phytomed. Clin Ther. 2014;2:442–54.
20. Kakarsulemankhel JK. Leishmaniasis in Pak-Afghan Region. Int J Agric Biol. 2011;13:611–20.
21. Ali N, Afrin F. Protection of mice against Visceral Leishmaniasis by immunization with promastigotes antigen incorporated in liposomes. J Parasitol. 1997;83:70–5.
22. Shah NA, Khan MR, Nadhman A. Antileishmanial, toxicity, and phytochemical evaluation of medicinal plants collected from Pakistan. BioMed Res Int. 2014. doi:10.1155/2014/384204.
23. Durrani AZ, Durrani HZ, Kamal N. Prevalence of *Leishmania* in sandfly in Pakistan. Pak J Zool. 2012;44:61–5.
24. Nasir E, Ali SI. Flora of Pakistan, vol. 175. Karachi: Fakhri Printing Press; 1986. p. 200.
25. Iqbal H, Khattak B, Ayaz S, Rehman A, Ishfaq M. Comparative efficacy of *Aloe vera* and *Tamarix aphylla* against cutaneous leishmaniasis. Int J Basic Med Sci Pharm. 2012;2:42–5.
26. Serakta M, Djerrou Z, Djaalab HM, Riachi FK, Hamimed S, Trifa W, Belkhiri A, Edikra N, Pacha YH. Antileishmanial activity of some plants growing in Algeria *Juglans Regia, Lawsonia Inermis* and *Salvia Officinalis*. Afr J Trad Complem Altern Med. 2013;10:427–30.
27. Perez SG, Ramos-lopez MA, Sanchez-miranda E, Fresan-Orozoco MC, Perez-Ramos J. Antiprotozoa activity of some essential oils. J Med Plants Res. 2012;6:2901–8.
28. Kirtikar KR, Basu BD. Indian medicinal plants. Allahad: Indian Press; 1981. p. 1031.
29. Weiner M, Weiner JA. Herbs that heal. Mill Valley. 1994;75:270–2.
30. Ali MI, Shalaby NM, Elgamal MH, Mousa AS. Antifungal effects of different plant extracts and their major components of selected *Aloe* species. Phytother Res. 1999;13:401–7.
31. Patel JP, Gami B, Patel K. Evaluation of in vitro Schizonticidal properties of acetone extract of Some Indian medicinal plants. Adv Biol Res. 2010;4:253–8.
32. Adebayoa JO, Krettli AU. Potential antimalarials from Nigerian plants: a review. J Ethnopharmacol. 2011;133:289–302.
33. Murad W, Azizullah A, Adnan M, Tariq A, Khan KU, Waheed S, Ahmed A. Ethnobotanical assessment of plant resources of Banda Daud Shah, District Karak. Pakistan. J Ethnobiol Ethnomed. 2013;9:1–10.

34. Khan MJ, Baloch NU, Nabi S, Ahmed N, Bazai Z, Yasinzai M, Yasser MSA, Kahraman A. Antileishmanial, cytotoxic, antioxidant activities and phytochemical analysis of *Rhazya stricta* Decne leaves extracts and its fractions. Asian J Plant Sci Res. 2012;2:593–8.

35. Baloch N, Nabi S, Kakar AM, Wajid Z, Alkharaman YMSA. In-vitro antileishmanial, antitumor, cytotoxic activities and phytochemical analysis of *Citrullus colocynthis* fruit extract. Int J Med Aroma Plants. 2013;3:78–84.

36. Abdullah IH, Farooq A, Shazia R, Poonam SN, Omar J, Satyajit DS. Composition, antioxidant and chemotherapeutic properties of the essentialoils from two *Origanum* species growing in Pakistan. Braz J Pharmacog. 2011;21:943–52.

37. Nabi S, Ahmed S, Khan MJ, Bazai Z, Yasinzai M, Yasser MSA, Kahraman A. In vitro antileishmanial, antitumor activities and phytochemical studies of methanolic extract and its fractions of *Juniperus Excelsa* Berries. World Appl Sci J. 2012;19:1495–500.

38. Khattak AA, Venkatesan M, Khatoon L, Ouattara A, Kenefic LJ, Nadeem MF, Nighat F, Malik SA, Christopher VP. Prevalence and distribution of human *Plasmodium* infection in Pakistan. Malaria J. 2013;12:297.

39. WHO. World malaria report 2012. Geneva: World Health Organization; 2013.

40. Willcox ML, Bodeker G. Traditional herbal medicines for Malaria. Br Med J. 2004;329:1156–9.

41. Willcox ML, Bodeker G, Rasoanaivo P. Traditional medicinal plants and Malaria. Boca Raton: CRC Press; 2004.

42. Mojarrab M, Shiravand A, Delazar A, Afshar, F.H. Evaluation of in vitro antimalarial activity of different extracts of *Artemisia aucheri* Boiss and *A. armeniaca* Lam and fractions of the most potent extracts. Sci World J. 2014. doi: 10.1155/2014/825370.

43. Azas N, Laurencin N, Delmas F, Di GC, Gasquet M, Laget M, Timon-David P. Synergistic in vitro antimalarial activity of plant extracts used as traditional herbal remedies in Mali. Parasitol Res. 2002;88:165–71.

44. Titanji VPK, Zofou DS, Ngemenya MN. The antimalarial potential of medicinal plants used for the treatment of malaria in Cameroonian Folk Medicine. Afr J Trad Complem Altern Med. 2008;5:302–21.

45. Sadia S, Khalid S, Qureshi R, Tagetes Bajwa AA, Minuta L. A useful underutilized plant of family Asteraceae: a Review. Pak J Weed Sci Res. 2013;19:179–89.

46. Luize PS, Tiuman TS, Morello LG, Maza PK, Nakamura TU, Filho PBD, Cortez DAG, Mello JCP, Nakamura CV. Effects of medicinal plant extracts on growth of *Leishmania* (L.) *amazonensis* sand *Trypanosoma cruzi*. Braz J Pharma Sci. 2005;41:85–94.

47. Ploypradith P. Development of artemisinin and its structurally simplified trioxane derivatives as antimalarial drugs. Acta Trop. 2004;89:329–42.

48. Mansoor A, Ibrahim MA, Zaidi MA, Ahmed M. Antiprotozoal activities of *Vincetoxicum stocksii* and *Carum copticum*. Bangladesh J Pharmacol. 2011;6:51–4.

49. Arab HA, Rahbari S, Rassouli A, Moslemi MH, Khosravirad F. Determination of artemisinin in *Artemisia sieberi* and anticoccidial effects of the plant extract in broiler chickens. Trop Anim Health Prod. 2006;38:497–503.

50. Romero MR, Serrano MA, Vallejo M, Efferth T, Alvarez M, Marin JJ. Antiviral effect of artemisinin from *Artemisia annua* against a model member of the Flaviviridae family, the bovine viral diarrhea virus (BVDV). Planta Med. 2006;72:1169–74.

51. Willoughby JA, Sundar SN, Cheung M, Tin MA, Modiano J, Firestone GL. Artemisinin blocks prostate cancer growth and cell cycle progression by disrupting Sp1 interactions with the cyclin-dependent kinase-4 (CDK4) promoter and inhibiting CDK4 gene expression. J Biol Chem. 2009;284:2203–13.

52. Mannan A, Ahmed I, Arshad W, Asim MF, Qureshi RA, Hussain I, Mirza B. Survey of artemisinin production by diverse *Artemisia* species in northern Pakistan. Malar J. 2010;9:310.

53. Sen R, Bandyopadhyay S, Dutta A, Mandal G, Ganguly S, Saha P, Chatterjee M. Artemisinin triggers induction of cell-cycle arrest and apoptosis in *Leishmania donovani* promastigotes. J Med Microbiol. 2007;56:1213–8.

54. Guimarães ET, Lima MS, Santos LA, Ribeiro IM, Tomassini TBC, Santos RR, Milena BPS. Effects of seco-steroids purified from *Physalis angulata* L., Solanaceae, on the viability of *Leishmania* sp. Braz J Pharmacog. 2010;20:945–9.

55. Elisalva T. Guimara, Milena S, Lima, Luana A, Santos, Ivone M, Ribeiro, Therezinha BC, Tomassini, Santos RR, Washington LC, Santos, Milena BPS. Activity of physalins purified from *Physalis angulata* in in vitro and in vivo models of cutaneous leishmaniasis. J Antimicrob Chemother. 2009;64:84–7.

56. Matheus SS, Menezes MND, Krettli AU, Ribeiro IM, Tomassini TC, Santos RR, Azevedo WF, Soares MB. Antimalarial activity of physalins B, D, F, and G. J Nat Prod. 2011;74:2269–72.

57. Priyanka BM, Vennila J, Ganesh S. An in-silicoapproach to identify drug targetable protein in visceral leishmaniasis using GC MS extracted active components from *Aloe vera*. Adv Appl Sci Res. 2011;2:426–31.

58. Nateghpour M, Sharbatkhori M, Edrissian GH, Souri E, Mohebali M, Akbarzadeh K, Haghi AM, Satvat M, Rahimi A. Assessment of in vitro activity of *Peganum harmala* extract on *Plasmodium falciparum* growth compared with chloroquine. Pak J Biol Sci. 2006;9:214–6.

59. Olasehinde GI, Ojurongbe O, Adeyeba AO. In-vitro studies on the sensitivity pattern of *Plasmodium falciparum* to anti-malarial drugs and local herbal extract. Malar J. 2014;13:63.

60. Monzote L. Current treatment of leishmaniasis. Open Antimicrob Agents J. 2009;1:9–19.

61. Marwat SK, Rehman FU, Khan MA, Ahmad M, Zafar M, Ghulam S. Medicinal folk recipes used as traditional phytotherapies in District Dera Ismail Khan. KPK Pakistan. Pak J Bot. 2011;43:1453–62.

62. Baloch N, Nabi S, Yasser MSA, Kahraman A. In-vitro antileishmanial, cytotoxic, antioxidant activities and phytochemical analysis of *Berberis baluchistanica* roots extracts and its fractions. J Phytopharmacog. 2013;4:282–7.

63. Baloch N, Nabi S, Bashir S, Yasser MSA, Kahraman A. In-vitro antileishmanial, cytotoxic activity and phytochemical analysis of *Nepeta praetervisa* leaves extract and its fractions. Int J Pharm Pharma Sci. 2013;5:475–8.

64. Ahmad B, Ali N, Bashir S, Choudhary MI, Azam S, Khan I. Parasiticidal, antifungal and antibacterial activities of *Onosma griffithii* Vatke. Afr J Biotechnol. 2009;8:5084–7.

65. Baloch N, Nabi S, Yasser MSA, Kahraman A. In-vitro antileishmanial, cytotoxic, antioxidant activities and their phytochemical analysis on methanolic extract and it is fractions of *Perotis hordeiformis* leaves. Int J Pharma Sci Rev Res. 2013;22:191–5.

66. Rahman AU. Samreen, Wahab A, Choudhary MI. Discovery of leishmanicidal agents from medicinal plants. Pure Appl Chem. 2008;80:1783–90.

67. Khan A, Khan MJ. *In vitro* antileishmanial, cytotoxic and antioxidant activities of *Salvia bucharica* leaves extract and its fractions. Int J Basic Appl Sci. 2013;13:74–8.

68. Choudhary MI, Adhikri A, Rehman AU. Antileishmanial steroidal alkaloids from roots of *Sarcococca coriacea*. J Chem Soc Pak. 2010;32:799–802.

69. Sher A. Antimicrobial activity of natural products from medicinal plants. Gomal J Med Sci. 2009;7:1–4.

70. Kakar AM, Khan AA, Nabi S, Kakar MA, Yasinzai M, Ymsa AK. *In vitro* antileishmanial, cytotoxic activity and phytochemical analysis of *Thuspeinanta Brahuica* leaves extract and its fractions. Int J Biol Pharm Appl Sci. 2013;2:520–8.

71. Bashir A, Ali N, Bashir S, Choudhary MI. Biological activities of aerial parts of *Tylophora hirsuta* Wall. Afr J Biotechnol. 2009;8:4627–31.

72. Wadood A, Ghufran M, Jamal SB, Naeem M, Khan A, Ghaffar R. Asnad. Phytochemical analysis of medicinal plants occurring in local area of Mardan. Biochem. Anal Biochem. 2013;2:1–4.

73. Ishtiaq M, Ahmed F, Maqbool M, Hussain T. Ethnomedicinal inventory of flora of Maradori Valley, district Forward Khahuta, Azad Kashmir. Pakistan. Am J Res Commun. 2013;1:239–61.

74. Khan RU, Mehmood S, Khan SU, Jaffar F. Ethnobotanical study of food value flora of district Bannu Khyber Pakhtunkhwa. Pakistan. J Med Plant Stud. 2013;1:93–106.

75. Hayat MQ, Khan MA, Ashraf M, et al. Ethnobotany of the Genus *Artemisia* L. (Asteraceae) in Pakistan. Ethnobot Res Appl. 2009;7:147–62.

76. Mahmood A, Mahmood A, Hussain I, Jabeen S. Indigenous medicinal knowledge of medicinal plants of Barnala area district Bhimber. Pakistan. Int J Med Arom Plants. 2011;1:294–301.

77. Azhar MF, Siddique MT, Ishaque M, Tanveer A. Study of ethnobotany and indigenous use of *Calotropis Procera* (Ait.) in Cholistan desert, Punjab. Pak J Agric Res. 2014;52:117–26.

78. Hadi F, Razzaq A, Rahman AU, Rashid A. Ethnobotanical notes on woody plants of Rech Valley, Torkhow, district Chitral, Hindu-Kush range, Pakistan. Scholarly J Agric Sci. 2013;3:468–72.

79. Zafar F, Jahan N, Rahman KU, Zafar WUI, Aslam S. Comparative evaluation of phytochemical, mineral and vitamin contents of Gemmo modified extracts and leaves of two indigenous medicinal plants. Int J Agric Biol. 2014;16:911–6.

80. Haq F. The ethno botanical uses of medicinal plants of Allai Valley, Western Himalaya Pakistan. Int J Plant Res. 2012;2:21–34.

81. Fatima T, Sajid MS, Hassan MJU, Siddique RM, Iqbal Z. Phytomedicinal value of *Moringa oleifera* with special reference to antiparasitics. Pak J Agric Sci. 2014;51:251–62.

82. Afzal S, Afzal N, Awan MR, Khan TS, Gilani A, Khanum R, Tariq S. Ethnobotanical studies from Northern Pakistan. J Ayub Med Coll Abbottabad. 2009;21:52–7.

83. Khan H, Saeed M, Muhammad N, Tariq SA, Ghaffar R, Gul F. Antimalarial and free radical scavenging activities of aerial parts of *Polygonatum Verticillatum* (L.) All and identification of chemical constituents by Gc-Ms. Pak J Bot. 2013;45:497–500.

84. Shahzadi I, Hassan A, Ummara W, Khan UW, Shah MM. Evaluating biological activities of the seed extracts from *Tagetes minuta* L. found in Northern Pakistan. J Med Plants Res. 2010;4:2108–12.

85. Awan ZI, Rehman HU, Minhas FA, Awan AA. Antiplasmodial activity of compounds isolated from *Viburnum nervosum*. Int J Pharma Sci Invent. 2013;2:19–24.

86. Gueye PEO, Diallo M, Deme AB. Tea *Artemisia annua* inhibited by *Plasmodium falciparum* isolates collected in Pikine. Senegal. Afr J Biochem Res. 2013;7:107–13.

87. Kakar AM, Khan AA, Nabi S, Kakar MA, Yasinzai M, Al-Kahraman YMSA. In-vitro Antileishmanial, Cytotoxic Activity and Phytochemical Analysis of *Thuspeinanta brahuica* leaves extract and its fractions. IJPBAS. 2013;2:520–8.

88. Soares MBP, Brustolim D, Santos LA, Bellintani MC, Paiva FP, Ribeiro YM, Tomassini TCB, Santos RRD. Physalins B, F and G, seco-steroids purified from *Physalis angulata* L., inhibit lymphocyte function and allogeneic transplant rejection. Int J Immunopharmacol. 2006;6:408–14.

89. Chaturvedula VSP, Prakash I. Isolation of Stigmasterol and β-Sitosterol from the dichloromethane extract of *Rubus suavissimus*. Int Curr Pharm J. 2012;1(9):239–42.

17

Patients with community-acquired bacteremia of unknown origin: clinical characteristics and usefulness of microbiological results for therapeutic issues: a single-center cohort study

Johan Courjon[1,2]*[iD], Elisa Demonchy[1], Nicolas Degand[3], Karine Risso[1], Raymond Ruimy[2,3,4] and Pierre-Marie Roger[1,2]

Abstract

Bacteremia of unknown origin (BUO) are associated with increased mortality compared to those with identified sources. Microbiological data of those patients could help to characterize an appropriate empirical antibiotic treatment before bloodcultures results are available during sepsis of unknown origin. Based on the dashboard of our ward that prospectively records several parameters from each hospitalization, we report 101 community-acquired BUO selected among 1989 bacteremic patients from July 2005 to April 2016, BUO being defined by the absence of clinical and paraclinical infectious focus and no other microbiological samples retrieving the bacteria isolated from blood cultures. The in-hospital mortality rate was 9%. We retrospectively tested two antibiotic associations: amoxicillin–clavulanic acid + gentamicin (AMC/GM) and 3rd generation cephalosporin + gentamicin (3GC/GM) considered as active if the causative bacteria was susceptible to at least one of the two drugs. The mean age was 71 years with 67% of male, 31 (31%) were immunocompromised and 52 (51%) had severe sepsis. Eleven patients had polymicrobial infections. The leading bacterial species involved were *Escherichia coli* 25/115 (22%), group D *Streptococci* 12/115 (10%), viridans *Streptococci* 12/115 (10%) and *Staphylococcus aureus* 11/115 (9%). AMC/GM displayed a higher rate of effectiveness compared to 3GC/GM: 100/101 (99%) vs 94/101 (93%) (p = 0.04): one *Enterococcus faecium* strain impaired the first association, *Bacteroides* spp. and *Enterococcus* spp. the second. In case of community-acquired sepsis of unknown origin, AMC + GM should be considered.

Keywords: Bacteremia, Empirical antibiotic treatment, Severe sepsis, Bacteremia of unknown origin, Antimicrobial resistance, Primary bacteremia

Background

Bacteremia is defined by the presence of viable bacterial agent in the bloodstream and is diagnosed in daily clinical practice with the use of blood cultures. The annual incidence of community-onset bacteremia is evaluated between 40 and 154/100000 [1]. The range of mortality rates is extremely large depending on the occurrence of septic shock, antimicrobial resistance, age, comorbidities and community or healthcare-acquired infections. Bacteremia corresponds to bacterial dissemination through the bloodstream from an initial infectious focus, among which urinary sepsis, pneumonia and intravascular catheter-related infection are the most frequent [2, 3]. Nevertheless, even with an exhaustive diagnostic procedure, this portal of entry sometimes remains unknown.

*Correspondence: courjon.j@chu-nice.fr
[1] Infectious Diseases Department, Hôpital Archet 1, Nice Academic Hospital, Infectiologie 151 Route de St Antoine de Ginestière, 06200 Nice, France
Full list of author information is available at the end of the article

The definitions of BUO vary significantly according to the different authors. In a study of Vallès et al. [4] the absence of a distal source documented is sufficient, whether other authors use a composite criterion [5] combining non-contributing physical exam, lack of microbiological investigations identifying the same bacteria as in bloodcultures and normal radiological exams.

BUO is associated with significant morbidity compared to bacteremic patients with an identified infectious focus [6]. Even in intensive care units (ICU) where huge risk factors as septic shock or ICU scoring systems often overshadow other clinical determinants, BUO has been associated with inappropriate antibiotic treatment [4] and poor outcome [7].

When empirical antibiotic treatment is required, the decision process usually includes the infection focus identified by physical exam or the first radiological results. During BUO, presenting as sepsis of unknown origin, these data are missing and could favour inappropriate antibiotic administration, which is known to increase mortality [8]. Nowadays, the challenge for empirical antibiotic prescription is to combine appropriate antibiotic use and to consider the risk of antimicrobial resistance in the community setting especially for 3rd generation cephalosporin resistant *Enterobacteriaceae* [9].

While studies focusing on BUO are scarce we present herein a cohort of 101 community-acquired BUO seen in our department. This study aims to describe clinical presentation and the main features of patients involved. On the basis of the microbiological results of our cohort we have tested the efficiency of two antibiotic associations which both include a beta-lactam with an aminoglycoside. The main objective is the characterization of a treatment that could be used, by extension, during sepsis of unknown origin.

Patients and method
Patients' selection and ethical approval
This retrospective cohort-study was conducted from July 2005 to April 2016 in the 34-bed infectious diseases department at Nice University Hospital (France). The medical dashboard of our ward records prospectively 28 characteristics of each hospitalization including hospitalization motive, final diagnosis, comorbidities, microbiological data including blood culture and all antibiotics prescribed [10]. Patients are classified regarding the site of infection; in case of bacteremia without any organ infection detected they are included in the BUO group. The dashboard classifies infective endocarditis or spondylodiscitis in other groups. In France no ethical approval is required for non-interventional study. The medical dashboard of the Infectious Diseases Department of Nice

University Hospital is authorized by the French National Commission on Informatics and Liberty (Number of Registration: 1430722). A signed consent form is used in our hospital for each patient in order to enable the use of the clinical data recorded during current care for medical research.

Definition of community-acquired BUO used for the study
The origin of the bacteremia was considered as unknown when clinical and paraclinical data failed to identify any infectious focus and when no other microbiological samples retrieved the bacteria isolated from blood cultures.

Inclusion and non-inclusion criteria
All patients classified in the BUO group were selected. After reviewing all the medical files, patients meeting the definition of community-acquired BUO used for the study were included.

Patients with coagulase-negative *Staphylococci* bacteremia and fungemia were excluded. Because of the difficulty to strictly rule out a cutaneous primary infection in case of chronic ulcers, pressure ulcers or in intravenous drug users, those patients were excluded. Health-care associated infections were also excluded.

Variable of interest
Symptoms leading to the emergency department before hospitalization were collected from the emergency department medical record. Fever was defined as a body temperature ≥ 38.3 °C. Inappropriate empirical treatment referred to an antibiotic administered before the blood cultures results, to which at least one bacteria isolate was resistant. The number of positive blood cultures bottles for each patient was recorded.

Results of the following exams were collected in the medical record: level of C-reactive protein (CRP) and/or procalcitonin (PCT) at day one, thoracic and abdominal CT-Scan, transthoracic and trans oesophageal echocardiography (TTE and TOE) and colonoscopy.

Duration of follow-up was determined by the date of the last visit in our hospital. Follow-up phone call was performed for the patients who did not visit our hospital after the treatment of the BUO in order to identify any recurrence of BUO. Unfavourable outcome included ICU transfer or death during in-hospital care.

Antibiotic combination evaluation
Based on the antimicrobial susceptibility testing, we retrospectively evaluated the efficiency of two antibiotic combinations for the treatment of BUO: amoxicillin–clavulanic acid + gentamicin (AMC/GM) and 3rd generation cephalosporin (cefotaxime or ceftriaxone) + gentamicin (3GC/GM). These associations were

considered as active if the causative bacteria were susceptible to at least one of the two drugs.

Severe sepsis and organ dysfunction

Sever sepsis was defined by the *Surviving Sepsis Cam-
paign*: systolic blood pressure <90 mmHg or mean arte-
rial pressure <70 mmHg, lactate above upper laboratory
limits, PaO_2 < 60 mmHg or pulse oximetry <90% in air,
creatinine >176.8 µmol/L, platelet count <100 G/L or
INR > 1.5, hyperbilirubinemia >70 µmol/L and also
altered mental status.

Microbiological findings

Blood samples were collected in a set of an aerobic and
an anaerobic bottles which were incubated in a BacT/
ALERT 3D (bioMérieux, Marcy l'étoile, France) automated blood culture system for 5 days. Bottles that
showed a positive signal in the BacT/ALERT 3D system
were routinely subjected to Gram staining and subcultured at least on blood agar plates and upon results of
Gram on Drigalski agar or on chocolate agar. Colonies
were identified using the API system (bioMérieux) and,
since 2013, MALDI-TOF MS Microflex LT (Bruker Dal-
tonics GmbH, Bremen, Germany) according to the manufacturer's recommendation. Antimicrobial susceptibility
testing was performed in accordance with the EUCAST
disk diffusion test methodology, as recommended [11].

Statistical analysis

The analysis was performed using StatView®F-4.5. The
relationship between variables were assessed with the
Chi2 test for categorical variables; Fisher's exact test was
used for number of variables <5. Continuous variables
were compared using the Mann–Whitney non-paramet-
ric test. Logistic regression was used for the multivariate
analysis of risk factors associated to in-hospital mortality or ICU transfer during BUO and results are presented
as adjusted odds ratios (AORs) with their 95% confidence
intervals (CIs). Variables were selected as candidates for
the multivariate analysis on the basis of the level of significance of the univariate (p < 0.1). Models were built
up sequentially, starting with the variable most strongly
associated with the outcome and continuing until no
other variable reached significance or altered the odds
ratios of variables already in the model. When the final
model was reached, each variable was dropped in turn to
assess its effect.

Results

Between July 2005 and April 2016 the medical dashboard
recorded 13,576 hospitalizations. A bacteremia was
detected among 1989 (15%) patients with 261/1989 (13%)
classified in the group BUO. After applying the inclusion

criteria to the 261 patients, 101 community-acquired
BUO were retained (Fig. 1). The characteristics of the
population studied are presented in Table 1. Thirty-one
(31%) patients were immunocompromised: 12 with neo-
plasms (diagnosed during the last year), six with cirrhosis, six HIV-infected (two with CD4 T-cells under 200/
mm³), three splenectomized patients, three with immu-
nosuppressor drugs and 1 chronic renal insufficiency
undergoing dialysis.

An antibiotic treatment had been prescribed the month
preceding the BUO in 11/101 (11%) patients. Fever was
detected at day 1 in 99/101 (98%) patients. The median
duration of symptoms leading to the emergency room visit
was 3 days. Severe sepsis was identified in 52/101 (51%)
patients. ICU management was required for 12/101 (12%)
patients. CRP and PCT values at admission were available
in 98/101 (97%) and 47/101 (46%) of the cases respectively.
The CRP value was below 20 mg/L in 17/98 (17%) patients
and PCT value below 0.5 ng/L in 10/47 (21%) patients. A
thoracic and abdominal CT-Scan was performed in 69/101
(68%) patients, colonoscopy in 37/101 (36%), TTE in
56/101 (55%) patients and TOE in 29/101 (28%).

Empirical antibiotic therapy was started in 55/101
(54%) patients and was inadequate in 9/55 (16%) cases.
Empirical antibiotic administration was significantly
associated with occurrence of organ dysfunction (70
vs 39%, p = 0.002). Unfavorable outcome occurred in
17/101 (17%) patients. In case of inadequate antibiotic
there was a trend toward unfavorable outcome (29 vs
13%, p = 0.16). *S. aureus* and diarrhea and/or vomiting
at admission were associated with unfavorable outcome
in multivariable analysis (Table 2). The in-hospital mortality rate was 9% (9/101) during community-acquired
BUO and 6.4% (862/13,475) for all the other patients
hospitalized during the study period. Among the nine
deaths three septic shocks occurred. The median follow-
up duration was 18 months and 13/101 (13%) of patients
were lost to follow up. Recurrence of BUO was observed
in 10/101 (10%) patients including five with bacteria presenting the same antibiotype than the first episode.

At least two blood culture bottles were positive for
94/101 (92%) BUO, eight patients had only one positive
bottle with the following bacteria: 2 *Streptococcus gallo-
lyticus*, 1 *Streptococcus oralis*, 1 *Escherichia coli*, 1 *Enterococcus faecalis*, 1 *Staphylococcus aureus* and 1 *Citrobacter
amalonaticus*. The 115 bacteria involved in the BUO are
presented in Table 3, 11/101 (11%) BUO were polymicrobial. The main species retrieved were *E. coli* 25/115
(22%), group D *Streptococci* 12/115 (10%), viridans *Streptococci* 12/115 (10%) and *S. aureus* 11/115 (9%). AMC/
GM displayed a higher rate of effectiveness compared to
3GC/GM: 100/101 (99%) vs 94/101 (93%) (p = 0.04). In
one patient a strain of *E. faecium* with modification of

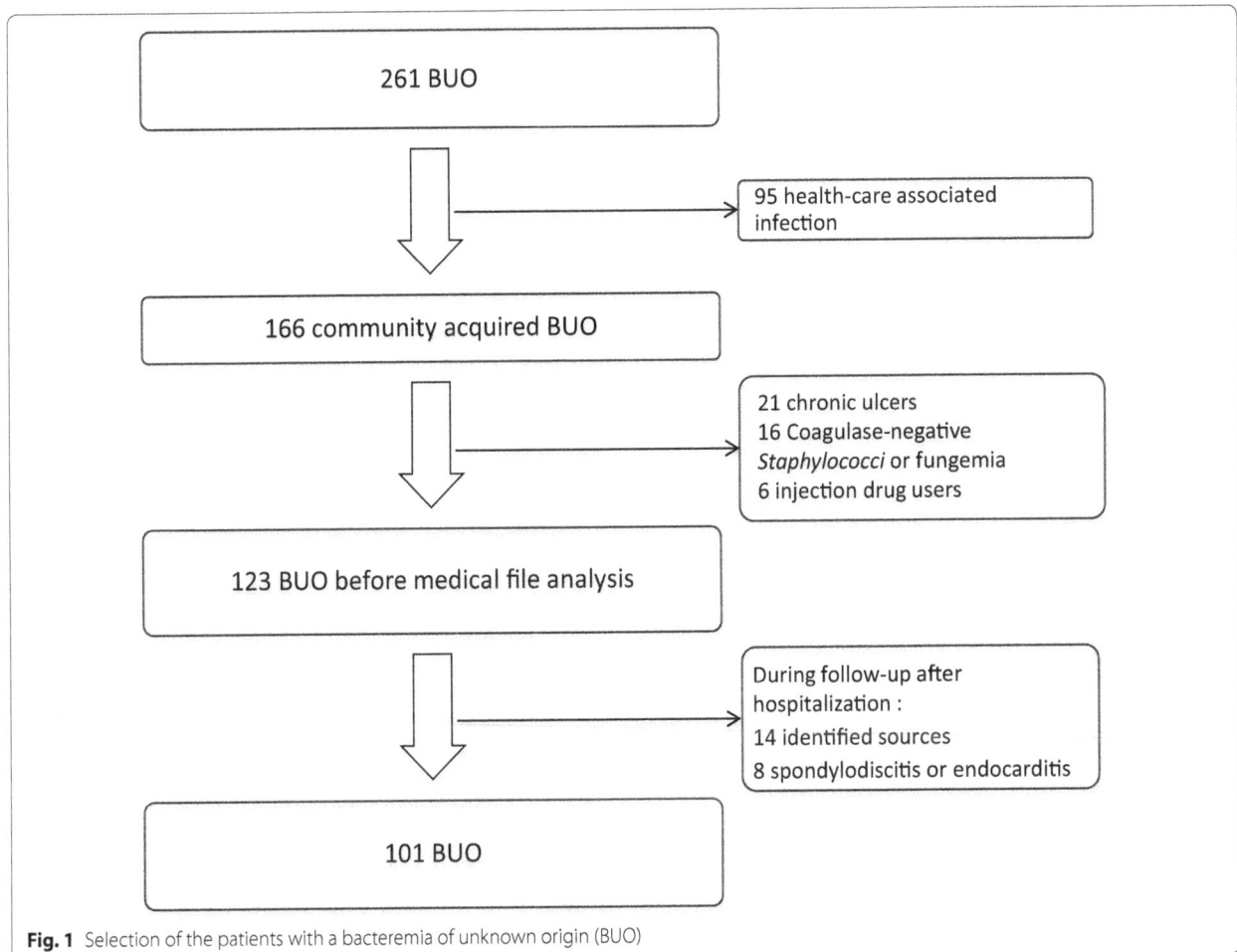

Fig. 1 Selection of the patients with a bacteremia of unknown origin (BUO)

penicillin-binding protein 5 impaired both associations. *Bacteroides* spp. (lack of aminoglycoside uptake + class A β-lactamase) in three patients and *E. faecalis* (intrinsic resistance to cephalosporins and aminoglycoside) in three patients impaired only 3GC/GM. All the natural or acquired resistance mechanisms of the bacteria to one of the drug of the associations are presented in Table 3.

Discussion

This study conducted in one French University Hospital shows that community BUO mainly involves old male patients, with half of them presenting at least one organ dysfunction and requiring ICU admission in 12% of the cases. Isolated fever with a recent onset (less than 3 days) represents the primary clinical feature for 22% of the patients whereas symptoms leading to emergency room visit vary widely for the rest of the patients. *S. aureus* BUO was associated to unfavourable outcome. Based on the analysis of the antibiotic susceptibility tests AMC + GM provided a higher rate of adequacy than 3GC + GM when used empirically.

The dashboard of our ward classifies infective endocarditis and vertebral osteomyelitis in other groups. Unfortunately in those groups i.e. bone and joint infections and vascular infections, the portal of entry is not recorded. So a number of BUO with vascular or bone secondary focus has not been included thus representing a selection bias. In the same way exclusion of chronic cutaneous conditions could have lead to selection bias. Bacteriological analysis of samples collected on chronic cutaneous conditions as pressure ulcers is often polymicrobial and variable over time. Deep tissue biopsies are not routinely performed for this purpose so the exclusion of a cutaneous primary focus is never obvious. Since the most frequent clinical presentation of coagulase-negative *Staphylococci* is device-associated health care-associated infections [12] BUO with those bacteria had been excluded from our work focusing on community-acquired infection. The choice of the two beta-lactams studied associated to an aminoglycoside results from the research for a spectrum broad enough but with consideration for appropriate antibiotic use and ecologic impact.

Table 1 Characteristics of the 101 patients with BUO

Clinical characteristics of patients	Values (%)
Age, years mean (SD)	71 (17)
Sex, men (%)	68 (67)
Comorbidities	
Cardiovascular	61 (60)
Immunosuppressed	31 (31)
Pulmonary	27 (27)
Diabetes mellitus	17 (17)
Dyslipidemia	14 (14)
Neurological	14 (14)
Medical device	17 (17)
Severe sepsis	52 (51)
Death	9 (9)
ICU transfer	12 (12)
Symptoms at admission	
Fever	99 (98)
Isolated fever	22 (22)
Dyspnea	14 (14)
Fatigue	13 (13)
Diarrhea/vomiting	13 (13)
Confusion	13 (13)
Loss of consciousness	11 (11)
Back pain	8 (8)
Arthralgia/myalgia	6 (6)
Fall	6 (6)
Chest pain	4
Abdominal pain	3
Neurological deficit	2
Jaundice	1
Cough	1
Headache	1

Table 2 Risk factors for unfavourable outcome (death or ICU transfer) during in-hospital care

Variables	Unfavourable outcome n = 17 (17)	Favourable outcome n = 84 (83)	p	OR [95% CI]
Age, years (mean)	70	74	0.335	
Sex (male)	9 (53)	59 (70)	0.165	
Comorbidities				
Cardiovascular	11 (65)	50 (60)	0.690	
Immunosuppressed	3 (18)	28 (33)	0.232	
Pulmonary	6 (35)	21 (25)	0.381	
Diabetes mellitus	3 (18)	14 (16)	0.921	
Dyslipidemia	4 (23)	10 (12)	0.205	
Neurological	3 (18)	11 (13)	0.620	
Medical device	5 (30)	13 (15)	0.170	
Symptoms at admission				
Dyspnea	2 (12)	11 (13)	0.881	
Diarrhea/vomiting	5 (30)	7 (8)	0.014	2.47 [1.62–26.78]
Confusion	2 (12)	11 (13)	0.881	
Loss of consciousness	4 (23)	8 (9)	0.103	
Bacteria				
Enterobacteriaceae	6 (35)	37 (44)	0.505	
Staphylococcus aureus	5 (29)	6 (7)	0.007	2.64 [1.42–22.17]
Streptococcus spp.	5 (29)	33 (39)	0.443	
Polymicrobial	2 (12)	9 (11)	0.899	

Univariate and multivariate analysis

In our dashboard, BUO corresponds to 13% of all the bacteremia. This result is close to the rates reported in a Spanish Emergency Department (12%) [13] and in a Spanish tertiary care center (16%) [5]. During the challenging management of BUO biomarkers may be helpful to the clinician. However, in our study, with a cut-off value of 0.5 ng/L the PCT yield a 21% rate of false negative. PCT is usually recognized as a biomarker able to rule out a bacteremia in patients presenting with fever in the emergency department [14]. In daily clinical practice a CRP value below 20 mg/L is usually considered not to be associated with a bacterial infection [15]. Compared to PCT, this cut-off provides a lower rate of false negative: 17%.

Bacterial epidemiology for *S. aureus*, *Enterobacteriaceae* and polymicrobial infections among the BUO are consistent with the few previously published data [5, 13,

16] while viridans *Streptococci*, *Enterococci* and group D *Streptococci* are more frequent in our study.

The high rate of patients presenting with at least one organ failure (51%) together with the 29% increase of the in-hospital mortality rate compare to the other patients hospitalized during the study period underscore the need to identify the best-suited empirical treatment. As in former studies, the definition of appropriate antibiotic used in our study considers monotherapy of aminoglycoside as efficient [17]. Compared to 3GC + GM, the use of AMC + GM enabled appropriate treatment in case of infection due to *Bacteroides* spp. and *E. faecalis*. ECDC antimicrobial resistance surveillance report [18] is the only tool providing resistance rate to antibiotic associations such as cephalosporins + aminoglycosides at an international level. Nonetheless those results include both community and health-care acquired infections and do not enable an assessment of our therapeutic strategy.

The fact that diarrhea and/or vomiting at admission is associated to unfavourable outcome remains unexplained. Similar to prior findings during BUO, *S. aureus* is associated with unfavourable outcome [5]. The use of beta-lactam/beta-lactamase inhibitor association for empirical treatment f *S. aureus* bacteremia has been associated with increased mortality rate compared to oxacillin or cefazolin [19]. Nevertheless in this study we propose the systematic use of a combination with an aminoglycoside known to significantly impact the course of *S. aureus* bacteremia [20].

Sepsis of unknown origin refers to a clinical situation encountered in the emergency room or just after ICU admission which includes: future BUO, sepsis with a primary source which will be documented in the following hours because of changes in clinical examination or results of paraclinical exams, sepsis which will never be documented and also non-infectious aetiologies [21]. So BUO represents only a subgroup of sepsis of unknown origin defined a posteriori on the basis of bloodcultures. Then our results regarding AMC + GM cannot be entirely and directly applied to sepsis of unknown origin. Our work based on patient hospitalized in an ID department aimed to use microbiological data of BUO as a surrogate marker to guide antimicrobial treatment during sepsis of unknown origin. As all surrogate markers it presents necessarily some drawbacks but to our knowledge no other work has intended to use a different one.

Table 3 Bacteria isolated and associated resistance to amoxicillin-clavulanic acid, gentamicin and 3rd generation cephalosporin

Bacteria	n	Natural resistance	n	Acquired resistance	n
Enterobacteriaceae					
Escherichia coli	25			High-level penicillinase (AMC-R)	3
Klebsiella pneumoniae	9			Inhibitor-resistant TEM (AMC-R)	2
Enterobacter spp.	5	ampC chromosomal inducible cephalosporinase (AMC-R[a])	5	Cephalosporinase hyperproduction (AMC-R and 3GC-R[b])	3
Proteus mirabilis	3			ESBL (AMC-R and 3GC-R)	1
Others	5				
Non-*Enterobacteriaceae* Gram-negative bacteria					
Pseudomonas aeruginosa	2	ampC chromosomal Inducible and low permeability (AMC-R and 3GC-R)	2		
Others	3				
Streptococcus spp.					
Group D *Streptococci*	12				
Viridans *Streptococci*	12				
Streptococcus milleri group	4				
Streptococcus pyogenes	3				
Streptococcus agalactiae	3				
Streptococcus pneumoniae	2				
Group C *Streptococci*	2				
Enterococcus spp.					
Enterococcus faecalis	3	PBP5 (3GC-R)	4		
Enterococcus faecium	1			High-level PBP5 (AMC-R)	1
Staphylococcus aureus	11			PBP2A (AMC-R and 3GC-R)	1
				APH 2″-AAC 6′ (GM-R[c])	2
Other Gram-positive					
Gemella haemolysans	1				
Listeria monocytogenes	2	PBP3 (3GC-R)	2		
Anaerobes		Lack of drug uptake (GM-R)	7		
Bacteroides spp.	4	Class A β-lactamase (3GC-R)	4		
Fusobacterium nucleatum	1				
Parvimonas micra	1				
Eubacterium spp.	1				

[a] Mechanism resulting in resistance to amoxicillin–clavulanic acid

[b] Mechanism resulting in resistance to ceftriaxone

[c] Mechanism resulting in resistance to gentamicin

Conclusion

When considering an empirical antibiotic treatment for community-acquired sepsis of unknown origin, microbiological features of BUO presenting half of the time with organ failure has to be integrated in the decision process. With our results, AMC + GM should be considered.

Authors' contributions

JC did the scientific literature search; JC and P-MR were responsible for the study design. JC, ED, ND, KR, RR and P-MR collected the data, all authors interpreted the data. JC, RR and P-MR analysed the data. JC created the figure and all authors were involved in the writing of the report. All authors read and approved the final manuscript.

Author details

[1] Infectious Diseases Department, Hôpital Archet 1, Nice Academic Hospital, Infectiologie 151 Route de St Antoine de Ginestière, 06200 Nice, France. [2] Université Côte d'Azur, Nice, France. [3] Department of Bacteriology, Archet 2 Hospital, Nice Academic Hospital, Nice, France. [4] INSERM U1065 (C3M), Bacterial Toxins in Host Pathogen Interactions, C3M, Archimed, Nice, France.

Acknowledgements

We would like to thank Marie-Hélène Schiano, Emilie Leroux, Sophie Leroux and Stephanie Caravel for the implementation of the dashboard of our ward.

Competing interests

The authors declare that they have no competing interests

Ethical approval

Not required, the medical dashboard of the Infectious Diseases Department of Nice university hospital is authorized by the Comission Nationale de l'Informatique et des Libertés (CNIL, Number of Registration: 1430722).

References

1. Viscoli C. Bloodstream infections: the peak of the iceberg. Virulence. 2016;7:248–51.
2. Weinstein MP, Towns ML, Quartey SM, et al. The clinical significance of positive blood cultures in the 1990s: a prospective comprehensive evaluation of the microbiology, epidemiology, and outcome of bacteremia and fungemia in adults. Clin Infect Dis. 1997;24:584–602.
3. Renaud B, Brun-Buisson C, Group IC-BS. Outcomes of primary and catheter-related bacteremia. A cohort and case-control study in critically ill patients. Am J Respir Crit Care Med. 2001;163:1584–90.
4. Valles J, Rello J, Ochagavia A, Garnacho J, Alcala MA. Community-acquired bloodstream infection in critically ill adult patients: impact of shock and inappropriate antibiotic therapy on survival. Chest. 2003;123:1615–24.
5. Hernandez C, Cobos-Trigueros N, Feher C, et al. Community-onset bacteraemia of unknown origin: clinical characteristics, epidemiology and outcome. Eur J Clin Microbiol Infect Dis. 2014;33:1973–80.
6. Pedersen G, Schonheyder HC, Sorensen HT. Source of infection and other factors associated with case fatality in community-acquired bacteremia—a Danish population-based cohort study from 1992 to 1997. Clin Microbiol Infect. 2003;9:793–802.
7. Adrie C, Garrouste-Orgeas M, Ibn Essaied W, et al. Attributable mortality of ICU-acquired bloodstream infections: impact of the source, causative micro-organism, resistance profile and antimicrobial therapy. J Infect. 2017;74:131–41.
8. Garnacho-Montero J, Gutierrez-Pizarraya A, Escoresca-Ortega A, Fernandez-Delgado E, Lopez-Sanchez JM. Adequate antibiotic therapy prior to ICU admission in patients with severe sepsis and septic shock reduces hospital mortality. Crit Care. 2015;19:302.
9. Canton R, Novais A, Valverde A, et al. Prevalence and spread of extended-spectrum beta-lactamase-producing Enterobacteriaceae in Europe. Clin Microbiol Infect. 2008;14(Suppl 1):144–53.
10. Roger PM, Farhad R, Leroux S, et al. Gestion de services, tarification à l'activité, recherche clinique et évaluation des pratiques professionnelles: un même outil informatique. Med Mal Infect. 2008;38:457–64.
11. Comité de l'antibiogramme de la société Française de Microbiologie. http://www.sfm-microbiologie.org/page/page/showpage/page_id/81.html.
12. Becker K, Heilmann C, Peters G. Coagulase-negative staphylococci. Clin Microbiol Rev. 2014;27:870–926.
13. Ortega M, Almela M, Martinez JA, et al. Epidemiology and outcome of primary community-acquired bacteremia in adult patients. Eur J Clin Microbiol Infect Dis. 2007;26:453–7.
14. Chirouze C, Schuhmacher H, Rabaud C, et al. Low serum procalcitonin level accurately predicts the absence of bacteremia in adult patients with acute fever. Clin Infect Dis. 2002;35:156–61.
15. Knudtzen FC, Nielsen SL, Gradel KO, et al. Characteristics of patients with community-acquired bacteremia who have low levels of C-reactive protein (</=20 mg/L). J Infect. 2014;68:149–55.
16. Leibovici L, Konisberger H, Pitlik SD, Samra Z, Drucker M. Bacteremia and fungemia of unknown origin in adults. Clin Infect Dis. 1992;14:436–43.
17. Marquet K, Liesenborgs A, Bergs J, Vleugels A, Claes N. Incidence and outcome of inappropriate in-hospital empiric antibiotics for severe infection: a systematic review and meta-analysis. Crit Care. 2015;19:795.
18. European Centre for Disease Prevention and Control (ECDC). Antimicrobial resistance surveillance in Europe 2014. Annual Report of the European Antimicrobial Resistance Surveillance Network (EARS-Net). Stockholm: ECDC; 2015. http://ecdc.europa.eu/en/publications/Publications/antimicrobial-resistance-europe-2014pdf.
19. Paul M, Zemer-Wassercug N, Talker O, et al. Are all beta-lactams similarly effective in the treatment of methicillin-sensitive *Staphylococcus aureus* bacteraemia? Clin Microbiol Infect. 2011;17:1581–6.
20. Lemonovich TL, Haynes K, Lautenbach E, Amorosa VK. Combination therapy with an aminoglycoside for Staphylococcus aureus endocarditis and/or persistent bacteremia is associated with a decreased rate of recurrent bacteremia: a cohort study. Infection. 2011;39:549–54.
21. Contou D, Roux D, Jochmans S, et al. Septic shock with no diagnosis at 24 hours: a pragmatic multicenter prospective cohort study. Crit Care. 2016;20:360.

18

Prevalence of multi drug resistant enteropathogenic and enteroinvasive *Escherichia coli* isolated from children with and without diarrhea in Northeast Indian population

Karuppasamy Chellapandi[1,2], Tapan Kumar Dutta[1*], Indu Sharma[2], Surajit De Mandal[3], Nachimuthu Senthil Kumar[3] and Lalsanglura Ralte[4]

Abstract

Background: Diarrheagenic *Escherichia coli* are associated with infantile diarrhea in the developing countries. The present study was conducted to determine the occurrence and antimicrobial resistance pattern of enteropathogenic and enteroinvasive *E. coli* associated with diarrhoea among the paediatric patients.

Methods: A total of 262 stool samples were collected from children with and without diarrhea from Mizoram, Northeast India. *E. coli* were isolated and subjected to multiplex PCR to detect virulent genes of EPEC (*eaeA* and *bfpA*) and EIEC (*ial*). Isolates were subjected to antimicrobial sensitivity assay using disc diffusion method. Selected *eaeA* genes were sequenced for identification and genetic relationship.

Results: A total of 334 *E. coli* was isolated, of which 17.37% were carrying at least one virulent gene. Altogether, 14.97 and 2.40% isolates were categorized as EPEC and EIEC, respectively. Among the DEC isolates, 4.79% were EPEC and 7.78% were EIEC. A total of 8 (2.40%) isolates were EIEC (*ial*+), of which 6 (1.80%) and 2 (0.60%) were from diarrhoeic and non-diarrhoeic patients, respectively. A total of 24 (41.40%) DEC isolates were MDR (resistance against ≥5 antimicrobials).

Conclusions: A high frequency of EPEC pathotypes associated with paediatric diarrhea was observed in Mizoram, Northeast India and majority of the isolates are resistant to antibiotics with a high frequency of MDR, which is a matter of concern to the public health. This also raises an alarm to the world communities to monitor the resistance pattern and analyse in a global scale to combat the problems of resistance development.

Keywords: EPEC, EIEC, Mizoram, Infants, MDR

Background

Infectious diarrheal disease is the second leading cause of morbidity and mortality among children under 5 years of age in developing countries [1]. Diarrhea is common in Indian children with an incidence of 334,000 of total 2.3 million annual deaths [2]. Diarrheagenic *Escherichia coli*, specifically enteropathogenic *E. coli* (EPEC) is the leading bacterial agent causing diarrhoea in children aged below 5 years [3, 4]. EPEC isolates are divided into two groups: typical EPEC (tEPEC), which contains an EPEC adherence factor (EAF) for bundle forming pili (BFP) encoded by *bfpA* gene and atypical EPEC (aEPEC) is devoid of EAF [5]. For many decades tEPEC isolates were considered as the major pathogen in infants in developing countries including India, but only a few sporadic reports indicated the association of aEPEC with children diarrhoea [6–8].

Enteroinvasive *E. coli* (EIEC) is known to develop symptoms, which are similar to those of shigellosis in

---

*Correspondence: tapandutta@rediffmail.com
[1] Department of Veterinary Microbiology, Central Agricultural University, Selesih, Aizawl, Mizoram 796 014, India
Full list of author information is available at the end of the article

adults and children. Despite being recognized as a human pathogen, little research has been conducted to identify the risk factors for this infection so far. The lack of epidemiological attention to EIEC is related to the low incidence of this pathogen as a cause of diarrhea in relation to other strains of diarrheal *E. coli*. The genes related to invasion of EIEC are located in virulence plasmid (pInv), which encodes a so-called type III secretion apparatus, the machinery required for the secretion of multiple proteins which are necessary for its full pathogenicity [9].

Apart from the conventional biochemical tests, the sensitive PCR based DNA assay helps in diagnosis of EIEC and detection of virulent genes like ipaH (Invasion plasmid antigen H) and *ial* (invasion-associated locus). The PCR based detection of *ial* gene for EIEC which is located on the pInv plasmid is a popular method, since it can also be effectively used to detect EIEC strains as well as other pathotypes of *E. coli* in a multiplex PCR [3, 10].

The emergence and spread of multi drug resistance (MDR) bacteria have been identified as a global burden in medical science and it stresses on surveillance monitoring to control the spread of MDR strains. Drug resistance in the developing countries has been attributed to the extensive uses of antibiotics and poor prescription practices. This problem may also affect the isolates recovered from children with diarrheal diseases. However, only a few studies have investigated the prevalence of diarrheagenic *E. coli* and their MDR patterns in India [8, 11, 12], where awareness and understating of MDR is still limited. Although sporadic reports on the association of EPEC and EIEC with children diarrhoea in India are available, the data is insufficient to understand the prevalence and strain variations to develop a National policy on management of the disease. The present study was formulated to investigate the prevalence of EPEC and EIEC from children with and without diarrhea in Northeast Indian Population. The other major aim of the study is to examine seasonal occurrence, multi drug resistance (MDR) pattern of the EPEC and EIEC isolates.

Methods
Clinical specimens and subjects
A total of 262 stool/rectal swab samples were collected from the childrens up to 5 years of age. Stool samples were collected using the sterile containers whereas rectal swab samples were collected using a sterile swab stick, preferably collected in the morning of the same day that the sample was processed. One sample from each patient was included in the present study and no repeated samples were collected from the same patient. Samples were collected between November 2013 to October 2015 from both inpatient and outpatient units of the major hospitals

(Civil Hospital Aizawl, Aizawl Hospital & Research Centre and Presbyterian Hospitals Durtlang) of Mizoram, Northeast India. The patients were primarily of urban and suburban residents. Out of 262 samples, 210 samples were collected from children suffering from diarrhea with or without blood or mucus and the rest 52 samples were obtained from apparently healthy children but were admitted to the hospital for non-diarrheal illness. Clinical samples from the patients treated with antibiotics or infected with *Salmonella, Shigella* and co-infected with parasites and were not included in this study.

Bacterial strains
All the samples were cultured on Mac Conkey's agar (HiMedia Laboratories Pvt. Ltd., India) and incubated at 37 °C for 24 h. At least five randomly selected lactose fermenting pink coloured colonies were selected from each plate and were subjected to routine microbiological and biochemical tests to identify *E. coli* [13]. All the isolates were stored in glycerol at −80 °C for further studies.

Serotyping
Serotyping of the *E. coli* isolates based on 'O' antigen was carried out at National Salmonella and Escherichia Centre, Central Research Institute (CRI), Himachal Pradesh, India as per the method of Edwards and Ewing [14].

Preparation of bacterial DNA for PCR assay
Bacterial DNA was prepared using boiled lysis method. The isolates were inoculated into Luria–Bertani (LB) broth (HiMedia, Mumbai, India) and incubated overnight at 37 °C. The broth was centrifuged at 3000 rpm for 5 min. and the pellet obtained was dissolved in autoclaved distilled water followed by boiling for 10 min. The bacterial lysate was centrifuged again and the supernatant was finally taken as template DNA for PCR assay [15]. The specificity of the multiplex PCR assay was determined by using locally available and or reference strains as positive control strains (*E. coli* O20 serotype positive for *eaeA, bfpA* genes of EPEC and *E. coli* ATCC® 43893 positive for *ial* gene of EIEC) for the standardization of multiplex PCR assay. The strains were subjected to both the multiplex and monoplex PCR assays. Both the multiplex and monoplex assays showed 100% specificity in identifying the reference strains and none of the reaction showed non-specific bands under UV-visualization.

Detection of virulence genes by multiplex PCR
A multiplex PCR assay was carried out and the following specific primers were used: *eaeA* F (5'-TGATAAGCTGC AGTCGAATCC-3'), *eaeA* R (5'-CTGAACCAGATCGT AACGGC-3'), *bfp*A F (5'-CACCGTTACCGCAGGTGT

GA-3′) *bfp*A R (5′-GTTGCCGCTTCAGCAGGAGT-3′) for the EPEC and *ial* F (5′-CTGGTAGGTATGGTGAGG-3′), *ial* R (5′-CCAGGCCAACAATTATTTCC-3′) for the EIEC as previously described [16]. The multiplex PCR reaction mixture contained 2.5 µl of 10× PCR buffer with 1.5 mM of MgCl₂, 1 µl each primer, 2 µl of 10 mM each of dNTPs, 0.2 µl of 5.0 U Taq DNA polymerase and 4.0 µl template DNA. The PCR reaction condition includes initial denaturation at 95 °C for 5 min, followed by 32 cycles of denaturation at 94 °C for 45 s, annealing at 57 °C for 45 s and extension at 72 °C for 1 min, followed by a final extension at 72 °C for 5 min. Amplified products were separated on 1.5% agarose gel and stained with ethidium bromide and were visualized under ultraviolet transilluminator and documented by a gel documentation system (Alpha Imager, Germany).

Cloning and sequence analysis

Selected PCR products were purified (QIAGEN kit) and cloned using TA cloning vector (MBI Fermentas) and sequenced in automated sequencer Applied Biosystems 3500 (USA) in the Dept. of Biotechnology, Mizoram University, India. Sequencing data were analysed using MEGA6 [17].

Antimicrobial susceptibility test

The isolates positive for at least one virulence marker gene by PCR were subjected to antimicrobial susceptibility test against the selected antimicrobials (ampicillin-10 µg, amikacin-10 µg, chloramphenicol-30 µg, ceftriaxone-10 µg, cephalexin-30 µg, ciprofloxacin-10 µg, co-trimoxazole-25 µg, cefoperazone-tazobactam-75 + 10 µg, meropenem-10 µg, norfloxacin-10 µg, gentamicin-10 µg, cefixime-5 µg, doxycycline hydrochloride-10 µg and ofloxacin-5 µg) (HiMedia, India) by disc diffusion method in Mueller–Hinton agar [18]. The performance of this test was checked by employing *E. coli* ATCC 25922 as a standard quality control strain. The results were expressed as sensitive, intermediate and resistant as per standard CLSI guidelines [19]. MDR was defined as "acquired non-susceptibility to at least one agent in three or more antimicrobial categories" [20].

Statistical analysis

Data were analysed using SPSS version 17.0 software. The significance (p < 0.05) of differences between the prevalence of EPEC and EIEC in age groups, Seasonal variations, the difference between MDR resistance occurrence and sample types were compared using a Chi square test for dependent samples or Fischer's exact test when appropriate. The *p* values less than 0.05 was considered statistically significant.

Results

Isolation and identification of *E. coli* pathotypes

A total of 334 *E. coli* isolates were recovered from 262 faecal samples derived from 262 patients. Based on culture, staining, colony characteristics as well as biochemical tests, 282 and 52 *E. coli* were isolated from diarrhoeic and non-diarrhoeic patients, respectively.

Clinical features of children affected with DEC

Occurrence of DEC among the female (10.3%) are little higher than male (11.8%) (p > 0.05 and 95% CI 0.456–9.86) though there is no role of sex factor as biological evidence, the mean age of the patients was 12 months (range from 2 to 36 months). Vomiting and abdominal pain were seen in 12.6 and 11.8% of children affected with EPEC and 1.5 and 1.9% in EIEC infected childrens, respectively. Childrens infected with EPEC (13%) and with EIEC (1.9%) showed fever at presentation (p > 0.05 and 95% CI 0.327–5.414). The consistency of the stool samples were mostly watery (68.7%), mucous (12.9%) and very few with blood (6.9%) with different number of episode per day and varied from mild to severe dehydration. Other clinical features with the pathotype are summarized in Table 1. The

Table 1 Clinical symptoms of subjects included in this study

Clinical characteristics	Total no. of subjects (n = 262)	EPEC (n = 50)	EIEC (n = 08)
Sex ratio			
Male	114 (43.5)	28 (10.69)	03 (1.14)
Female	148 (56.5)	22 (08.39)	05 (01.91)
Fever			
Febrile	123 (46.9)	34 (13.00)	05 (01.91)
Afebrile	139 (53.0)	13 (04.96)	02 (0.76)
Vomiting	91 (34.7)	33 (12.60)	04 (01.52)
Abdominal pain	48 (18.3)	31 (11.80)	05 (01.91)
Diarrhea and non-diarrhea			
Watery stool	158 (60.3)	40 (15.30)	01 (0.38)
Mucous	34 (12.9)	03 (01.15)	02 (0.76)
Bloody	18 (06.9)	01 (0.38)	04 (01.52)
No symptoms	52 (19.84)	03 (01.15)	–
Diarrheal frequency			
2–3 times a day	180 (68.7)	27 (10.31)	07 (02.67)
4–5 times a day	19 (07.25)	19 (07.25)	–
5–10 times a day	11 (04.2)	01 (0.38)	–
Dehydration			
Mild dehydration	37 (14.1)	13 (04.96)	01 (0.38)
Moderate dehydration	28 (10.7)	14 (05.34)	–
Severe dehydration	63 (24.0)	04 (01.53)	–
Unknown	134 (51.1)	16 (06.11)	06 (02.30)

Within parenthesis denotes the % of the samples

EPEC enteropathogenic *E. coli*, *EIEC* enteroinvasive *E. coli*

watery stool was found more common in EPEC infection (15.3%) than any other consistency such as mucous (1.1%) and blood (0.3%) with mild dehydration (4.96%) and only a few cases show severe dehydration (1.5%). When compared with EPEC infections, EIEC cases have shown more mucous stools (0.76%) and bloody stool (1.5%) than watery stools (0.3%) with mild dehydration (0.3%) only (p < 0.005 and 95% CI 5.70–631.59).

Distribution of DEC

As depicted in Table 2, of the total 334 *E. coli* isolates subjected for detection of EPEC (*eaeA*) and EIEC (*ial*) marker genes, 58 (17.36%) were positive for at least one of the target gene, of which 50 (14.97%) and 8 (2.33%) isolates were categorized as EPEC and EIEC, respectively. Among the 8 EIEC isolates, 6 (1.80%) and 2 (0.59%) were recovered from diarrhoeic and non-diarrhoeic patients, respectively. Similarly, amongst the EPEC isolates, 38 (11.38%) and 12 (3.59%) were isolated from the diarrhoeic and non-diarrhoeic patients, respectively (p > 0.05 and 95% CI 0.187–5.938). Among the EPEC isolates, 21 (6.29%) were also positive for *bfp*A gene, hence termed as typical EPEC (tEPEC) isolates and rest 29 (8.68%) were categorized as aEPEC. Among the aEPEC isolates, 22 (6.59%) were isolated from diarrhoeic patients and 7 (2.10%) were recovered from non-diarrhoeic patients.

Although the majority of the tEPEC were isolated from diarrhoeic patients, 5 (1.50%) isolates were also recovered from non-diarrhoeic patients (p > 0.05 and 95% CI 0.273–3.797). In case of EIEC, 2 (0.59%) isolates were recovered from children without diarrhea.

The incidence of acute diarrhea associated with EPEC and EIEC decreased significantly with the increasing age of the patient, and was highest (6.6%) in children aged 13–24 months and lowest among the age group of 37–48 months, which is significantly low (0.6%) compared with other age groups (Table 3) (p > 0.05 and 95% CI 0.043–28.547). Incidence in the age group of 0–12 months was lower (6.3%) than the weaning age group of children in Mizoram. The occurrence of aEPEC in children aged with 0–24 months (5.3%) was more than other age groups, and it's also found as not associated with diarrhea in 0–12 months children (0.9%) of the non-diarrheic group. Rate of tEPEC occurrence in the age group of 0–24 months (1.2%) is higher when compared with other age groups; occurrence in non-diarrheic cases shows the high prevalence of tEPEC carriers. All the EIEC pathotypes were recovered from the age group of 0–24 months except one isolate found in 49–60 group. Though the occurrence of EIEC in non-diarrheic group is meager (0.3%) its occurrence in non-diarrheic cases causes a confused state of the pathogenicity of this pathotype. Incidence of diarrhea

Table 2 Frequency of *E. coli* pathotypes isolated from fecal samples of children with and without diarrhea

S. no	*E. coli* pathotypes	*E. coli* isolates from non-diarrheic patients	*E. coli* isolates from diarrheic patients	Total (n = 334)
1.	EPEC	12 (3.59)	38 (11.38)	50 (14.97)
	a-EPEC	07 (2.10)	22 (6.59)	29 (8.68)
	t-EPEC	05 (1.50)	16 (4.79)	21 (6.29)
2.	EIEC	02 (0.59)	06 (1.80)	08 (2.33)
Total		14 (4.07)	44 (13.17)	58 (17.37)

Figures in parenthesis denotes the % of the samples

a-EPEC atypical enteropathogenic *E. coli*, *t*-EPEC typical enteropathogenic *E. coli*

Table 3 Age wise comparison of EPEC and EIEC from the stool samples of children

Age (months)	No. of isolates	Atypical EPEC (n = 29)		Typical EPEC (n = 21)		EIEC (n = 08)		Total (n = 334)
		Age	Non age	Age	Non age	Age	Non age	
0–12	176 (52.69)	07 (02.09)	03 (0.90)	06 (01.80)	01 (0.30)	03 (0.90)	01 (0.30)	21 (6.3)
13–24	98 (29.34)	11 (03.29)	–	05 (01.50)	03 (0.90)	02 (0.60)	01 (0.30)	22 (6.6)
25–36	37 (11.07)	05 (01.49)	–	01 (0.30)	01 (0.30)	–	–	7 (2.1)
37–48	14 (04.19)	01 (0.30)	–	01 (0.30)	–	–	–	2 (0.6)
49–60	09 (02.69)	02 (0.60)	–	03 (0.90)	–	01 (0.30)	–	6 (1.8)
Total	334	26 (7.8)	03 (0.9)	16 (4.8)	05 (1.5)	06 (1.8)	02 (0.5)	58 (17.4)

Figures in parenthesis denotes the % of the samples

AGE acute gastroenteritis, EPEC enteropathogenic *E. coli*, EIEC enteroinvasive *E. coli*

associated with EPEC/EIEC among the young infants and children of Mizoram was highest (8.08%) during summer followed by monsoon (5.09%) (p > 0.05 and 95% CI 0.275–2.589) and winter (4.20%) (Table 4).

Serotypes

The O serotypes detected in this study from diarrheagenic *E. coli* isolates were corroborating with the previously reported serotypes and association with childhood diarrhea with few novel serotypes. The majority of the isolates of typical and atypical EPEC belonged to the serogroups: O 84 (4), O 86 (4), O141 (4), O149 (4), Rough (7) and UT (7). All the isolates found to be EIEC belonged to O serogroups of O20 (1), O29 (1), O96 (2), O124 (1) O144 (1) and UT (2). The occurrence of these O serogroups in three different seasons was also studied to understand their occurrences and association with childhood diarrhea (Table 4).

Antimicrobial resistance of *E. coli* isolates

Antibiotics commonly used by local medical practitioners for the treatment of childhood diarrhea were included in this study for the antibiotic susceptibility tests. None of the diarrheagenic *E. coli* isolates were sensitive against all the antimicrobials used in this study. Altogether, 41.40% of DEC was recorded as multi drug resistant (MDR) of which >70% of aEPEC and 50% of tEPEC isolates were resistant to ampicillin, ceftriaxone, cefoperazone-tazobactam, cefixime and doxycycline. Similarly, the EIEC isolates also exhibited high rate (60–80%) of resistance to majority of the antibiotics used in the study (Table 5). The MDR isolates against the cephalosporin drugs (83%) still higher than other drugs including aminoglycosides, carbapenem, fluoroquinolone and sulphonamides (16.9%) used in this study (p > 0.05 and 95% CI 0.830–3.008).

Discussion

Escherichia coli is identified as an important cause of paediatric diarrhea in developing countries. Although DEC pathotypes are well recognized, they are not routinely sought due to lack of infrastructures such as antisera and advanced molecular techniques. Thus, the exact burden of *E. coli* diarrhea among the hospitalized children across India especially Northeast India is still unclear. In the present study, the samples were collected from Mizoram, located in the North Eastern part of India adjoining to Myanmar and Bangladesh where limited study has been conducted on the prevalence of diarrhea associated with DEC [15, 21]. This is the first report on an in-depth study on the prevalence of EPEC and EIEC associated with diarrhea in children less than 5 years of age in North-eastern Indian population. In the present study, children with DEC diarrhea were characterized by the presence of fever, profuse watery stools, more than 3–5 stools per 24 h, associated with vomiting and mild to severe dehydration as common clinical features. The occurrence of EPEC was much higher compared to EIEC and both the pathotypes were higher in febrile patients than afebrile patients. Similar clinical symptoms were observed in patients from other parts in India [6, 8].

Among all the DEC, EPEC found to be the most common pathotypes for diarrheal infection in Mizoram which is much higher than the previous report [15]. Recent studies from other part of India also found higher occurrence of EPEC compared to EIEC among diarrheal samples [8, 16, 22]. Of the 50 EPEC isolates from the present study, 11.38% were recovered from the diarrhoeic patients in comparison with the non-diarrhoeic patients 3.59%, which is probably good evidence for their role in development of diarrhea among the children. But at the same time presence of EPEC isolates from the

Table 4 Seasonal distribution of diarrheagenic *E. coli* among children

Seasons	*E. coli* isolates	'O' Serotypes (no. of isolates)	EPEC		EIEC (%)	Total (DEC) (%)
			Atypical (%)	Typical (%)		
Summer	138	EPEC (22): O2 (1), O26 (2), O84 (1), O86 (2), O91 (1), O116 (1), O 129 (1), O141 (4), O145 (1), O149 (3), Rough (2), UT (3)	12 (3.59)	10 (2.99)	05 (1.5)	27 (8.08)
		EIEC (05): O29 (1), O96 (2), O124 (1) UT (1)				
Rainy/autumn	96	EPEC (16): O2 (1), O 29 (1), O 83 (1), O84 (3), O86 (2), O91 (1), O126 (1), Rough (4), UT (2)	10 (2.99)	06 (1.8)	01 (0.3)	17 (5.09)
		EIEC (01): UT (01)				
Winter	100	EPEC (12): O 2 (1), O 35 (1), O83 (1), O 101 (1), O126 (2), O 145 (2), O 149 (1), Rough (1), UT (2)	07 (2.1)	05 (1.5)	02 (0.6)	14 (4.19)
		EIEC (02): O20 (1), O144 (1)				
Total	334	58	29 (8.68)	21 (6.29)	08 (2.4)	58 (17.37)

Figures in parenthesis denotes the % of the samples

EPEC enteropathogenic *E. coli*, *EIEC* enteroinvasive *E. coli*

Table 5 Antimicrobial resistance profile of diarrheagenic E. coli isolated from stool samples collected from children

DEC (n)	AMP	AK	C	CN	CI	CF	COT	CST	MRP	NX	G	CFM	DO	OF	MDR (%)
a-EPEC (29)	21 (72.4)	06 (20.7)	14 (48.3)	14 (48.3)	22 (75.9)	10 (34.5)	09 (31.0)	24 (82.8)	06 (20.7)	12 (41.4)	04 (13.8)	21 (72.4)	12 (41.4)	14 (48.3)	14 (48.3)
t-EPEC (21)	14 (66.7)	08 (38.1)	05 (23.8)	12 (57.1)	12 (57.1)	03 (14.3)	08 (38.1)	16 (76.2)	06 (28.6)	09 (42.6)	07 (33.3)	12 (57.1)	12 (57.1)	07 (33.3)	07 (24.1)
EIEC (08)	07 (87.5)	01 (12.5)	00 (0)	06 (75)	07 (87.5)	04 (50)	07 (87.5)	04 (50)	05 (62.5)	01 (12.5)	05 (62.5)	05 (62.5)	05 (62.5)	05 (62.5)	03 (37.5)
Total (58)	42 (72.4)	15 (25.9)	19 (32.8)	32 (55.2)	41 (70.7)	17 (29.3)	24 (41.4)	44 (75.9)	17 (29.3)	22 (37.9)	16 (27.6)	38 (65.5)	29 (50)	26 (44.8)	24 (41.4)

Figures in parenthesis denotes the % of the samples

MDR multi drug resistant, *a-EPEC* atypical enteropathogenic *Escherichia coli*, *t-EPEC* typical enteropathogenic *Escherichia coli*, *EIEC* enteroinvasive *Escherichia coli*, *µg* microgram, *Antibiotics* ampicillin (AMP10 = 10 µg), amikacin (AK10 = 10 µg), chloramphenicol (C 30 = 30 µg), cephalexin (CN30 = 30 µg), ciprofloxacin (CF10 = 10 µg), ceftriaxone (CI 10 = 10 µg), co-trimoxazole (COT25 = trimethoprim 1.25 µg and sulphamethoxazole 23.75 µg), cefoperazone-tazobactam (CST 75–10 µg), meropenem (MRP10 = 10 µg), norfloxacin (NX10 = 10 µg), gentamicin (G10 = 10 µg), cefixime (CFM 5 = 5 µg), doxycycline hydrochloride (DO10 = 10 µg) and ofloxacin (OF 5 = 5 µg)

Prevalence of multi drug resistant enteropathogenic and enteroinvasive Escherichia coli...

151

population of the non-diarrhoeic patients also indicates their role as potent carrier of the organism, which may infect the other vulnerable population of the locality. In non-diarrheic group, both atypical 2.1% and typical 1.5% EPEC were detected which is very less than the previous reports in India [7, 16]. For many decades tEPEC isolates were considered as the major pathogen in infants in developing countries including India [6, 22], but few sporadic reports indicated the association with aEPEC with children diarrhea [6, 7, 22]. In contrast to typical EPEC, atypical EPEC strains appear to be common in domestic animals, raw meats and have been reported in food borne and water borne outbreaks [5, 9, 15]. This might be the possible source of transmission of this pathogen among children through mother, baby sitter or other members of the family.

In India, very few reports are available the occurrence of EIEC associated with children diarrhea. In the present study, a total of 2.33% E. coli isolates were confirmed as EIEC, of which 0.59 and 1.80% were from non-diarrhoeic and diarrhoeic patients, respectively. Other studies in India also reported less percentage of EIEC (1–1.5%) only in diarrheal patients [8, 16, 22]. The presence of EIEC strains in non-diarrheic group suggests that their prevalence is high in this study region among other age groups or sources including contaminated food and water [9]. Detection of EIEC in association with infants or children is a paramount important issue for effective treatment and control of the disease. Given the potential importance of this invasive pathogen, more work should be focused on why EIEC is prevalent in children of non-diarrheic group of this study region.

Considering the age groups, the EPEC ad EIEC strains were detected in almost all the age groups, but significantly higher prevalence was seen in children over 12 months of age (p < 0.05). Almost similar rate of occurrence was seen in 0–12 month age group, where the children's are completely dependent on mother. Thus, a proper hygienic condition of mother prior to breastfeeding could significantly reduce mother-to-infant transmission of this DEC. Of the 2.3% EIEC strain all of them occurred in the age group of 0–24 month except one single strain detected in the age group of 49–60 month. Occurrence of these age groups children as a pathogen indicates there might be some immune related issues in the particular individual as there are studies reported that these pathogens infecting the children enhance immunity as they grow into adults and then they act as carriers of this pathogen [9]. Seasonal distribution of the DEC in Aizawl, Mizoram showed that most of the cases occurred in summer probably owing to the increase in temperature, followed by rainy and winter seasons. Similar results were found in other parts of India and outside India [11,

23, 24]. Serotype associated with a particular pathotypes was similar with the previous studies [7, 9]. Occurrence of serotypes in different seasons was also considered in this study and no seasonal variation was observed.

Many factors play a role related to the high prevalence of diarrhea, including lack of education of mother, lack of exclusive breastfeeding, breastfeeding for less than 1 year, roundworm infestation, nutritional status, immunization status, night blindness, personal hygiene, overcrowding, garbage disposal, source of water supply and toilet facility. Earlier studies has reported that occurrence of diarrhea is higher (31.57%) in children who were breastfed for less than 6 months compared to exclusively breastfed children (20.33%) and bottle-fed children (26.08%). It was found that mixed-fed infants aged between 0 and 11 months tend to have a higher risk of diarrhea than fully breastfed children [25].

As per WHO protocol, paediatric diarrheal patients should be treated with rehydration solution, intravenous fluids, oral zinc suspensions, but failure of this protocol lead to MDR in bacterial pathogens [26]. High prevalence of MDR-EPEC strains was recorded in different parts of the world [27–29]. In the present study, antimicrobial resistance pattern was performed for all the DEC. Both tEPEC and aEPEC showed high levels of resistance to almost all the generic drugs used in this study such as aminoglycosides, cephalosporin, fluoroquinolone and tetracycline, but a very low level of resistance to carbapenem drugs. And the EIEC isolates were not only resistant to the commonly used genera drugs, but also to the fluoroquinolone and carbapenem. The aEPEC showed a significantly higher rate of resistance to antimicrobials than tEPEC against the selective antibiotics. It may be due to the fact that aEPEC was circulating in the human environment for a longer period in this region than the tEPEC, which got lesser exposure to the commonly used antimicrobials. In contrast to our result Sunaifa et al. [12] reported the higher antimicrobial resistance to the tEPEC than aEPEC from paediatric patients. The rate of adaptive mutation in E. coli is high which might be a cause of emergence of resistant varieties of aEPEC [6, 30]. The result of the present study indicates that aEPEC is the major DEC in Mizoram and also showing higher level of resistance against antimicrobials. The EIEC isolates recovered from this region showed high level of resistance against commonly used antimicrobials including fluoroquinolone and carbapenem, which is a clear indication of indiscriminate use of antimicrobials in clinical practice and sale across the counter in this region.

This is the first report on drug resistance EIEC isolated from Children in India. The emergence of widespread resistance to quinolone and other cephalosporin antimicrobials like cefixime, cefoperazone, and cephalexin etc. among diarrheal isolates is an important concern in this region. But the resistance rates against some of the broad spectrum antibiotics like gentamicin, amikacin, ciprofloxacin and meropenem were limited and can be used for the treatment of MDR diarrheal pathogens.

Therefore, it may be concluded that antibiotic resistant DEC is highly prevalent among the young population of Mizoram, India. Atypical EPEC are more prevalent compared to the typical EPEC and the aEPEC showed high level of resistance against the commonly used antimicrobial agents. High level of resistance development towards common antibiotics as well as quinolone and carbapenem in the EIEC isolates from human patients from North Eastern Region of India has been reported for the first time in the study. This study highlights the need for proper microbial diagnosis before antibiotic treatment, especially in the developing and under-developed regions of the world, where antibiotic abuse is widespread and a major growing concern.

Authors' contributions
TKD and IS made substantial contribution to conception and design of the study. KC and SDM was involved in data collection and interpretation. KC, SDM and NSK drafted the manuscript. KC, TKD, IS, SDM, NSK and LR critically revised the manuscript. All authors are accountable to the accuracy and integrity of all parts of the paper. All authors read and approved the final manuscript.

Author details
[1] Department of Veterinary Microbiology, Central Agricultural University, Selesih, Aizawl, Mizoram 796 014, India. [2] Department of Microbiology, Assam University, Silchar, Assam, India. [3] Department of Biotechnology, Mizoram University, Aizawl, Mizoram, India. [4] Department of MLT, Regional Institute of Paramedical and Nursing Sciences, Aizawl, Mizoram, India.

Acknowledgements
Authors are highly thankful to the Dean, C.V.Sc & AH, CAU, Selesih, Aizawl for granting permission to carry out the work and to the Director, RIPANS, Zemabawk, Aizawl for their constant support. The authors are also thankful to the DBT, New Delhi, India funded project on ADMaC for financial support and Advanced State Level Biotech Hub, Mizoram University for the infrastructural facility to conduct the work. The authors are thankful to National Salmonella and Escherichia Centre, Central Research Institute (CRI), Kasuali—Himachal Pradesh, India for assisting in serotyping of all the E. coli isolates.

Competing interests
The authors declare that they have no competing interests.

References
1. Bryce J, Boschi-Pinto C, Shibuya K, Black RE, WHO Child Health Epidemiology Reference Group. WHO estimates of the causes of death in children. Lancet. 2005;365(9465):1147–52.
2. Bassani DG, Kumar R, Aswathi S, Morris SK, Paul VK, Shet A, Ram U, Gaffey MF, Black RE, Jha P, Million death study collaborators. Causes of neonatal and child mortality in India: a nationality representative mortality survey. Lancet. 2010;376(9755):1853–60.
3. Nataro JP, Kaper JB. Diarrheagenic *Escherichia coli*. Clin Microbiol Rev. 1998;11:142–201.
4. Clarke SC, Haigh RD, Freestone PPE, Williams PH. Virulence of enteropathogenic *Escherichia coli*, a global pathogen. Clin Microbiol Rev. 2003;16(3):365–78.
5. Yanmei X, Xiangning B, Ailan Z, Wang Z, Pengbin B, Kai L, Yujuan J, Hong W, Quisheng G, Hui S, Jianguo X, Yanwen X. Genetic diversity of intimin gene of atypical enteropathogenic *Escherichia coli* isolated from human, animals and raw meats in China. PLoS ONE. 2016;11(3):1–14.
6. Ghosh PK, Ali A. Isolation of atypical enteropathogenic *Escherichia coli* from children with and without diarrhea in Delhi and the National Capital Region, India. J Med Microbiol. 2010;59:1156–62.
7. Wani SA, Asifa N, Iffiat F, Irfan A, Yoshikazu N, Khursheed Q, Khan MA, Chowdhary J. Investigation of diarrheic faecal samples for enterotoxigenic, Shiga toxin-producing and typical or atypical enteropathogenic *Escherichia coli* in Kashmir, India. FEMS Microbiol Lett. 2006;261:238–44.
8. Rajeshwari K, Beena U, Singh R, Tiwari G, Ajay KM. Multi drug resistant enteropathogenic *E. coli* diarrhea in children. Am J Res Commun. 2015;3(9):27–48.
9. Vieira N, Bates SJ, Solberg OD, Ponce K, Howsmon R, Cevallos W, Trueba G, Riley L, Eisenberg JN. High prevalence of enteroinvasive *Escherichia coli* isolated in a remote region of Northern Costal Ecuador. Am J Trop Med Hyg. 2007;76(3):528–33.
10. Lanjewar M, Anuradha SD, Mathur M. Diarrheagenic *E. coli* in hospitalized patients: special reference to Shiga-like toxin producing *Escherichia coli*. Indian J Pathol Microbiol. 2010;53(1):75–8.
11. Sudershan RV, Kumar RN, Bharathi K, Kashinath L, Bhaskar V, Polasa K. *E. coli* pathotypes and their antibiotic resistance in young children with diarrhea in Hyderabad, India. Int J Curr Microbiol App Sci. 2014;3(9):647–54.
12. Sunaifa SM, Roy S, Dhanashree B. Prevalence of enteropathogenic *Escherichia coli* (EPEC) in adult diarrhoea cases and their antibiotic susceptibility pattern. Br Microbiol Res J. 2015;8(5):560–6.
13. Collee JG, Miles RS, Wan B. Tests for the identification of bacteria. In: Collee JG, Fraser AG, Marmion BP, Simmons A, editors. Mackie and McCartney practical medical microbiology. 14th ed. Edinburgh: Churchill Livingstone; 1996 **(Reprint-2014)**.
14. Edwards PR, Ewing WH. Identification of Enterobacteriaceae. 4th ed. Minneapolis: Burgess Publishing Company; 1986.
15. Begum J, Dutta TK, Chandra R, Chodhury PR, Varte Z, Bitew M. Molecular and phenotypic characterization of shiga toxigenic *Escherichia coli* (STEC) and enteropathogenic *E. coli* from piglets and infants associated with diarrhoea in Mizoram, India. Afr J Biotechnol. 2014;13(13):1452–61.
16. Hegde A, Ballal M, Shenoy S. Detection of diarrheagenic *Escherichia coli* by multiplex PCR. Indian J Med Microbiol. 2012;30(3):279–84.
17. Tamura K, Stecher G, Peterson D, Filipski A, Kumar S. MEGA6: molecular evolutionary genetics analysis version 6.0. Mol Biol Evol. 2013;30(12):2725–9.
18. Bauer AW, Kirby MD, Sherries JC, Truck M. Antibiotic susceptibility testing by a standardized single disk method. Am J Clin Pathol. 1966;45:493–6.
19. Clinical Laboratory Standards Institute. M100-S22 (2012). Clinical and Laboratory Standards Institute: performance standards for antimicrobial susceptibility testing. 22nd informational supplement, vol. 31, no. 1. (M100-S22). Villanova: Clinical and Laboratory Standards Institute; 2012.
20. Magiorakos AP, Srinivasan A, Carey RB, Carmeli Y, Falagas ME, Giske CG, et al. Multidrug-resistant, extensively drug-resistant and pandrug-resistant bacteria: an international expert proposal for interim standard definitions for acquired resistance. Clin Microbiol Infect. 2012;18(3):268–81.
21. Dutta TK, Warjri L, Roychoudhury P, Lalzampuia H, Samanta I, Joardar SN, Bandyopadhyay S, Chandra R. Extended-spectrum β-lactamase producing *Escherichia coli* isolate possessing the shiga toxin gene (stx1) belonging to the O 64 serogroup associated with human diseases in India. J Clin Microbiol. 2013;51(6):2008–9.

22. Rajendran P, Ajjampur SS, Chidambaram D, Chandrabose G, Thangaraj B, Sarkar R, Samuel P, Rajan DP, Kang G. Pathotypes of diarrheagenic *Escherichia coli* in children attending a tertiary care hospital in south India. Diagn Microbiol Infect Dis. 2010;68(2):117–22.

23. Jafari F, Shokrzadeh L, Hamidian M, Salmanzadeh AS, Zali MR. Acute diarrhea due to enteropathogenic bacteria in patients at Hospitals in Iran. Jpn J Infect Dis. 2008;61:269–73.

24. Dallal MMS, Khorramizadeh MR, Ardalan KM. Occurrence of enteropathogenic bacteria in children under 5 years with diarrhea in south Tehran. East Mediterr Health J. 2006;12:792–7.

25. Gupta A, Gautam S, Arup JR, Tanushree M, Ranabir P. Risk correlates of diarrhea in children under 5 years of age in slums of Bankura, West Bengal. J Glob Infect Dis. 2015;7(1):23–9.

26. World Health Organization. Treatment of diarrhea—a manual for physicians and other senior health workers, WHO/CAH/03.1. Geneva: World Health Organization. http://whqlibdoc.who.int/publications/2005/9241593180.pdf.

27. Scaletsky ICA, Souza TB, Aranda KRS, Okeke IN. Genetic elements associated with antimicrobial resistance in enteropathogenic *Escherichia coli* (EPEC) from Brazil. BMC Microbiol. 2010;10:2–5.

28. Dhanashree B, Mallya PS. Molecular typing of enteropathogenic *Escherichia coli* from diarrheagenic stool samples. J Clin Diagn Res. 2012;6:400–4.

29. Farthing M, Salam MA, Lindberg G, Dite P, Khalif I, Salazar-Lindo E, Krabshuis J. Acute diarrhea in adults and children: a global perspective. J Clin Gastroenterol. 2013;47(1):12–20.

30. Perfeito L, Fernandes L, Mota C, Gordo I. Adaptive mutations in bacteria: high rate and small effects. Science. 2007;317:813–5.

19

Enzyme-mediated formulation of stable elliptical silver nanoparticles tested against clinical pathogens and MDR bacteria and development of antimicrobial surgical thread

Rupak Thapa[1], Chintan Bhagat[2], Pragya Shrestha[1], Suvash Awal[1] and Pravin Dudhagara[2*]

Abstract

Background: Silver nanoparticles (AgNPs) are believed to be emerging tool against various infectious diseases including multi-drug resistant (MDR) bacteria. In the present study, in vitro synthesis of AgNPs was optimized using 1:50 ratio of macerozyme (25 µg/µl) and 1 mM $AgNO_3$ incubated at 80 °C for 8 h. AgNPs were characterized by UV–Visible spectroscopy, dynamic light scattering (DLS), scanning electron microscopy, energy-dispersive X-ray spectroscopy, transmission electron microscopy (TEM) and X-ray diffraction (XRD).

Results: Characterization studies suggest the synthesis of elliptical, stable and crystalline AgNPs with an average size of 38.26 ± 0.4 nm calculated using TEM. The XRD pattern revealed the face-centered-cubic (fcc) form of metallic silver. Good shape integrity and dispersion of AgNPs after 1 year of incubation confirmed their stability. AgNPs were exibited the antimicrobial property against ten pathogenic bacteria, three molds and one yeast. The AgNPs also revealed remarkable antimicrobial activity against three MDR strains i.e. Extended spectrum beta-lactamase positive *Escherichia coli*, *Staphylococcus aureus* (MRSA) and Teicoplanin resistant *Streptococcus Pneumoniae*. The AgNPs coated surgical threads (suture) were revealed the remarkble antibacterial activity against three MDR strains. This is the first report to synthesize antimicrobial elliptical AgNPs using enzymes.

Conclusion: The results suggest the possibilities to develop the nanoparticles coated antimicrobial medical fabric to combat against MDR infection.

Keywords: Silver nanoparticles (AgNPs), Antimicrobial activity, Multi-drug resistant (MDR), Surgical thread

Background

The silver and gold nanoparticles have been largely explored in biomedical sector due to its great potential as a broad spectrum antimicrobial agent [1–4]. Despite of its wide use, antibacterial activity of silver nanoparticles is poorly understood with few implicit mechanisms including (1) generations of reactive oxygen species (ROS) intracellularly and/or extracellularly, (2) cellular uptake of silver ions (3) cascade of intracellular reactions and (4) interactions between nanoscale silver and cell membranes [5, 6]. Recently, Hsueh et al. [7] reported the release of Ag+ ions intracellular or extracellular from the AgNPs, highlights the precise antimicrobial mechanism. Based on these mechanisms, AgNPs have been employed and established as an antibacterial agent in wound treatment, medical devices, cosmetics, water purification, air treatment and clothing [8, 9]. Presently, >30% of AgNPs are utilized by the healthcare sector due to impressive demand of antimicrobial consumable stuff. Thus, the

*Correspondence: dudhagarapr@gmail.com
[2] Department of Biosciences (UGC-SAP-DRS-II), Veer Narmad South Gujarat University, Surat, Gujarat 395007, India
Full list of author information is available at the end of the article

growing demand of antimicrobial materials in health-care applications is projected to drive silver nanoparticles market to reach USD 2.45 billion by 2022 (http://www.grandviewresearch.com/press-release/global-silver-nanoparticles-market). This ongoing demand of the AgNPs will promote the exploration of various new synthesis routes.

Nanobiotechnological production of nanoparticle using biomolecules offers the characteristic of specificity, benign nature, viability and conceivability for functionalization [2]. Biocatalysis dependent nanoparticles synthesis was found to be more pharmacologically active than chemical route formulation and holds promise for amended biocompatible nanoparticles production [10]. Few green approaches have been tested for metal nanoparticles synthesis, which includes the use of plant extract, enzyme, biomolecule, biosurfactant and micro-organisms [11–15]. In vitro synthesis process is new developed concept which eliminates the culturing of the microorganisms and extraction of their metabolites/macromolecules. Several enzymes have been explored for lab scale as well as bulk production of AgNPs including keratinase, nitrate reductase, alpha-amylase and sulfite reductase [16–19]. Enzyme-mediated nanoparticle formation is widely utilized methods as it is simple, eco-friendly, inexpensive and easily scaled-up process for bulk production of functionalized and stable nanoparticles [16–18]. The size and shape controlled synthesis of the AgNPs is the key issues to determined their efficacy and applications. Such controlled synthesis of AgNPs can be formulated through the optimization of process variables including pH, temperature, reaction time, enzyme concentration and substrate concentration.

Biosynthesis of the size and shape controlled nano-particles are yet the challenging task for the nano-technologiest. The size of the AgNPs determines their effectiveness against pathogenic bacteria. Smaller than 50 nm of AgNPs are reported as a best antimicrobial weapon against bacterial pathogens [20]. The shape of AgNPs also play the significant role to kill the microorganisms, sphere-shaped nanoparticles are considered to be the best-suited for antimicrobial applications in either colloidal form or immobilized state [21]. Elliptical or oval AgNPs may also more antimicrobial than other reported shape due to more surface area to interact with cell membrane and ease to inter into cell. Morphological variation of the AgNPs is not only the determinant of microbial susceptibility, but the microbial cell structure and type (i.e. Gram positive and negative), are also play a significant role [22]. Earlier studies of AgNPs as bactericides have been largely explored through the model microbial species—*Escherichia coli* [23]. The outputs of such experiments are not adequate to confirm the AgNPs as

antimicrobials. Additionally, the susceptibility of MDR bacteria against antimicrobials is very negligible than the non-MDR bacteria. So the multiple non-MDR and MDR bacterial species need to test against the AgNPs to establish it as antimicrobials.

Currently, the outbreak of various MDR strains globally at the alarming rate resulted in treatment difficulties which have imposed a burden on health care systems and simultaneously intensifying the need for new antimicrobial agents [24]. Recently, WHO list out the 12 MDR bacterial species (http://www.who.int/mediacentre/news/releases/2017/bacteria-antibiotics-needed/en/) that pose a greatest threat to human health suggest the prompt need of new therapy to manage this antimicrobial crisis. The discovery of the new antimicrobials is quite slower than the emerging rate of the antimicrobial resistance among the bacteria. Provisionally, the use of the metal nanoparticles to achieve the success in antimicrobial crisis can be a viable option. Due to the interaction of nano-silver with multiple microbial target sites, it is expected to be feasible and promising alternative against most common MDR strains such *E. coli, Staphylococcus aureus* and *Streptococcus pneumoniae*. Moreover, the synergistic activity of AgNPs coupled with antibiotics is also an advisable approach to combat against various MDR strains. Therefore, stable AgNPs are effective bactericidal materials due to its combined effects with antibacterial agents and are the robust ammunition against the MDR strains [25].

In present research, attempt was made to in vitro synthesis of AgNPs using macerating enzymes. AgNPs characterization was investigated to confirm the size, shape, and nature. The antimicrobial activity of AgNPs was studied against pathogenic bacteria, yeast and molds. The key investigation was carried out by testing the antimicrobial activity against three MDR bacterial species *E. coli, S. aureus* and *S. pneumoniae*.

Methods
Materials
Macerating enzymes, Macerozyme R-10, Nutrient agar, Blood agar, Chocolate agar and MacConkey agar, Mueller–Hinton (MH) agar and potato dextrose agar (PDA) were purchased from Hi-Media Laboratories Pvt. Ltd. Mumbai, India. Silver nitrate (AgNO$_3$) was acquired from S.D. Fine-Chem. Ltd. Mumbai, India. Throughout the experiment, MiliQ (Millipore®) water was used for solutions preparation. The antibiotics sensitivity tests were verified using antibiotics disc purchased from Hi-Media Laboratories Pvt. Ltd. Mumbai, India. The identification of clinical cultures was carried out by VITEK®2 system (Biomerieux Inc. Hazelwood, Mo.) at Anand Laboratory, Surat, India.

Synthesis of AgNPs

Total 20 reaction systems were prepared using different concentration of macerozymes and AgNO$_3$. Different volumes of macerozyme (25 µg/µl solution) i.e. 20, 100, 200, 500, and 1000 µl were added separately in 5 ml AgNO$_3$ solution of varying concentration of 0.1, 0.5, 1 and 2 mM and were incubated at 37, 60, 80, and 90 °C for 2–8 h. The pH of all the reaction systems was adjusted 7.2 ± 0.2. After every 2-h interval, a reduction of silver ions was confirmed by the color changes and verifies the time required for the formation of AgNPs.

Characterization of nanoparticles
UV–Vis spectroscopy

Formation of AgNPs indicated by the color changes of the reaction mixture from colorless to pinkish-red due to the bioreduction of the silver ions using enzymes. The synthesis of AgNPs was assured by scanning the absorption spectra of the reaction mixture over the range of 300–800 nm wavelengths with UV–Vis spectrophotometer (UV-1800, Shimadzu, Japan) using dual beam operated at 1 nm resolution. The optimum result indicated reaction was subjected to further analysis.

Dynamic light scattering

Zetasizer (Nano-ZS, Malvern Instruments, USA) was used to monitor the size distribution profile of synthesized colloidal AgNPs using MiliQ water as a dispersant (refractive index = 1.330, viscosity = 0.8872 cP). The size calculation was carried out using colloidal sample and means value of three readings was considered.

Scanning electron microscopy and elemental analysis

Colloidal AgNPs dried at 60 °C, and analyzed by SEM (JEOL JSM-6360LV), operating at an accelerating voltage of 15.0 kV under high vacuum. The dried AgNPs sample was applied to the carbon-coated copper grid for measurement of elemental composition profile of the sample using EDX equipped with SEM.

TEM analysis

Colloidal AgNPs were further analyzed by the TECNAI G^2 TEM instrument (FEI Corp. Hillsboro, USA) operating at 80 kV, and the image was taken using TIA software after drop coating with 50 µl of nanoparticles on a carbon-coated copper grid of 300 mesh size. After 1 year storage at 37 °C, colloidal AgNPs were again visualized using TEM to check the agglomeration.

X-ray diffraction analysis

Dried powder of synthesized AgNPs analyzed by diffractometer on X'Pert Pro PANaltyical, USA operated at 45 kV and 40 mA current at 25 °C temperature and diffraction pattern was recorded by CuKα1 radiation with λ of 1.54 Å, step size 0.017 in the region of 2θ from 20 to 100.

Evaluation of antimicrobial activity

Out of six Gram-positive bacteria, four i.e. *Micrococcus luteus* NCIM 5262, *Bacillus subtilis* NCIM 2920, *Bacillus cereus* NCIM 5557, and *Bacillus megaterium* NCIM 5334 as well as four molds include *Aspergillus niger* NCIM 1358, *Mucor racemosus* NCIM 1334, *Penicillium chrysogenum* NCIM 1333, *Rhizopus stolonifer* NCIM 1139 were purchase from National Collection of Industrial Microorganisms (NCIM), Pune, India. These laboratory control strains of bacteria and molds were maintained on Nutrient agar and PDA respectively. *S. aureus* and *S. pneumoniae* were isolated on Blood agar from the blood and throat swab respectively. *E. coli*, *Klebsiella pneumoniae*, *Proteus vulgaris*, *Pseudomonas aeruginosa*, were isolated using Blood agar, Chocolate agar and MacConkey agar from urine, throat swab, urine and sputum respectively. The *Candia albicans* was isolated form viginal swab on PDA.

Antimicrobial activity of AgNPs was analyzed using disc diffusion method against clinical pathogenic bacteria, yeast and molds. The pure cultures of all bacteria and yeast were grown on MH liquid medium. The active culture of bacteria and yeast were uniformly swabbed onto the MH agar plates using sterile cotton swabs, pre-soaked with 20 µl of each culture (A$_{620 nm}$ = 0.85). After incubation at 37 °C for 24 h, the zone of inhibition (ZOI) was measured in millimeter and result was recorded in triplicate experiments. Whereas, each sporulated mold were grown on PD agar plates using spores sprinkling method by placing the plate containing one week old growth of mold and tapped ten times on fresh PD agar plate aseptically and incubate 5 days at 30 °C to obtain an adequate growth. Subsequently, paper discs were impregnated with 20 µl of AgNPs, AgNO$_3$, and sterile H$_2$O and laid aseptically over the pre-inoculated agar plates.

Activity against MDR bacteria

The ESBL positive *E. coli*, *S. aureus* (MRSA), Teicoplanin resistance *S. pneumoniae* were isolated from urine, blood and throat swab of pediatric sample respectively. Blood agar Chocolate agar and MacConkey agar were used for the isolation. Identification were carried out by using VITEK®2 system. For the verification of the MDR, the antibiotic susceptibility of each strain was performed using disc diffusion test on MH agar against various antibiotics suggested by guideline (2016) of National Committee for Clinical Laboratory Standards (NCCLS), now Clinical and Laboratory Standards

Institute (CLSI). Susceptibility of 20 µl of AgNPs, $AgNO_3$, and sterile H_2O was also tested as discussed in earlier section.

Development of nano-coated surgical threads

The nanocoated surgical threads were developed by dipping 30 mm long threads into colloidal AgNPs followed by drying at 45 °C and wash aseptically with sterile distilled water. Nanocoated threads were placed in MH agar plates, pre-streaked with three MDR strains and antimicrobial activities were tested as explained earlier section.

Result

Synthesis of AgNPs formation

Out of 20 different reactions, four reactions containing 100 µl of macerozyme solution (25 µg/µl) and 5 ml of 1 mM $AgNO_3$ incubated at four different temperature i.e. 37, 60, 80 and 90 °C were selected and among them the best AgNPs synthesis was observed at 80 °C temperature after 8 h. As the time and temperature increased in all four reaction mixtures, the reduction of the silver ions was increased and corresponding orange color was also intensify. However, UV–Vis spectroscopic analysis indicated the narrow bell shaped graphs with highest absorbance at 425 nm after 8 h treatment at 80 °C was selected as a best reaction (Additional file 1).

Characterization of AgNPs

Optimized reaction based on UV-Vis spectroscopic analysis, AgNPs were subjected for particle size analysis. The average size of ~90% AgNPs was 63.65 ± 12.71 nm by DLS with a good dispersity (Fig. 1). SEM results suggest the elongated morphology of the AgNPs. Energy dispersive X-ray spectrum of AgNPs revealed the clear and heightened peak at 3 keV correspond to the binding energies of Ag Lα, which is the characteristics peak of nano-silver (Fig. 2) [26]. Elemental composition profile indicates the relatively high purity of the particles with high concentration of silver i.e. 39.50% by weight. The result of the TEM confirmed elliptical shape of individual particles with average diameter of 38.26 ± 0.4 nm in fresh and 1-year-old sample (Fig. 3). A very slight clump was observed in old sample; however, the visible clumps were absent. To the best of our knowledge, this is

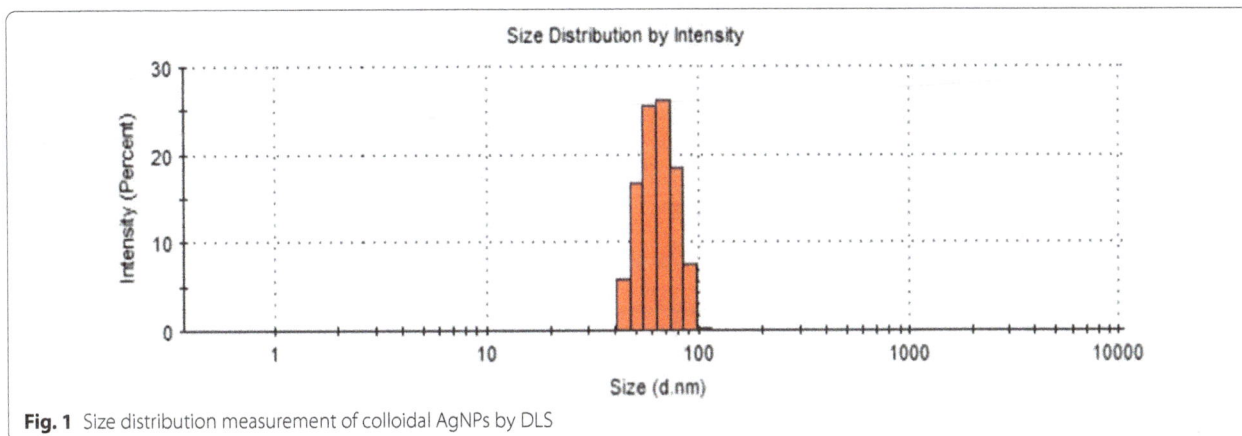

Fig. 1 Size distribution measurement of colloidal AgNPs by DLS

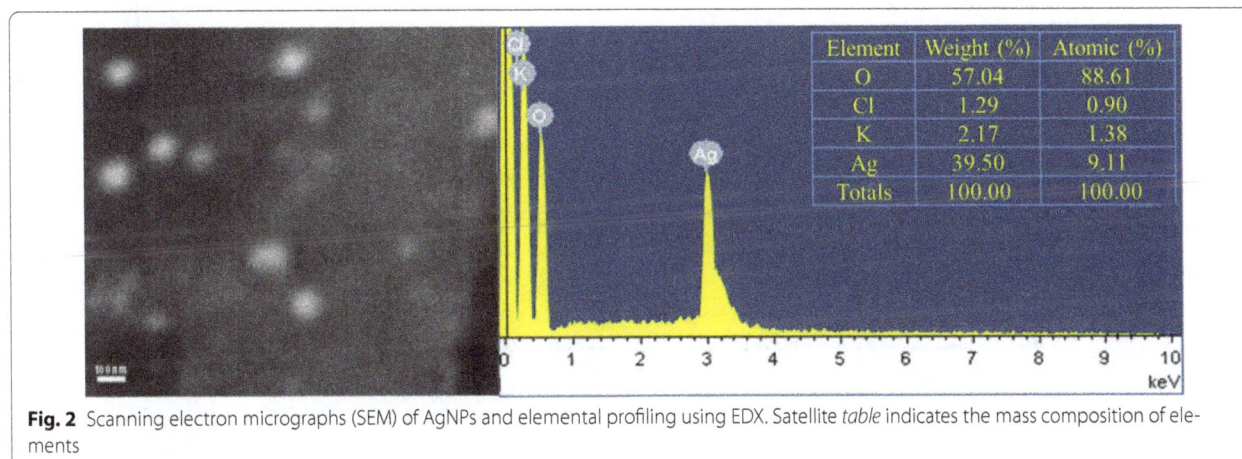

Element	Weight (%)	Atomic (%)
O	57.04	88.61
Cl	1.29	0.90
K	2.17	1.38
Ag	39.50	9.11
Totals	100.00	100.00

Fig. 2 Scanning electron micrographs (SEM) of AgNPs and elemental profiling using EDX. Satellite *table* indicates the mass composition of elements

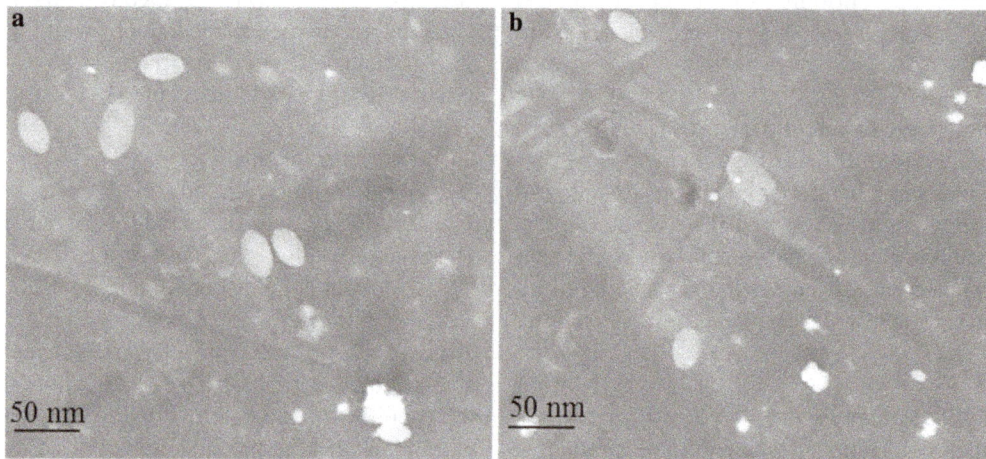

Fig. 3 Confirmation of elliptical shape of AgNPs by TEM **a** in fresh and **b** 1-year-old colloidal sample

the first report to formulat the elliptical shaped particles using biological route. The XRD analysis confirmed the presence of peaks at $2\theta = 38°, 44°, 64°, 77°$ and $81°$, which coincide to (111), (200), (220), (311) and (222) indicating planes of silver respectively (JCPDS, standard file no. 04-0783) (Fig. 4). To calculate the crystalline (grain) size form the XRD data, we use standard Debye–Scherrer method for better conformation of crystalline size. The average crystalline size of our prepared sample was 36.01 ± 1.4 nm (Table 1). The size of AgNPs measured by TEM and XRD are supportive but differs from the DLS analysis due to the brownian motion and elliptical shape

of particles that lead to the more diverse results of DLS than TEM and XRD.

Antimicrobial activity

The efficiency of antibacterial activity of AgNPs was assessed as size of ZOI against the ZOI of $AgNO_3$ solution and sterile H_2O. AgNPs were found to have better antimicrobial activity against *B. subtilis, M. leutus, P. aeruginosa, B. megaterium* and *S. aureus* having a zone of inhibition of more than 15.0 ± 0.0 mm. The AgNPs showed remarkable antifungal activity against all the tested strains among which, maximum activity was

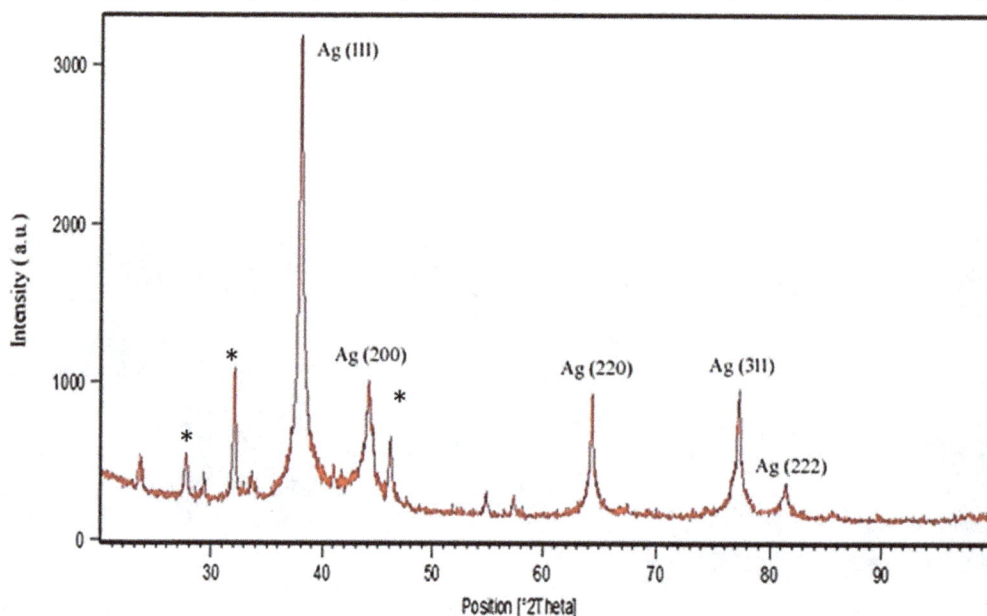

Fig. 4 XRD pattern of AgNPs

Enzyme-mediated formulation of stable elliptical silver nanoparticles tested against...

159

Table 1 Crystalline size of AgNPs calculated using Debye–Scherrer's equation

2θ (deg)	θ	Planes-hkl	FWHM (deg)	Crystalline size (nm)	Average crystalline size (nm)
38	19	111	0.041	35.70	36.01 ± 1.4
44	22	200	0.043	34.76	
64	32	220	0.047	34.77	
77	38.5	311	0.048	36.89	
81	40.5	222	0.048	37.97	

seen against *R. stolonifer* with 14.0 ± 1.0 mm ZOI and minimum activity was seen against *C. albicans* with 12.0 ± 0.0 mm ZOI. The percentage increases in inhibition zone area for the AgNPs against *P. chrysogenum* NCIM 1333 was highest i.e. 96% followed by *A. niger* NCIM 1358 (43.12%), *E. coli* (32.45%) and *P. aeruginosa* (31.82%). For other tested microorganisms, the percent of increases of inhibition zone area were ranging from 15.62 to 31.65% (Table 2). AgNPs ZOI against ESBL positive *E. coli* was 10.5 ± 0.50 mm, which is far greater than the most of the tested antibiotics. *S. aureus* (MRSA) showed the 13.5 ± 0.5 mm zone which is 2.5 ± 0.5 mm greater than the AgNO₃. Teicoplanin resistant *S. pneumoniae* was exibited the 13.16 ± 0.28 mm ZOI (Table 3). From the study, the comparative effectiveness of AgNPs and AgNO₃ against MDR strains was clearly observed.

AgNPs showed clear zone of inhibition that was greater than various tested first and second generation antibiotics. The remarkable antimicrobial activity of AgNPs treated surgical threads against ESBL positive *E. coli*, *S. aureus* (MRSA) and Teicoplanin resistant *S. pneumoniae* indicates the firmly coating of AgNPs on the threads (Fig. 5).

Discussion

AgNO₃ reduction and AgNPs formation was found to temperature and time dependent. The increase in the reaction temperature and the time, increase the accessibility of the silver ions for the rapid reduction. The synthesis of AgNPs at elevated temperature is due to the accessibility of thiol groups of macerating enzymes. High temperature unfolds the structure of enzymes and makes an easy availability of thiol groups for the bioreduction of metal (i.e. silver) [27, 28]. However, there are many possibilities for reduction using enzymes. The optimum temperature was 80 °C and time was 8 h. The further increase up to 90 °C caused the broadening of the peak suggesting the bigger and heterogeneous particles formation that led the decrease in absorption [29]. The sharpness of the absorbance peak is dependent to size of the AgNPs because the particle size may be smaller at the higher temperature consequently narrow and sharp SPR band of AgNPs was observed [30]. Beside temperature, reaction time is another factor to determine the controlled synthesis. The steady increasing of

Table 2 Antimicrobial activity of colloidal AgNPs against various species of pathogenic bacteria, yeast and molds

Sr. no.	Microorganisms	ZOI of 20 µl of AgNPs (mm) (y)	ZOI of 20 µl of 1 mM AgNO₃ (mm) (x)	ZOI of 20 µl of H₂O (mm)	Increase in the ZOI area (%)[a]
1	*E. coli*	12.66 ± 0.28	11.00 ± 0.0	0 ± 0	32.45
2	*S. pneumoniae*	14.33 ± 0.57	13.16 ± 0.28	0 ± 0	18.57
3	*K. pneumonia*	14.16 ± 0.28	13.0 ± 0.5	0 ± 0	18.64
4	*P. vulgaris*	14.00 ± 0.5	12.33 ± 0.28	0 ± 0	28.92
5	*S. aureus*	15.0 ± 0.0	13.16 ± 0.28	0 ± 0	29.91
6	*P. aeruginosa*	15.5 ± 0.5	13.5 ± 0.5	0 ± 0	31.82
7	*B. cereus* NCIM 5557	12.50 ± 0.5	11.16 ± 0.28	0 ± 0	25.45
8	*B. megaterium* NCIM 5334	15.33 ± 0.28	13.5 ± 0.5	0 ± 0	28.94
9	*M. luteus* NCIM 5262	15.5 ± 1.0	14.0 ± 0.5	0 ± 0	22.57
10	*B. subtilis* NCIM 2920	16.0 ± 1.0	14.0 ± 0.5	0 ± 0	30.61
11	*C. albicans*	12.0 ± 0.0	11.16 ± 0.28	0 ± 0	15.62
12	*A. niger* NCIM 1358	13.16 ± 0.28	11.0 ± 0.5	0 ± 0	43.12
13	*M. racemosus* NCIM 1334	13.0 ± 0.5	11.33 ± 0.28	0 ± 0	31.65
14	*P. chrysogenum* NCIM 1333	14.0 ± 1.0	10.0 ± 0.5	0 ± 0	96.00
15	*R. stolonifer* NCIM 1139	14.0 ± 1.0	12.5 ± 1.0	0 ± 0	25.44

All experiments were performed in triplicate

[a] The mean surface area of the growth inhibition zone (mm²) was calculated for AgNPs and AgNO₃ from the mean diameter. The percent of increases of inhibition zone area for the AgNPs against different microorganism were calculated as $(y^2-x^2)/x^2 \times 100$, where x and y are the inhibition zone for 20 µl of AgNO₃ and 20 µl of AgNPs respectively

Table 3 Antibiotic-resistance profile of MDR strains and AgNPs susceptibility test

Bacteria	Tested antibiotics	Disk content (µg)	ZOI (mm)	Antibiotics susceptibility interpretation[a]
ESBL+ve *E. coli*	Nalidixic acid	30	6.0 ± 0.50	R
	Doxycycline	30	16.16 ± 0.28	S
	Norfloxacin	10	8.0 ± 0.50	R
	Nitrofurantoin	30	15.0 ± 0.50	I
	Cefixime	30	6.0 ± 0.50	R
	Cefixime/clavulanate	5/10	8.0 ± 0.50	R
	Cefoperazone	75	6.0 ± 0.0	R
	Cefoperazone/tazobactam	75/10	19.5 ± 1.0	S
	Ceftazidime	30	7.0 ± 1.0	R
	Cetazidime/clavulanate	30/10	14.0 ± 0.0	I
	Chloramphenicol	30	15.16 ± 0.28	I
	Cefprozil	30	6.5 ± 0.50	R
	Cefepime	30	10.5 ± 0.50	R
	AgNPs	2.16[b]	10.5 ± 0.50	–
	AgNO$_3$	3.4	9.16 ± 0.28	–
	Sterile H$_2$O	20 µl	0 ± 0	–
S. aureus (MRSA)	Oxacillin	1	6.66 ± 0.28	R
	Cefoxitin	30	19.33 ± 0.57	R
	AgNPs	2.16[b]	13.5 ± 0.5	–
	AgNO$_3$	3.4	11.0 ± 0.0	–
	Sterile H$_2$O	20 µl	0 ± 0	–
S. pneumoniae MDR	Teicoplanin	30	10.0 ± 0.0	R
	AgNPs	2.16[b]	13.16 ± 0.28	–
	AgNO$_3$	3.4	11.0 ± 0.0	–
	Sterile H$_2$O	20 µl	0 ± 0	–

All experiments were performed in triplicate

R resistant, *I* intermediate, *S* susceptible

[a] The antibiotics susceptibility interpretation was based on CLSI guideline-2016

[b] 20 µl of 1 mM AgNO$_3$ (MW 169.87) contains 3.4 µg AgNO$_3$ and the percentage of silver is 63.5% in nanoparticles (i. e 2.16 µg)

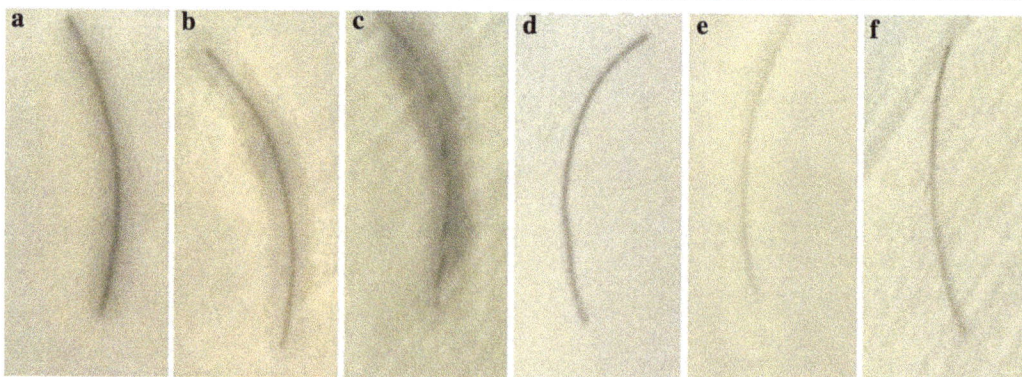

Fig. 5 Antimicrobial activity of AgNPs coated surgical suture against **a** ESBL positive *E. coli*, **b** *S. aureus* MRSA, **c** Teicoplanin resistant *S. pneumoniae*. Control: Sterile H$_2$O treated suture tested against **d** ESBL positive *E. coli* (E) *S. aureus* MRSA **f** Teicoplanin resistant *S. pneumoniae*

absorbance spectrum with increasing the reaction time resulted in the colorless reaction mixture shifts to pinkish-orange with the duration of incubation indicates the increased concentrations of the AgNPs. Thus, the rate of synthesis can be accelerated by increasing the temperature and contact time [31].

Size distribution profile of the colloidal nanoparticles showed narrow monodispersity with an average size of 63.65 ± 12.71 nm by DLS. Nucleation of the silver ions and growth of nanoparticles is the key processes to determine the size. In biosynthesis route the amino and carboxyl group are usually involved into nucleation process. However, the mechanism of biogenic AgNPs is poorly understood. Earlier reports of enzymes assisted AgNPs synthesis suggested the involvement of various amino acids and their functional groups for the AgNPs formation [32, 33]. The result of EDX proved the presence of nearly 40% silver and 60% other trace metals (O, K, Cl) by weight; this is primarily due to the biogenic root of synthesis. Biological derived impurities like carbon, oxygen, potassium are usually involves in stabilizing the particles by capping on the surface of AgNPs [34]. Absence of oxides indicated the sample contain pure silver. TEM image confirmed elliptical shape and average size of particles is 38.26 ± 0.4 nm. TEM also indicate the good stability of particles with negligible aggregation after 1 year may be due to the presence of Cl ions. The XRD pattern reveals the AgNPs correspond to face-centered cubic (fcc) crystalline phase. Few minor unassigned peaks (*) were due to the formation of the crystalline bioorganic compounds by the enzyme [35].

Antimicrobials resistance (AMR) in pathogenic microorganisms is ever challenging global issue. A wide range of antimicrobial compounds and their combination are used to control AMR in the MDR bacteria and the searching of new antimicrobials for MDR species are yet ongoing practices. One of the best substitutions to combating the resistant problem in different microbes is use of metal nanoparticles due to the multifaceted antimicrobial mechanisms of metals nanoparticles against wide range of microbes [36, 37]. Silver is known to be used for centuries as a potent antimicrobial weapon because of its growth hindrance abilities against a diverse microorganism by exerting its effect at multiple site. AgNPs synthesized by various routes and of different size and shape was tested against diverse clinical pathogenic MDR strains [4, 8, 12, 13, 16, 25, 31]. Due to failure of first and second line antibiotics, the exploration of AgNPs against various MDR strains is the new emerging trend. These suggest the further exploration of silver or other nanoparticles for treatment of various MDR, extensively drug-resistant (XDR) and pan drug resistance (PDR) pathogens. The remarkable antimicrobial activity of 2.1 µg of AgNPs was reported against *S. aureus*, *B. subtilis*, *P. aeruginosa*, *P. vulgaris*, *M. racemosus*, *P. chrysogenum* and *R. stolonifer*. The minimum inhibitory concentration of AgNPs is found to be varies in literature and it depends on coating medium, route of synthesis, types of strains, different size and shape of nanoparticles [4, 8, 16, 30, 38–40]. Result of antimicrobial activity against *E. coli* ESBL positive,

S. aureus (MRSA) and MDR *S. pneumoniae* were also very excellent. The antimicrobial activities against all the Gram-negative and Gram-positive bacteria are more than 12.50 ± 0.5 which is far better than the earlier report [20]. The toxicity of AgNPs is due to the release of intracellular Ag ions in bacterial cell but its orders of magnitude is different into different bacterial species because the intracellular bioavailability of Ag ions liberated from AgNPs is bacterial strain-specific [41]. Moreover, extracellular secretion i.e. organic acids, peptides, biosurfactants and cellular uptake of Ag ions via cell-nanoparticles interaction my affects the toxicity. Additionally, the AgNPs-cell contact is the key phenomenon to determine the toxicity of nanoparticle [41]. The formation of biocorona by hydrogen bonding and hydrophobic interactions between cellular peptides/proteins and AgNPs may varies on cell to cell, consequently the toxicity will be varies among the different microbial cell [42]. Thus, the binding behaviors and kinetics of AgNPs with proteins are important aspects in realizing the toxicity of AgNPs in biosystem [43]. The size and shape determine the surface-to-volume ratio of AgNPs and impacting on its effectiveness. AgNPs are readily interact with organic materials and mounted in fabric for slow release to exert their long-lasting antimicrobial effect. Thus, the safe use and enduring antimicrobial properties can be achieved by tethering the AgNPs on organic nanosheets [44]. Antimicrobial property of nano-coated surgical threads is a key outcome of the present study which is promising tool to control the spreading of MDR infections over a long time. The nano-silver coated nylon thread is useful in the healing process as AgNPs not allows the tissue adherence and thereby helps in healing process [45, 46]. The antimicrobial dressing materials developed through the tethering of the AgNPs can be easily use for biomedical application.

Although, the AgNPs are broad spectrum antimicrobials, it is hard to conclude using clinical and laboratory control strains that it can be substitutes the antibiotics as their toxicity is still a big challenge for their clinical and biomedical applications. Furthermore, there are few controversies related to safe use of AgNPs in human diseases treatment and health care. In the present study, use of only three MDR strains may be inadequate and in future we will conduct the study with few more MDR strains. Nevertheless, the study provides the baseline information to develop the prototype for antimicrobial medical materials.

Conclusion

Macerating enzymes are good reductant of AgNO$_3$ for in vitro synthesis of silver nanoparticles. The adopted process was environment-friendly, simple, rapid, and easy to perform. Bioformulated AgNPs were well dispersed, small in size, elliptical and stable over a year suggest promising application in the biomedical and healthcare sector. Synthesized AgNPs showed antimicrobial activity against various non-MDR and MDR bacteria, yeast and molds. This study confirms the biologically synthesized AgNPs are safe and viable option against pathogens. So it is proved that the AgNPs has a great potential to be used as an antimicrobial agent. The nano-silver treated nylon thread can be useful especially for the stitching the surgery cuts to avoids the secondary infection.

Abbreviations

$AgNO_3$: silver nitrate; AgNPs: silver nanoparticle; AMR: antimicrobials resistance; CLSI: Clinical and Laboratory Standards Institute; DLS: dynamic light scattering; EDX: energy-dispersive X-ray spectroscopy; ESBL: extended-spectrum beta-lactamases; fcc: face-centered cubic; JCPDS: Joint Committee on Powder Diffraction Standard; MDR: multi-drug resistant; MH: Mueller-Hinton agar; mm: millimeter; mM: millimolar; MRSA: methicillin-resistant *staphylococcus aureus*; NCCLS: National Committee for Clinical Laboratory Standards; NCIM: National Collection of Industrial Microorganisms; PDA: potato dextrose agar; PDR: pan drug resistance; SEM: scanning electron microscopy; TEM: transmission electron microscopy; WHO: World Health Organization; XDR: extensively drug-resistant; XRD: X-ray diffraction; ZOI: zone of inhibition; µg: microgram; µl: microliter.

Authors' contributions

All author contributed equally. All authors read and approved the final manuscript.

Author details

[1] Department of Biotechnology, Veer Narmad South Gujarat University, Surat, Gujarat 395007, India. [2] Department of Biosciences (UGC-SAP-DRS-II), Veer Narmad South Gujarat University, Surat, Gujarat 395007, India.

Acknowledgements

Authors are thankful to Department of Biosciences (UGC-SAP-DRS-II), Veer Narmad South Gujarat University for providing infrastructure support. Authors also acknowledge to Dr. Vandhana Lad, Chief Microbiologist, Anand Microbiology Laboratory, Surat, India for providing the clinical isolates and allowing the use of laboratory facilities.

Competing interests

The authors declare that they have no competing interests.

Funding

The authors declare that they did not have any funding source or grant to support their research work.

References

1. Radulescu M, Andronescu E, Dolete G, Popescu R, Fufă O, Chifiriuc M, et al. Silver nanocoatings for reducing the exogenous microbial colonization of wound dressings. Materials. 2016;9:345.
2. Nath D, Banerjee P. Green nanotechnology—A new hope for medical biology. Environ Toxicol Pharmacol. 2013;36:997–1014.
3. Victor S-U, José Roberto V-B. Gold and silver nanotechology on medicine. J Chem Biochem. 2015;3:21–33.
4. Geetha R, Ashokkumar T, Tamilselvan S, Govindaraju K, Sadiq M, Singaravelu G. Green synthesis of gold nanoparticles and their anticancer activity. Cancer Nanotechnol. 2013;4:91–8.
5. Prabhu S, Poulose EK. Silver nanoparticles: mechanism of antimicrobial action, synthesis, medical applications, and toxicity effects. Int Nano Lett. 2012;2:32.
6. Durán N, Durán M, de Jesus MB, Seabra AB, Fávaro WJ, Nakazato G. Silver nanoparticles: a new view on mechanistic aspects on antimicrobial activity. Nanomed Nanotechnol Biol Med. 2016;12:789–99.
7. Hsueh Y-H, Lin K-S, Ke W-J, Hsieh C-T, Chiang C-L, Tzou D-Y, et al. The antimicrobial properties of silver nanoparticles in *Bacillus subtilis* are mediated by released Ag^+ ions. PLoS ONE. 2015;10:e0144306.
8. Rai M, Yadav A, Gade A. Silver nanoparticles as a new generation of antimicrobials. Biotechnol Adv. 2009;27:76–83.
9. Lee KJ, Jun BH, Kim TH, Joung J. Direct synthesis and inkjetting of silver nanocrystals toward printed electronics. Nanotechnology. 2006;17:2424–8.
10. Singh P, Kim Y-J, Zhang D, Yang D-C. Biological synthesis of nanoparticles from plants and microorganisms. Trends Biotechnol. 2016;34:588–99.
11. Mangrola MH, Joshi VG, Dudhagura PR, Parmar BH. Two step synthesis and biophysical characterization of silver nanoparticles using green approach. J Environ Res Dev. 2012;7:1021–5.
12. Dudhagara P, Maniar N, Anjana G, Mangrola M. Plant leaf assisted synthesis and application evaluation of silver nanoparticles. Int J Res Advent Technol. 2014;2:112–21.
13. Wu Q, Cao H, Luan Q, Zhang J, Wang Z, Warner JH, et al. Biomolecule-assisted synthesis of water-soluble silver nanoparticles and their biomedical applications. Inorg Chem. 2008;47:5882–8.
14. Farias CBB, Silva AF, Rufino RD, Luna JM, Souza JEG, Sarubbo LA. Synthesis of silver nanoparticles using a biosurfactant produced in low-cost medium as stabilizing agent. Electron J Biotechnol. 2014;17:122–5.
15. Prakash A, Sharma S, Ahmad N, Ghosh A, Sinha P. Bacteria mediated extracellular synthesis of metallic nanoparticles. Int Res J Biotechnol. 2010;1:071–9.
16. Lateef A, Adelere IA, Gueguim-Kana EB, Asafa TB, Beukes LS. Green synthesis of silver nanoparticles using keratinase obtained from a strain of *Bacillus safensis* LAU 13. Int Nano Lett. 2015;5:29–35.
17. Hebbalalu D, Lalley J, Nadagouda MN, Varma RS. Greener techniques for the synthesis of silver nanoparticles using plant extracts, enzymes, bacteria, biodegradable polymers, and microwaves. ACS Sustain Chem Eng. 2013;1:703–12.
18. Mishra A, Sardar M. Alpha-amylase mediated synthesis of silver nanoparticles. Sci Adv Mater. 2012;4:143–6.
19. Gholami-Shabani M, Shams-Ghahfarokhi M, Gholami-Shabani Z, Akbarzadeh A, Riazi G, Ajdari S, et al. Enzymatic synthesis of gold nanoparticles using sulfite reductase purified from *Escherichia coli*: a green eco-friendly approach. Process Biochem. 2015;50:1076–85.
20. Agnihotri S, Mukherji S, Mukherji S. Size-controlled silver nanoparticles synthesized over the range 5–100 nm using the same protocol and their antibacterial efficacy. RSC Adv. 2014;4:3974–83.
21. Agnihotri S, Mukherji S, Mukherji S. Immobilized silver nanoparticles enhance contact killing and show highest efficacy: elucidation of the mechanism of bactericidal action of silver. Nanoscale. 2013;5:7328–40.
22. Martínez-Castañón GA, Niño-Martínez N, Martínez-Gutierrez F, Martínez-Mendoza JR, Ruiz F. Synthesis and antibacterial activity of silver nanoparticles with different sizes. J Nanoparticle Res. 2008;10:1343–8.
23. Sondi I, Salopek-Sondi B. Silver nanoparticles as antimicrobial agent: a case study on E. coli as a model for Gram-negative bacteria. J Colloid Interface Sci. 2004;275:177–82.

24. Dudhagara PR, Ghelani AD, Patel RK. Phenotypic characterization and antibiotics combination approach to control the methicillin-resistant *Staphylococcus aureus* (MRSA) strains isolated from the hospital derived fomites. Asian J Med Sci. 2011;2:72–8.

25. Rai MK, Deshmukh SD, Ingle AP, Gade AK. Silver nanoparticles: the powerful nanoweapon against multidrug-resistant bacteria: activity of silver nanoparticles against MDR bacteria. J Appl Microbiol. 2012;112:841–52.

26. Khan MAM, Kumar S, Ahamed M, Alrokayan SA, AlSalhi MS. Structural and thermal studies of silver nanoparticles and electrical transport study of their thin films. Nanoscale Res Lett. 2011;6:434.

27. Faramarzi MA, Forootanfar H. Biosynthesis and characterization of gold nanoparticles produced by laccase from *Paraconiothyrium variabile*. Colloids Surf B. 2011;87:23–7.

28. Sharma B, Mandani S, Sarma TK. Biogenic growth of alloys and core-shell nanostructures using urease as a nanoreactor at ambient conditions. Sci Rep. 2013;3:2601.

29. Amin M, Anwar F, Janjua MRSA, Iqbal MA, Rashid U. Green synthesis of silver nanoparticles through reduction with *Solanum xanthocarpum* L. berry extract: characterization, antimicrobial and urease inhibitory activities against *Helicobacter pylori*. Int J Mol Sci. 2012;13:9923–41.

30. Philip D. Green synthesis of gold and silver nanoparticles using *Hibiscus rosasinensis*. Physica E. 2010;42:1417–24.

31. Khalil MMH, Ismail EH, El-Baghdady KZ, Mohamed D. Green synthesis of silver nanoparticles using olive leaf extract and its antibacterial activity. Arab J Chem. 2014;7:1131–9.

32. Kumar U, Ranjan KA, Sharan C, AA Hardikar, Pundle A, Poddar P. Green approach towards size controlled synthesis of biocompatible antibacterial metal nanoparticles in aqueous phase using lysozyme. Curr Nanosci. 2012;8:130–40.

33. Raju D, Mendapara R, Mehta UJ. Protein mediated synthesis of Au–Ag bimetallic nanoparticles. Mater Lett. 2014;124:271–4.

34. Devadiga A, Shetty KV, Saidutta MB. Timber industry waste-teak (*Tectona grandis* Linn.) leaf extract mediated synthesis of antibacterial silver nanoparticles. Int Nano Lett. 2015;5:205–14.

35. Philip D, Unni C, Aromal SA, Vidhu VK. Murraya koenigii leaf-assisted rapid green synthesis of silver and gold nanoparticles. Spectrochim Acta Part A Mol Biomol Spectrosc. 2011;78:899–904.

36. Dakal TC, Kumar A, Majumdar RS, Yadav V. Mechanistic basis of antimicrobial actions of silver nanoparticles. Front Microbiol. 2016;7:1831.

37. Cheng G, Dai M, Ahmed S, Hao H, Wang X, Yuan Z. Antimicrobial drugs in fighting against antimicrobial resistance. Front microbiol. 2016;7:470.

38. Zhou Y, Kong Y, Kundu S, Cirillo JD, Liang H. Antibacterial activities of gold and silver nanoparticles against *Escherichia coli* and *Bacillus Calmette-Guérin*. J Nanobiotechnol. 2012;10:19.

39. Dos Santos CA, Seckler MM, Ingle AP, Gupta I, Galdiero S, Galdiero M, et al. Silver nanoparticles: therapeutical uses, toxicity, and safety issues. J Pharm Sci. 2014;103:1931–44.

40. Shrivastava S, Bera T, Singh SK, Singh G, Ramachandrarao P, Dash D. Characterization of antiplatelet properties of silver nanoparticles. ACS Nano. 2009;3:1357–64.

41. Bondarenko O, Ivask A, Käkinen A, Kurvet I, Kahru A. Particle-cell contact enhances antibacterial activity of silver nanoparticles. PLoS ONE. 2013;8:e64060.

42. Shannahan JH. Nanoparticle biocorona. Encyclopedia of nanotechnology. Berlin: Springer; 2015. p. 1–4.

43. Wang G, Lu Y, Hou H, Liu Y. Probing the binding behavior and kinetics of silver nanoparticles with bovine serum albumin. RSC Adv. 2017;7:9393–401.

44. Su H-L, Lin S-H, Wei J-C, Pao I-C, Chiao S-H, Huang C-C, et al. Novel nanohybrids of silver particles on clay platelets for inhibiting silver-resistant bacteria. PLoS ONE. 2011;6:e21125.

45. Konop M, Damps T, Misicka A, Rudnicka L. Certain aspects of silver and silver nanoparticles in wound care: a minireview. J Nanomater. 2016;2016:1–10.

46. Choi HJ, Thambi T, Yang YH, Bang SI, Kim BS, Pyun DG, et al. AgNP and rhEGF-incorporating synergistic polyurethane foam as a dressing material for scar-free healing of diabetic wounds. RSC Adv. 2017;7:13714–25.

20

Effect of the 2014 Clinical and Laboratory Standards Institute urine-specific breakpoints on cefazolin susceptibility rates at a community teaching hospital

Daniel B. Chastain[1,2]*⓪, Ijang Ngando[3], Christopher M. Bland[4], Carlos Franco-Paredes[2,5] and W. Anthony Hawkins[1,2,6]

Abstract

Background: Enterobacteriaceae, which include *Escherichia coli, Klebsiella pneumoniae,* and *Proteus mirabilis*, are identified as the infectious etiology in the majority of urinary tract infections (UTIs) in community hospitals across the United States. The minimum inhibitory concentration (MIC) is a useful tool when choosing an appropriate antibacterial agent. Recent changes to the 2014 Clinical and Laboratory Standards Institute (CLSI) guidelines included reporting a urine-specific cefazolin breakpoint for enterobacteriaceae (susceptible $\leq$16 mcg/mL). The purpose of this study was to determine the clinical and financial impact of implementing the 2014 CLSI urine-specific breakpoints for cefazolin in a community-based teaching hospital in the Southern U.S.A.

Methods: A retrospective review of patients hospitalized from January 1, 2010 through October 1, 2014 was performed. Patients that met inclusion criteria had a documented initial clinical isolate of *E. coli, K. pneumoniae,* or *P. mirabilis* from urine cultures during each year. Descriptive statistics and two-proportion test of hypothesis were used in the analysis to compare susceptibility rates before and after implementation of the updated CLSI breakpoints for cefazolin.

Results: A total of 190 clinical isolates from patients were included in the study. *E. coli* was the most common organism isolated (63.7%), followed by *K. pneumoniae* (22.1%), and *P. mirabilis* (14.2%). 86% of the included isolates were susceptible to cefazolin using the 2010 breakpoints. Implementation of the 2014 breakpoints did not significantly impact susceptibility results for *E. coli, K. pneumoniae,* or *P. mirabilis*.

Conclusion: Modification of breakpoints did not significantly impact susceptibility rates of cefazolin. Substituting cefazolin may decrease the overall drug cost by 77.5%. More data is needed to correlate in vitro findings with clinical outcomes using cefazolin for UTIs.

Keywords: Antibiotic susceptibility, Microbiology, Urinary tract infections (UTI)

*Correspondence: daniel.chastain@uga.edu
[1] University of Georgia College of Pharmacy, 1000 Jefferson Street, Albany, GA 31701, USA
Full list of author information is available at the end of the article

Background

Urinary tract infections (UTIs) account for over 7 million healthcare provider visits annually as well as 1 million emergency visits which result in 100,000 hospitalizations [1, 2]. The majority of microorganisms that cause UTIs in community hospitals across the United States are enterobacteriaceae, which include *Escherichia coli, Klebsiella pneumoniae,* and *Proteus mirabilis* [1, 3]. UTIs are diagnosed by assessing patient symptoms (e.g. dysuria, increased urinary frequency) in combination with urinalysis. A urine culture is typically used to identify the responsible pathogen(s). Following organism identification, determination of antimicrobial susceptibility is crucial in determining appropriate targeted antimicrobial therapy [3].

Minimum inhibitory concentrations (MICs) provide quantitative information about the antibacterial agents' in vitro activity against the isolated organism [4]. The MIC value must therefore be interpreted in combination with clinical parameters, including pharmacokinetic (PK) and pharmacodynamic (PD) properties of the drug and the site of infection. Certain antibacterial agents, such as β-lactams and fluoroquinolones (FQs), achieve higher urinary concentrations than others. However, clinically some β-lactams have been shown to not be as effective as FQs despite adequate urinary concentrations [5]. Despite these discordant outcomes, most studies have shown that urine concentrations of antimicrobials are better predictors of treatment success than are serum concentrations.

The Clinical and Laboratory Standards Institute (CLSI) publishes guidelines for conducting and interpreting in vitro antibiotic susceptibility testing (AST) [6]. AST is an indispensable component of the microbiology laboratory and is often used to aid clinicians in identifying susceptible and resistant antibacterial agents [7]. In January 2010, CLSI updated the MICs for cefazolin when enterobacteriaceae are isolated from blood cultures [6] (Table 1). These changes were to account for the mechanisms of drug-resistance observed in documented treatment failures in patients with enterobacteriaceae bacteremia treated with cephalosporins. The primary concern was that the new MICs for cefazolin (susceptible [≤1 mcg/mL], intermediate [2 mcg/mL], and resistant [≥4 mcg/mL]) could eventually eliminate its use in the treatment of organisms lacking the expression of AmpC β-lactamases [3].

The 2014 CLSI guidelines retained the current MICs for cefazolin against enterobacteriaceae, but specified that susceptible results were based on a dosing regimen of 2 grams intravenously every 8 h and is specific for non-urine isolates [8]. One of the major changes included in these guidelines involves the reporting of a urine-specific cefazolin MIC for enterobacteriaceae

Table 1 Comparison of susceptibility breakpoints for cefazolin

Cefazolin	Susceptible (mcg/mL)	Intermediate (mcg/mL)	Resistant (mcg/mL)
CLSI guidelines: revisions to serum breakpoints			
Pre-2010	≤8	16	≥32
2010–2014	≤1	2	≥4
CLSI guidelines: addition of urine-specific breakpoint			
2014	≤16	–	≥32

(susceptible ≤16 mcg/mL). Furthermore, for uncomplicated UTIs caused by *E. coli, K. pneumoniae,* and *P. mirabilis,* cefazolin may be used as a surrogate to predict susceptibility to oral cephalosporins such as cephalexin and cefpodoxime. The purpose of this study was to determine the potential impact of implementing the 2014 CLSI urine-specific MICs for cefazolin.

Methods

This was a single-center retrospective cohort study of hospitalized patients at a 671-bed community-based teaching hospital in Southwest Georgia, U.S.A. The study was approved by the institutional review boards of the hospital and affiliated university. Microbiology data was obtained from January 2010 to October 2014. Urinary isolates were identified using the Siemens MicroScan® kits. Patients were included if they were 18 years of age or older, admitted between January 1, 2010 and October 1, 2014 with a urinary isolate positive for enterobacteriaceae, limited to *E. coli, K. pneumoniae,* and *P. mirabilis.* Only the first isolate of a certain bacterium per patient during the specified year was utilized in the analysis. Patients with repeated clinical isolates or polymicrobial urine cultures were also excluded.

A Siemens MicroScan® query report was generated for urinary isolates of the specified pathogens during the time frame. Patients were included if the bacteria isolated was treated as clinically significant UTI. Urinalysis was not included in the patient selection due the retrospective nature of the study. Data collected included demographic information, past medical history, type of UTI, date and type of urine sample, organism isolated, susceptibility profile, empiric antibacterial agent(s) chosen for treatment, and intended duration of therapy. Infections were categorized as uncomplicated or complicated according to the Infectious Diseases Society of America (IDSA) consensus definitions [9].

Determinations of antibiotic susceptibilities for enterobacteriaceae were carried out by an overnight microdilution method with commercial dehydrated panels provided by Siemens MicroScan® (Negative Urine

Combo Panel Type 62). Breakpoints for the following drugs were also reported: amikacin, ampicillin/sulbactam, ampicillin, aztreonam, cefazolin, cefoxitin, ceftazidime, ceftriaxone, cefuroxime, ciprofloxacin, gentamicin, levofloxacin, nitrofurantoin, tobramycin, and trimethoprim/sulfamethoxazole [10].

The primary outcome was assessed by evaluating the change in susceptibility patterns for enterobacteriaceae (*E. coli*, *K. pneumoniae*, and *P. mirabilis*) isolated from urine cultures. We compared susceptibility rates before and after implementation of the updated CLSI breakpoints for cefazolin. MICs reported by the microbiology laboratory were based on the 2010 CLSI breakpoints, at the time the research was conducted. The MICs were then extrapolated to determine susceptibility based breakpoints published in the 2014 update. The secondary outcome was measured by comparing the total drug costs associated with the UTI for the hospital admission with that of cefazolin versus levofloxacin which was the most common agent used for complicated UTIs at our facility. Pricing for cefazolin was determined based on our contract through a Group Purchasing Organization (GPO).

Statistical analysis was completed using SAS v9.3 (SAS Institute, Inc., Cary, NC). Statistical significance for the primary outcome was assessed by implementing the two-proportion test of hypothesis, which was set at a *p* value less than 0.05 (5% level of significance) with a 95% confidence interval.

Results

Baseline demographics
Of the 204 patients screened, 14 were excluded as a result of not meeting the age criteria. The majority of patients were elderly females (n = 154) [67.3 ± 21.2 years old] (Table 2). Patients had a complicated UTI (78.4%) with

Table 2 Baseline demographics

Female, n (%)	154 (80.6)
Age (year), mean ± SD	67.3 ± 21.2
Race, n (%)	
Black	79 (41.4)
White	110 (57.6)
UTI classification, n (%)	
Complicated	149 (78.4)
Uncomplicated	41 (21.6)
Type 2 diabetes mellitus, n (%)	56 (29.3)
ESRD, n (%)	13 (6.8)
NH residents, n (%)	31 (16.2)
Penicillin/cephalosporin allergy, n (%)	56 (29.3)
ESBL-producing, n (%)	13 (6.5)

ESRD end stage renal disease, *NH* nursing home, *ESBL* extended-spectrum β-lactamase

majority of them having a documented past medical history significant for type 2 diabetes mellitus (29.3%) or end-stage renal disease (6.8%). Approximately 29% of patients (n = 56) had a documented allergy to penicillins and/or cephalosporins.

Microbiology data
Escherichia coli was the most common organism isolated (63.7%), followed by *K. pneumoniae* (22.1%) and *P. mirabilis* (14.2%). This frequency distribution reflected the historical pattern seen in previous years.

Primary outcome
Prior to the 2014 CLSI cefazolin urine-specific breakpoints, a total of 163 isolates (85.8%) were susceptible to cefazolin, 7 (3.7%) were intermediate, and 20 (10.5%) were determined to be resistant (Fig. 1). After implementing the updated breakpoint of ≤16 mcg/mL (susceptible), the following changes were noted: 166 (87.4%) were susceptible, none were intermediate, and 24 (12.6%) were resistant. There was a non-statistically significant increase in the susceptibility rates for *E. coli* and *P. mirabilis*, from 80 to 88% (p = 0.077) and from 96 to 100% (p = 0.313), respectively. The susceptibility rate for *K. pneumoniae* was unchanged at 95% (p = 1.00). Susceptibility rates for ceftriaxone were 95% for *K. pneumoniae*, 91% for *E. coli*, and 100% for *P. mirabilis*. Similar rates were also observed for ceftazidime (95, 93, and 100%, respectively).

Secondary outcome
Intravenous levofloxacin was the most common agent used for both empiric and definitive treatment. Patients received approximately 6 doses of levofloxacin intravenously during the inpatient visit. The direct medication cost of levofloxacin compared to cefazolin was based on the average duration of inpatient therapy. Total acquisition cost of intravenous levofloxacin was $20.04 whereas cefazolin was $8.82. An additional 33 isolates would be expected to be cefazolin susceptible based on the updated breakpoints, which could represent a reduction in drug acquisition cost by approximately $370.

Discussion
Globally, FQs are frequently used as the first-line therapy for uncomplicated and often complicated UTIs [11, 12]. Concomitantly, there is rising antimicrobial resistance and increasing awareness of their potential side effects, toxicities, and their frequent association with *Clostridium difficile* infection. FQ resistance rates continue to increase both locally and nationally especially to *E. coli* where our susceptibility has decreased by 11.3% in the last 2 years. In this context, the use of β-lactams offers

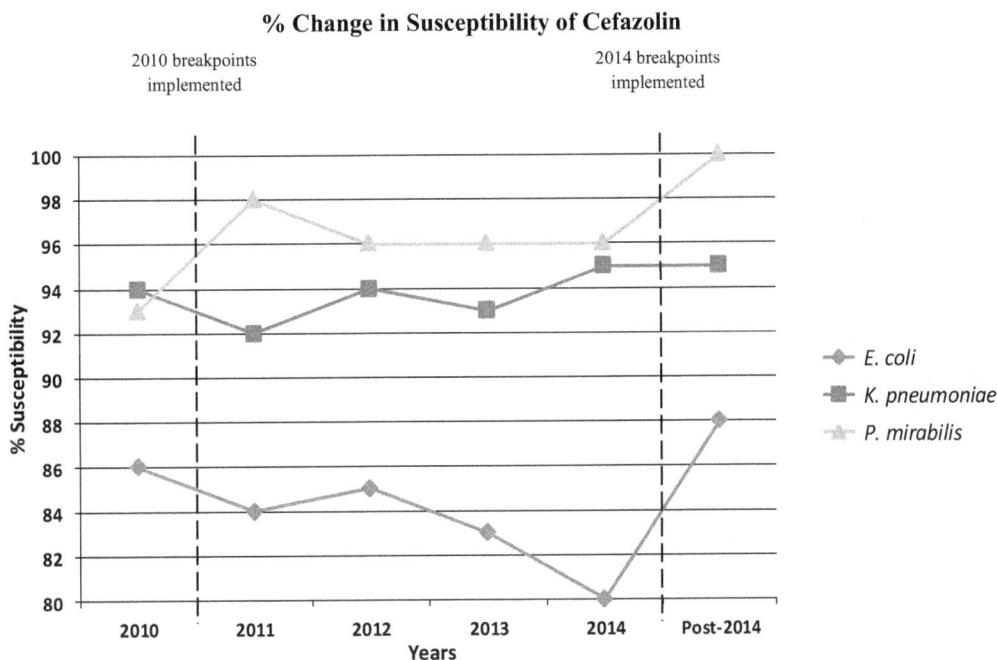

Fig. 1 The change in percentages of susceptibility patterns for *E. coli*, *K. pneumoniae*, and *P. mirabilis* to cefazolin with CLSI breakpoint update

many advantages, especially in patients who are not candidates for trimethoprim/sulfamethoxazole therapy. In particular, the use of cefazolin remains as an affordable and effective antimicrobial that may potentially be considered in many settings as a first-line therapy for the treatment of UTIs. Our study provides further evidence to support the use of cefazolin as a first-line therapy in the management of UTIs in some settings even after implementing the new urine-specific breakpoints among *E. coli* and *P. mirabilis* isolates. We did not observe any statistical difference for any of the organisms when comparing the 2010–2014 and post-2014 results. Indeed, compared to baseline, in vitro susceptibility rates remain high despite implementing the new urine specific breakpoint. In addition to preventing potential side effects and toxicities associated with the use of FQs, the substitution of cefazolin for treatment of both complicated and uncomplicated UTIs may decrease drug costs by approximately 60% [11]. Finally, after implementation of the updated cefazolin breakpoints, susceptibility rates were comparable between first and third generation cephalosporins.

Current UTI and pyelonephritis guidelines, published in 2011, do not recommend cefazolin as a first-line choice for treatment of UTIs [9]. Recently, there has been renewed interest in repurposing older or narrower-spectrum antibiotics due to increasing rates of resistance and paucity of novel agents [3, 7, 12, 13]. Greater knowledge

of antimicrobial PK, PD, and resistance mechanisms will allow modifications to susceptibility breakpoints. From an antimicrobial stewardship perspective, evaluation and use of cefazolin is potentially of great interest. Data for cefazolin use in UTIs remains limited despite increasing use at some facilities. A recent study however demonstrated noninferiority of cefazolin compared to ceftriaxone for acute pyelonephritis [12]. High rates of susceptibility to cefazolin, comparable to those observed with third generation cephalosporins, as presented by our data, suggest that empirical use of cefazolin may be warranted. Avoiding widespread use of third generation cephalosporins for UTIs in patients requiring hospitalization may limit development of resistance. Third generation cephalosporins have been associated with subsequent infections caused by vancomycin resistant enterococci (VRE), extended spectrum β-lactamase (ESBL) producing *K. pneumoniae*, and *C. difficile* [11].

The ability to transition patients from cefazolin to oral cephalosporins to complete therapy represents an area of uncertainty [13]. A recent in vitro study was conducted in an attempt to determine whether cefazolin could be used as a surrogate marker for cefpodoxime for urinary tract isolates. The authors found significantly higher categorical agreement with cefazolin compared to cefuroxime. Cefuroxime was noted to have better major and very major error rates than cefazolin. This data may allow clinicians to convert patients to an oral cephalosporin much sooner, potentially decreasing length of stay related to UTI diagnoses. For patients with an uncomplicated UTI who require treatment in an outpatient setting, cefazolin urine-specific MICs may be used as a surrogate for oral cephalosporins such as cephalexin and cefpodoxime. Although efficacious, FQs are not benign, as they were once considered. The Food and Drug Administration (FDA) recently strengthened warnings on FQs urging clinicians to avoid their use in uncomplicated UTIs due to serious toxicities and potentially irreversible adverse events [14]. Avoidance of FQs in patients with uncomplicated UTIs may be achieved with increased use of oral cephalosporins in the outpatient setting.

There are several limitations to this study. The small sample size from a single center institution limits its external validity. In addition, our cost analysis did not account for indirect cost (such as nursing time, insertion and maintenance of an intravenous line, or frequency of cefazolin administration). Furthermore, the cost analysis did not account for patients with a penicillin allergy, which would likely decrease the usage of cefazolin in this population.

Conclusion

The institution of newer urinary breakpoints along with increasing antimicrobial resistance to first-line UTI agents such as FQs or trimethoprim/sulfamethoxazole may require instead the use of β-lactams for treating UTIs. Third-generation cephalosporins should be avoided if possible due to their frequent association with VRE, ESBL producing *K. pneumoniae*, and *C. difficile*. The use of cefazolin and potentially other first-generation cephalosporins offers an affordable, safe, and efficacious antimicrobial alternative as a first-line therapy in the management of complicated and uncomplicated UTIs. Further research is needed to ascertain in vitro effect as well as clinical effect in settings that may be significantly affected by the updated urine-specific breakpoints.

Abbreviations

UTI: urinary tract infections; MIC: minimum inhibitory concentrations; CLSI: Clinical and Laboratory Standards Institute; PK: pharmacokinetic; PD: pharmacodynamics; FQs: fluoroquinolones; AST: antibiotic susceptibility testing; IDSA: Infectious Diseases Society of America; VRE: vancomycin resistant enterococci; ESBL: extended-spectrum β-lactamase; FDA: Food and Drug Administration; ESRD: end stage renal disease; NH: nursing home.

Authors' contributions

DBC, IN, and WAH conceived and designed the study. IN collected clinical data. DBC, IN, and WAH analyzed the data. IN wrote the first draft. All authors contributed with subsequent versions. All authors read and approved the final manuscript.

Author details

[1] University of Georgia College of Pharmacy, 1000 Jefferson Street, Albany, GA 31701, USA. [2] Phoebe Putney Memorial Hospital, Albany, GA 31701, USA. [3] Beaufort Memorial Hospital, Beaufort, SC 29902, USA. [4] University of Georgia College of Pharmacy, Savannah, GA 31405, USA. [5] Hospital Infantil de Mexico, Federico Gomez, Mexico City, Mexico. [6] Medical College of Georgia at Augusta University, Albany, GA 31701, USA.

Acknowledgements

Not applicable.

Competing interests

Christopher M. Bland is on the speaker's bureau for Merck Pharm, and has received grant funding for research from ALK Pharm. Others authors have no competing interests.

Consent for publication

A waiver of consent and waiver of written documentation of consent were granted due to the retrospective nature of this research study. A waiver of HIPAA Authorization was granted as the use or disclosure of PHI involves no more than minimal risk to the privacy of individuals, and the research could not be practically conducted without the waiver. All authors agreed the publication of data presented in this manuscript.

Funding

No funding was provided for the completion of this work.

References

1. Kumar S, Dave A, Wolf B, Lerma EV. Urinary tract infections. Dis Mon. 2015;61(2):45–59.
2. Foxman B. Epidemiology of urinary tract infections: incidence, morbidity, and economic costs. Am J Med. 2002;118(Suppl 1A):5S–13S.
3. Turnidge JD. Subcommittee on antimicrobial susceptibility testing of the clinical and laboratory standards institute. Cefazolin and enterobacteriaceae: rational for revised susceptibility testing breakpoints. Clin Infect Dis. 2011;52(7):917–24.
4. Turnidge JD, Paterson DL. Setting and revising antibacterial susceptibility breakpoints. Clin Microbiol Rev. 2007;20(3):391–408.
5. Hooton TM, Scholes D, Gupta K, et al. Amoxicillin–clavulanate vs ciprofloxacin for the treatment of uncomplicated cystitis in women: a randomized trial. JAMA. 2005;293:949–55.
6. Clinical and Laboratory Standards Institute (CLSI). Performance Standards for Antimicrobial Susceptibility Testing -Twentieth Informational Supplement (Update). CLSI document. Wayne: CLSI; 2010. pp. M100–S22.
7. Ambrose PG, Bhavnani SM, Rubino CM, et al. Pharmacokinetics–pharmacodynamics of antimicrobial therapy: it's not just for mice anymore. Clin Infect Dis. 2007;44:79–86.
8. Clinical and Laboratory Standards Institute (CLSI). Performance standards for antimicrobial susceptibility testing-fourth informational supplement (Update). CLSI document. Wayne: CLSI; 2014. pp. M100–S24.
9. Gupta K, Hooton TM, Naber KG, et al. International clinical practice guidelines for the treatment of acute uncomplicated cystitis and pyelonephritis in women: a 2010 update by the infectious diseases Society of America and the European society for microbiology and infectious diseases. Clin Infect Dis. 2011;52(5):e103–20.

Effect of the 2014 Clinical and Laboratory Standards Institute urine-specific...

169

10. MicroScan Package Insert. http://www.healthcare.siemens.com/microbi-ology-testing/microscan-panels. Accessed 19 Sept 2014.

11. Paterson DL. "Collateral Damage" from cephalosporin or quinolone antibi-otic therapy. Clin Infect Dis. 2004;38(Suppl 4):s341–5.

12. Hobbs AL, Shea KM, Daley MJ, et al. Are first-generation cephalospor-ins obsolete? A retrospective, non-inferiority, cohort study comparing empirical therapy with cefazolin versus ceftriaxone for acute pyelonephri-tis in hospitalized patients. J Antimicrob Chemother. 2016;71(6):1665–71.

13. Bookstaver DA, Bland CM, Arroyo MA. Evaluation of cefazolin as a sur-rogate marker for cefpodoxime susceptibility for urinary tract isolates. J Med Microbiol. 2015;64(10):1170–3.

14. US Food and Drug Administration. Fluoroquinolone antibacterial drugs. Drug Safety Communication-FDA advises restricting use for certain uncomplicated infections. http://www.fda.gov/Safety/MedWatch/Safe-tyInformation/SafetyAlertsforHumanMedicalProducts/ucm500665.htm. Accessed 5 May 2017.

21

Parasitological and biochemical studies on cutaneous leishmaniasis in Shara'b District, Taiz, Yemen

Qhtan Asmaa[1], Salwa AL-Shamerii[2], Mohammed Al-Tag[3], Adam AL-Shamerii[4], Yiping Li[1*] and Bashir H. Osman[5]

Abstract

Background: The leishmaniasis is a group of diseases caused by intracellular haemoflagellate protozoan parasites of the genus Leishmania. Leishmaniasis has diverse clinical manifestations; *cutaneous leishmaniasis* (CL) is the most common form of leishmaniasis which is responsible for 60% of disability-adjusted life years. CL is endemic in Yemen. In Shara'b there is no reference study available to identify the prevalence of endemic diseases and no investigation has been conducted for diagnosing the diseases.

Methods: This study was conducted in villages for CL which collected randomly. The study aimed at investigating the epidemiological factors of CL in Shara'b by using questioner. Symptoms of lesions in patients suffering from CL, confirmed by laboratory tests, gave a new evidence of biochemical diagnosis in 525 villagers aged between 1 and 60 years old. Venous bloods were collected from 99 patients as well as from 51 control after an overnight fast.

Results: The percentage prevalence of CL was found 18.8%. The prevalence rate of infection among males (19.3%) was higher than females (18.40%). Younger age group (1–15) had a higher prevalence rate (20.3%) than the other age groups. Furthermore, the population with no formal education had the higher rate of infection (61% of the total). A significant increase of serum malondialdehyde (P < 0.001) in CL patients was obtained. The highest level of MDA may be due to over production of ROS and RNS results in oxidative stress and the acceleration of lipid peroxidation in CL patients.

Conclusions: There were high prevalence rates of CL in Shara'b. The patient who had CL has been found with many changes in some biochemical levels. This study provides a clear indication on the role of MDA as an early biochemical marker of peroxidation damage occurring during CL. Increased uric acid, and catalase activity was provided of free radical.

Keywords: Leishmaniasis, Prevalence, Malondialdehyde, Free radicals scavengers, Yemen

Background

Leishmaniasis is a diseases caused by obligatory and intracellular haemoflagellate protozoan parasites of the genus *Leishmania* (family trypanosomatidae). Human leishmaniasis is a compound disease with numerous clinical forms, which variety from mild self-healing cutaneous lesions to fatal visceral disease and neotropics [1]. It is overwhelmingly referred to as a group of diseases in view of the fact that the varied spectrum of clinical manifestations, which has the scope from small cutaneous nodules to overall mucosal tissue destruction. CL can be caused by a number of *Leishmania* spp. and is transferred to human beings and animals by sandflies. Cutaneous leishmaniasis is predominant in 88 countries including 77 of developing, tens of millions of people are at hazard of getting this disease and it is estimated that each year 1–1.5 million new cases appear. CL was endemic in Yemen [2, 22]. It has been recognized as a public health problem predominated by infection with the highest burden of leishmaniasis, but has not been fully documented.

---

*Correspondence: liyiping_hhu@163.com
[1] College of Environment, Hohai University, Nanjing 210098, China
Full list of author information is available at the end of the article

Parasitological and biochemical studies on cutaneous leishmaniasis in Shara'b District...

171

Cutaneous leishmaniasis is endemic and most of the cases are registered in Lahg, Abun, Hagga and Sa'adah Taiz Governorates [3].

CL is transmitted by the bite of an infected sand fly. When the parasites enter the Polymorph nuclear neutrophils (PML) and the monocyte macrophage cells play an important role in the host defense [4]. These cells are capable to generating a large amounts of extremely toxic molecules, such as reactive oxygen species (ROS), comprise superoxide radicals (O_2^-), hydrogen peroxide (H_2O_2) and hydroxyl radicals (OH), and reactive nitrogen species (RNS), inclusive nitric oxide (NO) Bogdan C Rolling off Bacteria, parasites and tumor cells motivate macrophages to synthesize considerable amounts of NO which has cytotoxic effects on these activators.

ROS and RNS are capable of degrading many biomolecules, including DNA, carbohydrates and proteins. Furthermore, ROS and RNS can assault the polyunsaturated fatty acids of membrane lipids causing lipid peroxidation and the disorder of cell construction and function [5]. Lipid peroxidation is a well-recognized mechanism of cellular injury and is used as a marker of oxidative stress in cells and tissues [6].

Polyunsaturated fatty acid derived that are not stable, can decay hence forming many series of complex products [7]. They are degraded such as carbonyl compound which are plentiful Malondialdehyde (MDA) that is widely used as marker of lipid peroxidation [8]. High levels of lipid peroxidation products are accompanying with a variety of chronic diseases with parasitic infections [9]. The serum concentration of MDA was dignified in humans with cutaneous leishmaniasis to establish its connection in the pathological mechanism of the disease [10].

To avoid potential oxidative damage there are defense mechanisms systems which classified as enzymatic [superoxide dismutase (SOD), catalase, glutathione peroxidase (GSH peroxidase), glutathione reductase and GSH reductase] and non-enzymatic (vitamins and uric acid). The estimation of MDA level and antioxidant enzyme activity are the main standards in relation to the severity of probable peroxidation, which occur in the cell membrane [11]. Anti-oxidant vitamins for instance E, C, and A protect the cells from destruction in contradiction of free oxygen radicals generated consequently of parasites.

Antioxidant systems including vitamins have a cellular protective action against oxidative stress subsequent in cell, organ, and tissue damage because of parasitic invasion [12]. This study aimed to determine the prevalence of CL in some villages in Shara'b district, Taiz, Yemen, to investigate the risk factors that increase the prevalence of CL, and explore the evidence of free radicals and antioxidants during CL.

Methods

Study area

Shara'b is a district with an area of about 61,700 km² and population of about 393, 425, forms about 12,000 km² faraway from Taiz Governorate. Shara'b is divided into two districts: Shara'b Salam district with an area of 20,000 km² and population of 146,650, and Shara'b Ar Rawnah district with area of 41,700 km² and population about 18, 6955. Shara'b district has mountains and Aqueducts. Mountains are located on the northwest side of Taiz governorate and is about 2000 m above sea level. Aqueducts is meant by the valleys where the water is held permanently throughout the year such as Nobaqe, Rasan valleys. The climate where there is the mountain and highland is predominately a cold climate with mild winters in winter and warm to relatively warm in the summer. The abundance of vegetation and variety of the most important trees are available in the province of Samar, *Frangula alnus*, *Acacia nilotica* and *Ziziphus spina-christi*, *Acacia drepanolobium*, *Acacia ehrenbergiana*, *Tunb*, *Ficus benjamina*, *arabic-tree—Acacia*, *Salvadora persica*, *Tamarix aphylla*, *Cactaceae* and other medical plants some weeds and small plants. Animals and birds: There are many species of wild animals and the most important of these animals hyenas, foxes, tigers, lions, *Lycaon pictus*, rabbits, hedgehogs.

The samples were collected from eleven villages located in the above mentioned districts. These villages were chosen for collection from this district. These villages are Banny ziad, Alhosia, Almakhabeer and Nakhla which belong to Shara'b Ar Rownah. Other villages are belong to Shara'b As Salam which include Alamgod, Alzakarer, Banny Sarry, Alafuch, Alshahna, Banny Wahban and Mekhlaf a'ala, as shown in Taiz map (Fig. 1).

Study population

To assess the prevalence of cutaneous leishmaniasis, 525 villagers ranging between 1 and 60 old years were examined. The survey was conducted of orients as recommended by the World Health Organization (WHO) [13]. Samples of 11 villages in each ecologically homogenous area were considered adequate to evaluate prevalence of Leishmanial infection in an endemic area. Materials used in the present study were collected from eleven villages of Shara'b district. All cases were investigated included: response to the questionnaire containing the required information such as age, sex, education level, house type, defense type, treatment before, drug type and scar sites.

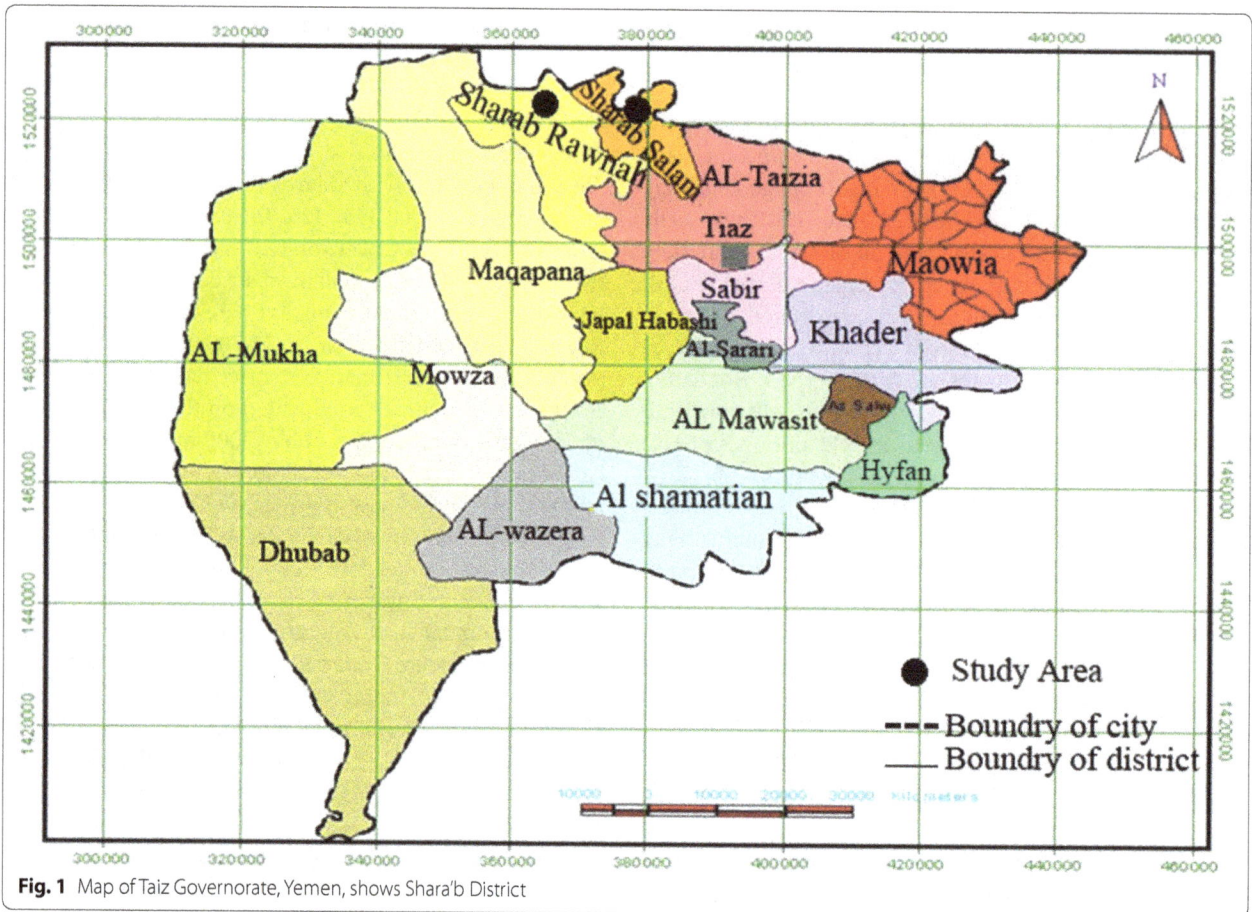

Fig. 1 Map of Taiz Governorate, Yemen, shows Shara'b District

Cases preparation and blood collection

The samples were collected from April 2012 to October 2013. Cases were collected at Banny Ziad Health Center in Shara'b. Diagnosis was confirmed clinically, as well as by laboratory demonstration of the parasite in the lesions by direct smears using microscopic examination. Tissue scrapings performed with staining the specimen with by Giemsa stain. The lesions cleaned and any eschars or exudates was removed. 1% lidocaine used to decrease bleeding, optimize debridement, and obtain and improve tissue scraping quality. For tissue scrapings, ten scalpel blade was used. Scraping was performed with a pressure that is adequate to obtain exudates, without evoke bleeding. The dermal tissue was spread in a 2–3 cm diameter on a glass slide then fixed briefly with methanol, Giemsa stained, and examined for the presence of amastigotes.

In the second day 10 ml of venous blood were collected from 91 patients as well as from 51 control after an overnight fast and it was positive. The aspirated blood was immediately put into two different test tube (T.T) the other fraction of blood was clotted in plain T.T., then the serum was separated by centrifugation at $1000 \times g$ and used for the quantitation of the biochemical reaction [14]. This transported by hole freezer immediately to Palestine hospital laboratory and other parts to Alborehee hospital laboratory in Taiz governorate to complete the analysis. Uric acid reagent, MDA reagents [0.5% (W/V) tricholoroacetic acid (BDH), 0.5% (W/V) 2-thiobarbituric acid, 70% tricholoroacetic acid, chloroform (BDH)]. Catalase reagents (ammonium molybdate, hydrogen peroxide, sodium–potassium phosphate buffer), spectrophotometer and waterbath.

Examination of samples

Microscopic examination

Lesions were cleaned with ethanol and punctured at the margins of the lesion with a sterile lancet. Smears were made from exudating material, air dried and fixed in methanol. Then they were stained with Giemsa's stain for examination by light microscopy [13].

Biochemical tests

Measurement of catalase activities

Intracellular catalase enzyme activity was determined according to the modified technique of Goth et al. [15]. A simple method for the determination of serum catalase which included the use of optimized conditions for enzymatic degradation of hydrogen peroxide, spectrophotometric assay of hydrogen peroxide based on formation of its stable complex with ammonium molybdate and measuring the reaction by reading the absorbance by spectrophotometer.

Measurement of serum lipid peroxide (MDA) levels

Measurement of serum MDA, secondary product of lipid peroxidation was based on the colorimetric reaction with thiobarbituric acid (TBA). The molar extinction coefficient of MDA is 1.56×105 M/cm and the results were expressed as nM of MDA/ml [16].

Determination of uric acid

Determination of uric acid was by reaction with uricase. The formed H_2O_2 reacts under catalysis of peroxidase with 3,5-dichloro-hydroxybenzene-sulfonic acid (DCHBS) and 4-aminophenazone 9 PAP0 to give red–violet quinone-monoimine as indicator [17]. Reaction principle

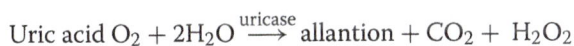

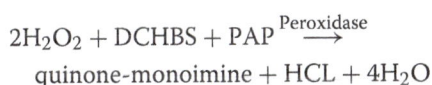

$$\text{Uric acid } O_2 + 2H_2O \xrightarrow{\text{uricase}} \text{allantion} + CO_2 + H_2O_2$$

$$2H_2O_2 + DCHBS + PAP \xrightarrow{\text{Peroxidase}}$$
$$\text{quinone-monoimine} + HCL + 4H_2O$$

Statistical analysis

The statistical package for social sciences (SPSS) program on the computer was used. Results were expressed as mean ± stander error of mean (SEM). The data were analyzed by linear regression, paired t test, and two-ways analysis of variances (ANOVA) which was applied for the comparison among different groups. The level of significance was taken as the 0.05.

Results

Epidemiological study

Prevalence of cutaneous leishmaniasis infection

Among 525 of a total cases studied, the percent of infected cases are 18.87% and not infected are 81.13% (Fig. 2). Most prevalence rate which were positive collected from Shara'b district was in Nakhla with percent to (25.2%), and the lowest percent in Almakhabeer (11.10%) (Fig. 3).

According to sex, the highest prevalence of CL infection were recorded in males (19.3%) with account (47) and the negative (196) from total male (243) examined. Whereas the lowest prevalence in females with account (52) with a percent of (18.40%) and a negative number (230) from total females (282) cases (Fig. 3; Table 1).

Prevalence of CL infection according to the sex and age

The distribution of 525 skin scraping samples infection (19.3% males and 18.4% females) shown in Fig. 4.

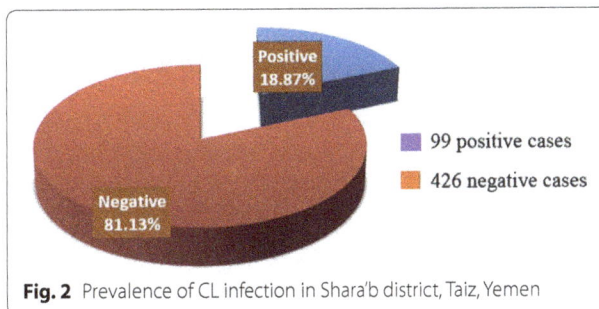

Fig. 2 Prevalence of CL infection in Shara'b district, Taiz, Yemen

Legend: 99 positive cases / 426 negative cases

In relation to sex, the prevalence of infection in males (19.3%) was slightly higher than in females (18.4%) there is high significant difference (P < 0.05) Table 1.

In relation to cutaneous leishmaniasis infection among cases examined, according to age and sex groups in Shara'b, district, there was high significant (P < 0.05) between age group 1–15. The males is high 22.7% than in females 18.4% and also there was high significant (P < 0.05) in group 46–60 the high prevalence were in females group 23.5% than in males group 13.6% (Table 2). The rate of Cutaneous leishmaniasis infection in relation to age groups, the age group (1–15) has high significant (OR = 0.458, P < 0.05) than other groups (Table 2).

Types and distribution of lesions

Distribution of lesions on various parts on various parts of body in patients shows the highest percent of infection was in hands (36%), and the lowest on the ear and hands (1%) (Fig. 5). In relation to type of scars on body description in infection with cutaneous leishmaniasis in this study the dry scars have were the highest percentage (14%), and the lowest percent with an extensive scars (3.2%) (Fig. 6).

Also, in relation to the type of scars single lesions were observed in most of the patients. Figures 7 and 8 showed pictures of lesions, of patients with CL in Shara'b, district (a) Typical lesion sever inflammatory reaction, (b) dry lesion on nose, (c) local and dry lesion on right ear, (d) extensive lesion on cheek, (e) dry lesion after skin scraping, (f) dry lesion on upper lip, (g) large lesion on right hand, (h) mucocutaneous infection in mucose of nose with more lesions under lower lip (I); 1 dry lesion; (j) cancerous lesion. In relation to distribution of lesions by site of lesions and age groups, in adult group, the highest percent present in hands (91%) and the lowest lesions in the eras (7.1%), but it is opposite in the child group the highest percent in ears (92.9%) and lowest in hands (8.7%) (Table 3). Leishmaniasis is a diseases caused by obligatory and intracellular haemoflagellate protozoan parasites of the genus *Leishmania* (family trypanosomatidae). Human leishmaniasis is a

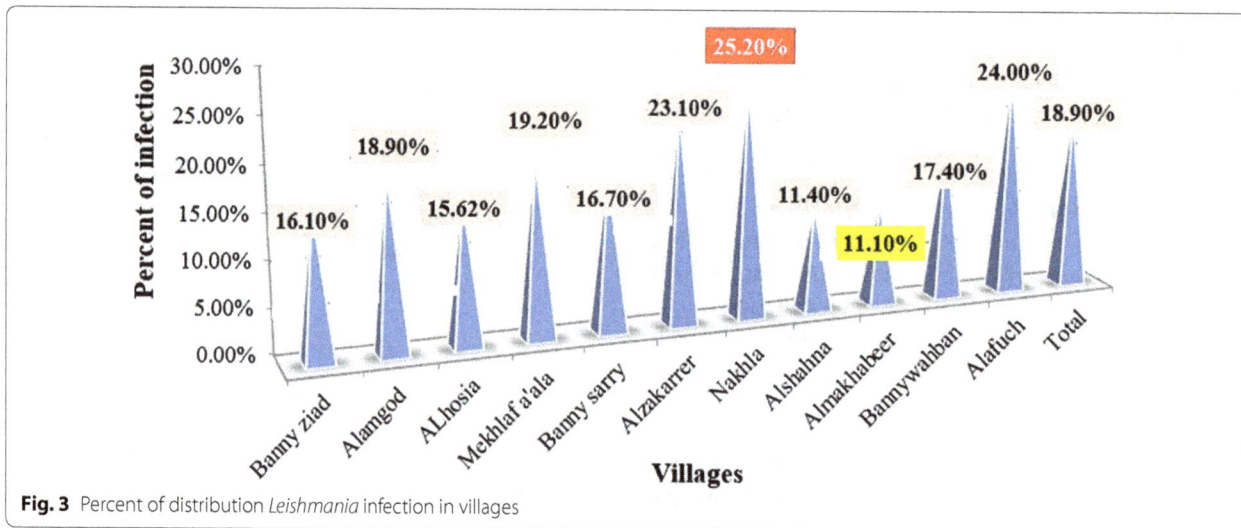

Fig. 3 Percent of distribution *Leishmania* infection in villages

Table 1 Rate of CL infection in relation to sex

Sex	No. examined	Overall infection		Odds ratio	(95% CI)	P value
		No.	%			
Male	243	47	19.3	0.011	0.833–0.813	0.044*
Female	282	52	18.4			

* Significant (P < 0.05)

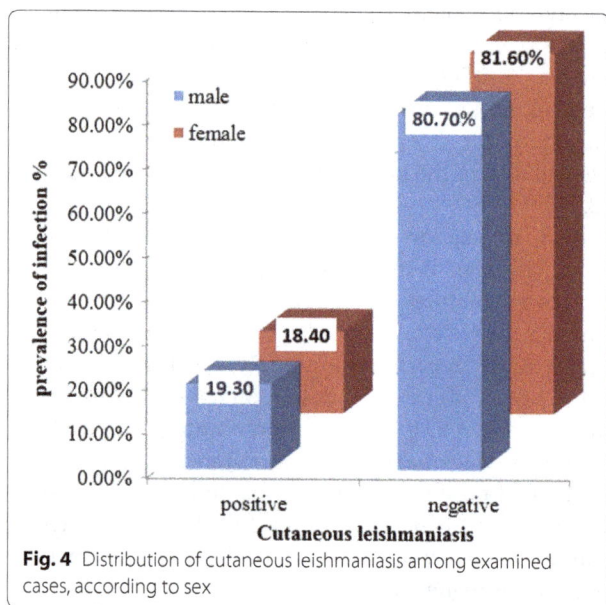

Fig. 4 Distribution of cutaneous leishmaniasis among examined cases, according to sex

compound disease with numerous clinical forms, which variety from mild self-healing cutaneous lesions to fatal visceral disease [1].

Cutaneous leishmaniasis is endemic in the tropics and neotropics. Leishmaniasis was endemic in Yemen [2].

It has been recognized as a public health problem predominated by infection with the highest burden of Leishmaniasis, but has not been fully documented [18]. CL is endemic and most of the cases are registered in Lahg, Abun, Hagga and Sa'adah Taiz Governorates [3]. CL is transmitted by the bite of an infected sand fly. When the parasites enter the polymorph nuclear neutrophils (PML) and the monocyte macrophage cells play an important role in the host defense [5]. These cells are capable to generating a large amounts of extremely toxic molecules, such as reactive oxygen species (ROS), comprise superoxide radicals (O_2^-), hydrogen peroxide (H_2O_2) and hydroxyl radicals (OH), and reactive nitrogen species (RNS), inclusive nitric oxide (NO). Bogdan C Rolling off Bacteria, parasites and tumor cells motivate macrophages to synthesize considerable amounts of NO which having cytotoxic effects on these activators [19]. ROS and RNS are capable of degrading many biomolecules, including DNA, carbohydrates and proteins. Furthermore, ROS and RNS can assault the polyunsaturated fatty acids of membrane lipids causing lipid peroxidation and the disorder of cell construction and function [4]. Lipid peroxidation is a well-recognized mechanism of cellular injury and is used as a marker of oxidative stress in cells and tissues [6]. Polyunsaturated fatty acid derived that are not stable, can

Table 2 Prevalence of CL infection among cases examined, in relation to age and sex groups

Age group	Gender						P value	Odds ratio	(95% CI)	Overall infection P value
	Male			Female						
	No examined	No +ve	% +ve	No examined	No +ve	% +ve				
1–15	88	20	22.7	114	21	18.4	0.013*	0.458	0.943–0.933	0.024*
16–30	90	16	17.8	86	16	18.6	0.373[n]			
31–45	43	8	18.6	65	11	16.9	0.410[n]			
46–60	22	3	13.6	17	4	23.5	0.002*			
Total	243	47	19.3	282	52	18.4	0.555[n]			

[n] non-significant

* Significant difference at (0.05)

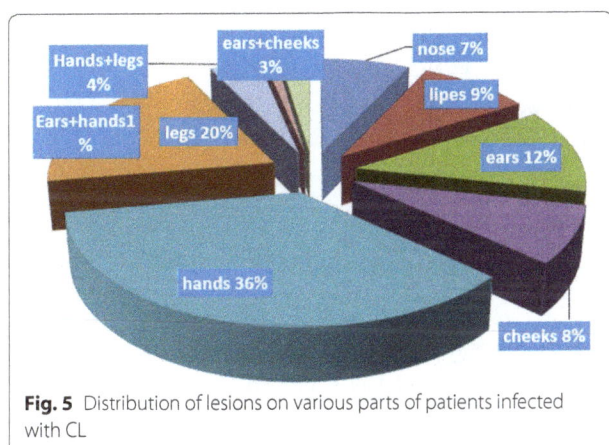

Fig. 5 Distribution of lesions on various parts of patients infected with CL

decay hence forming many series of complex products [7]. They are degraded such as carbonyl compound which are plentiful malondialdehyde (MDA) that is widely used as marker of lipid peroxidation [20]. High levels of lipid peroxidation products are accompanied with a variety of chronic diseases with parasitic infections [3]. The serum concentration of MDA was dignified in humans with *cutaneous leishmaniasis* to establish its connection in the pathological mechanism of the disease [9].

To avoid potential oxidative damage there are mechanisms defense systems which are classified as enzymatic [superoxide dismutase (SOD), catalase, glutathione peroxidase (GSH peroxidase), glutathione reductase and GSH reductase] and non-enzymatic (vitamins and uric acid). The estimation of MDA level and antioxidant enzyme activity are main standards in relation to the severity of probable peroxidation, which occur in cell membrane [10]. Anti-oxidant vitamins for instance E, C, and A protect the cells from destruction in contradiction of free oxygen radicals generated consequently of parasites. Antioxidant systems including vitamins have a cellular protective action against oxidative stress subsequent in cell, organ, and tissue damage because of parasitic invasion [11].

Rate of cutaneous leishmaniasis infection in relation to certain environmental and social factors

The rate of CL infection in relation to education was showed in Table 4. This table shows that the high rate (54.6%) of infection was seen in cases who have not any level of education, followed by the primary school level (18.2%), secondary school level (18.2%), Diploma (4.0%), Bachelor (5.9%), but it does not give any significant differences (OR = 3.955, P > 0.05).

In relation to certain environmental conditions and the rate of CL infection, Table 5 showed that there was a significant correlation (OR = 0.002, P < 0.05) between infection and animals found in houses, which have no protective defenses. Also, our results show significant correlation between infection and types of residents (OR = 0.035, P < 0.05). The high rate of infection was (19.8%) in populist building than of new building (17.6%) that bullied with mud, cracks and dampness in Table 5. Also, it showed a significant correlation between infection and sitting on the first floor of the house (P < 0.05, OR = 5.50) (Table 6).

Free radical scavengers
Enzymatic scavenger's catalase

The mean of catalase activity in the present study decrease (72.53 ± 4.5 K/Ul), but this value did not reach a statistically significant in the patient as compared to control (83.11 ± 4.91 K/Ul) in Table 6. In relation to age (Table 7) and sex effects (Table 8) on catalase levels among patients groups and control groups (Table 9) show no significant effect of age on catalase levels among patient and control groups.

Non enzymatic scavenger uric acid

Our study shows that uric acid level has high significant (P < 0.001) increase in patients groups than those of control groups (Table 7).

In relation to the effect of age on uric acid, Table 10 shows that there is no significant increase of serum

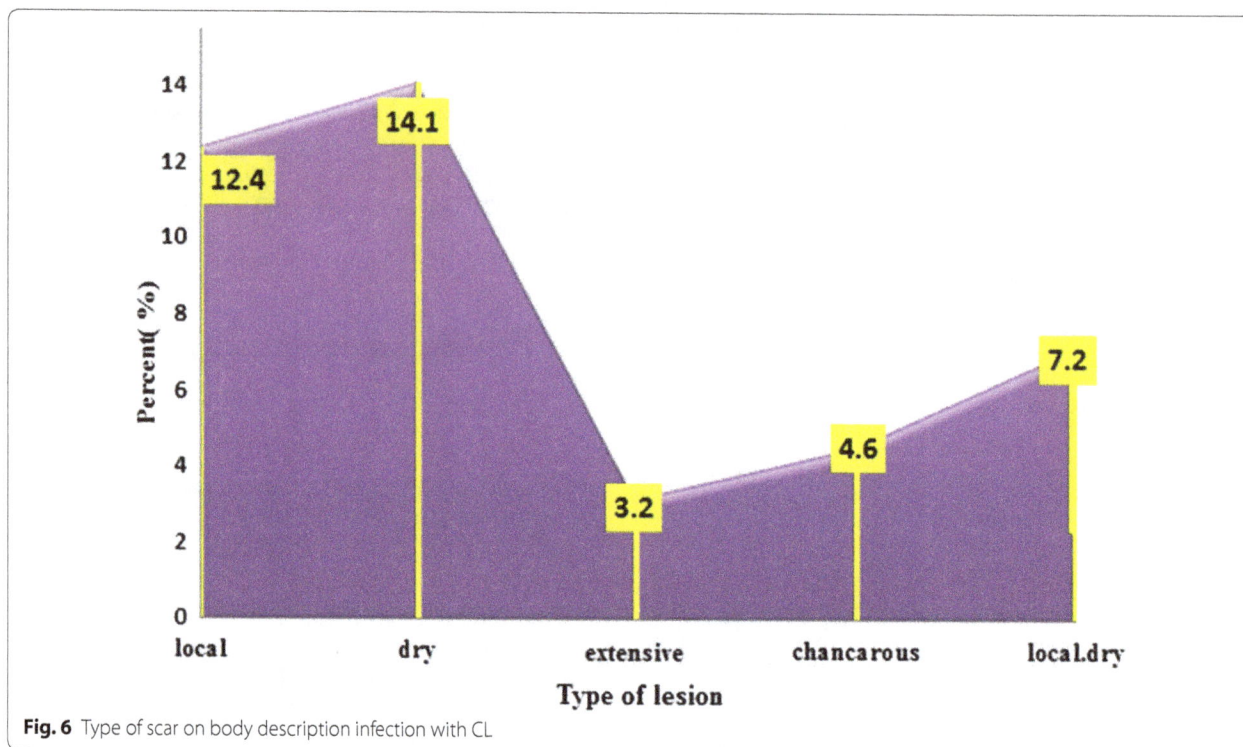

Fig. 6 Type of scar on body description infection with CL

levels of uric acid and catalase in age groups of patients infected with CL. Table 11 shows that there is significant (P < 0.05) increase of uric acid in male than in female comparing to healthy groups.

Discussion

Cutaneous leishmaniasis

According to results obtained, among 525 of total cases was studied, 99 cases with a percentage of 18.87% was infected with CL and 426 cases not infected with percent of 81.13%. The prevalence of infection was higher in males (19.3%) than in females (18.40%). The same results were reported by AL-Jawabreh et al. [20], and Silva et al. [21].

Cutaneous leishmaniasis (CL) is a social problem in the tropics and subtropics [22] and the North Western [23]. CL reported in the most decade in Yemen, mostly among young children, including the Governorates of Sana'a, Taiz, Ibb, Alhodeidah, Hajjah, Damar, Sa'adah, Al-Mahweet, Ma'arab, and Aljawf [24]. Differences were seen between males and females, overly more males were infected. This is probably happened due to the cultural habits of these areas, as they are exposing themselves to sand flies bites [25] there was a slightly increased positive percent of infection in females group. This may be due to the females staying in these epidemic villages with sand flies all the time to make all jobs including cultures activities. The highest percent of infection was in

Nakhla (25.2%) due to the geographical site which was near mountains and has water stream flow all year and abundant of fresh water holes which provide sand flies with a suitable environment to complete its life cycle and increase agriculture activities. Similar results found by Al-Qubaty [3] in the Western area of Yemen. The low percent of infection in Almakhabeer (11.10%) was due to the decrease water sources and decreased of agricultural activity and the geographical site of these village have many mountains, which play in distribution of sand fly [26] that may explain the lowest rate of infection.

The most infected cases in the present study were increased from April 2012 to October 2013. The climate has many subtropical features; the mean annual temperature lying between 20 and 30 °C with little seasonal variation. The relative humidity ranging between (40–60%) in the Western Yemen with relatively high rainfall in summer and its sub humid warm-temperature climate with a distinct dry period during the winter months. The annual rainfall from approximately 800–1200 mm, and most of this falls from April to October. The middle heights are well watered by perennial streams (Wadies) and small irrigation channels, temporary streams and pools are plentiful during the rainy seasons [27]. The majority of the populations are engaged in agriculture near their houses where sand flies are found, which the primary source of income is, so this climate may explain why the leishmanias is has wide spreads in this village.

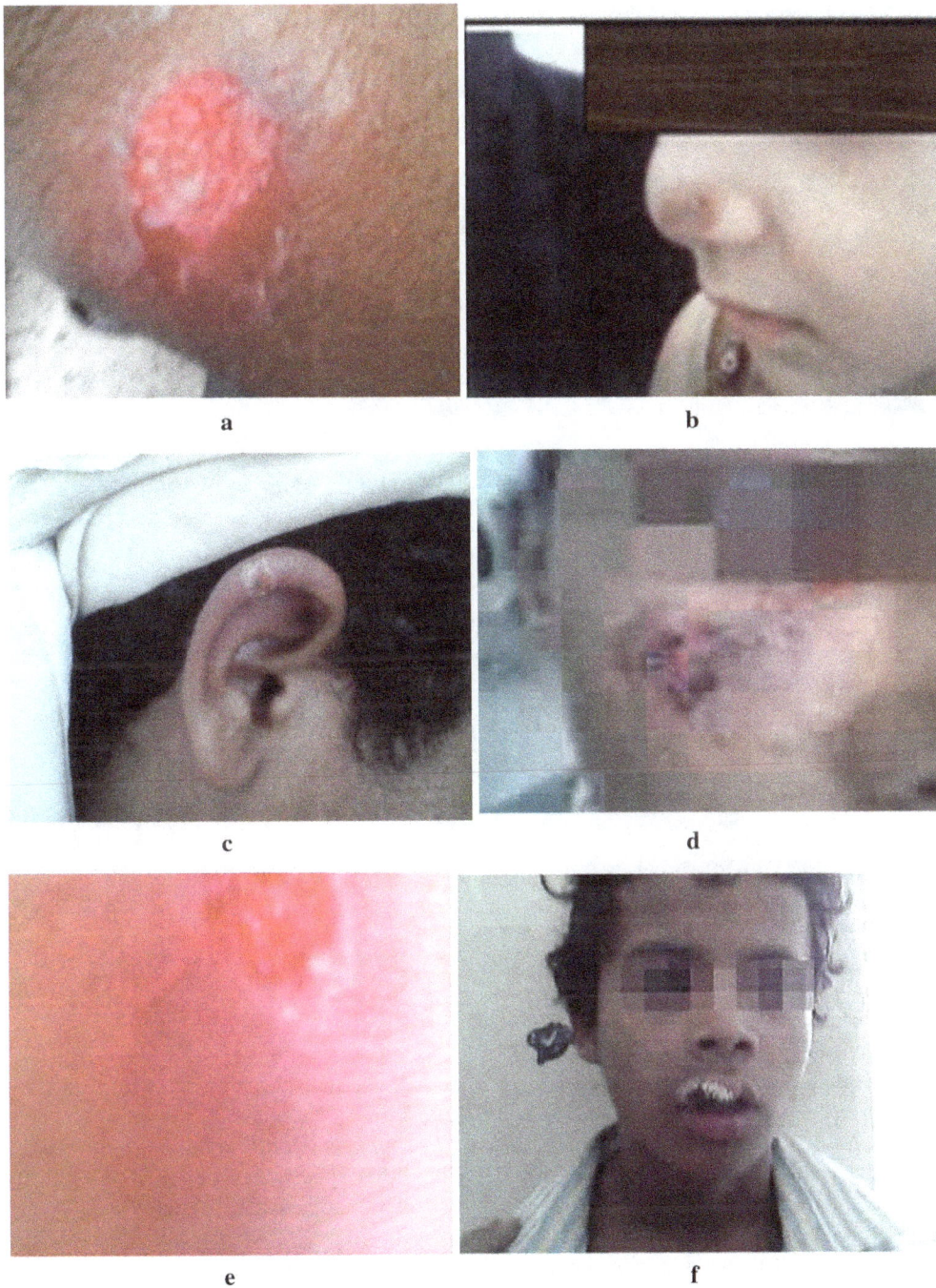

Fig. 7 Pictures of lesions in patients with CL. **a** Typical lesion sever inflammatory. **b** Dry lesion on nose. **c** Local and dry lesion on ear. **d** Extensive lesion on cheek. **e** Dry lesion after skin scraping. **f** Dry lesion on upper lip

These results show that the highest infection is significant ($P < 0.05$) among males aged group of (1–15), but not in females of the same aged group. This may be due to the increased activity of males aged than females during this age. Wearers the significant ($P < 0.05$) increased is observed in females aged (46–60 years) than males that may due to low immunity of females in this age.

The reasons of high significant and higher prevalence rate (OR = 0.458, $P < 0.05$) in younger age is probably due to the fact that they have poorly developed an

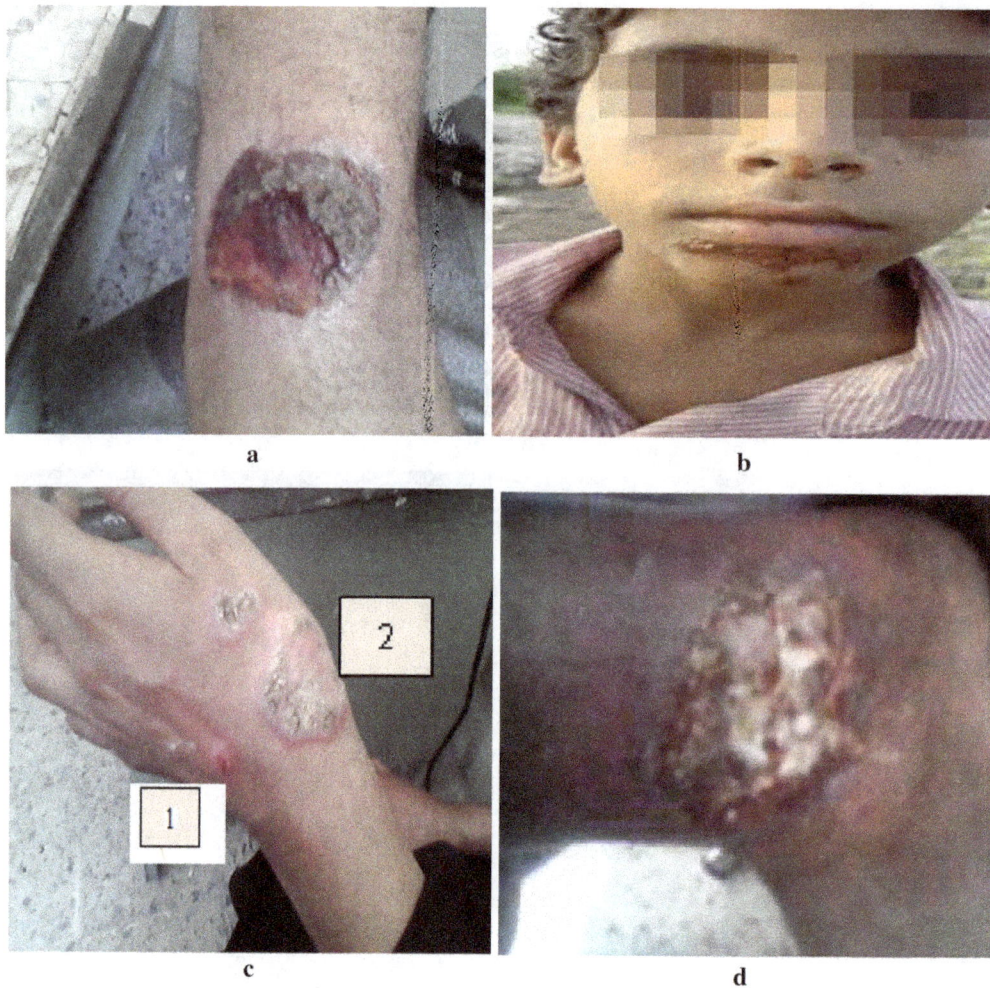

Fig. 8 Pictures of lesions in patients with CL. **a** Large lesion on right hand. **b** Lesion under lower lip. **c** *1* Dry lesion and *2* fungi infection. **d** Chancrous lesion on left leg

immune system. They cannot prevent themselves from bites of sand flies and do not have cultural knowledge of defending themselves. Similar results and discussion were observed by [21]. As most of the people residing in the endemic areas are not aware of disease, public health education is of great importance. They were not taught to change their sleeping habit to avoid cracks, dampness in their houses, and did not to keep the surrounding free of sand fly. Although animals seem to be reservoirs, this possibility should not be ruled out by carrying our surveillance in the most likely domestic and wild animals. Similar results and discussion found by [26].

These results showed that there is a significant correlation (OR = 0.002, P < 0.05) between infection and animals found in houses, which have not protective defenses (OR = 0.010, P < 0.05). Human and domestic animals are accidental hosts for any *Leishmania* spp. which are maintained in cycles between wild animals and sand flies [28].

Leishmania infantum, Leishmania peruviana and possibly other species can be found in dogs, increasing the risk of transmission to people. [29] Other domesticate animals might be involved as secondary maintenance hosts. *Leishmania donovani* and *Leishmania tropica* are adapted to humans, but animals can also be infected occasionally [28]. The occurrence of this outbreak of Zoonotic cutaneous leishmaniasis in the district seems to be the results of construction of buildings near colonies of rodents and also travelling to the other infected foci of Shara'b. This result was the same by Alkhavan et al. [30]. This study shows a significant correlation (P < 0.05) between infection and types of residents. The high percent of the infection is 19.8% in populist building than of new building (17.6%) that bullied with mud, cracks and

Table 3 Distribution of CL lesions according to site of lesion and age groups

Infected groups		Site of lesions										Total
		No describe	Hands	Legs	Hands and legs	Ears	Cheeks	Lips	Nose	Ear and hands	Ear and cheek	
Child (1–15)	% of total count	1	2	1	1	13.1	9.1	10.1	1	1	2	41.4
	% with site scars	50.0	8.7	20.0	50.0	92.9[a]	37.5	58.8	25.0	25.0	50.0	41.4
	Count	1	2	1	1	13	9	10	1	1	2	41
Adult (16–60)	% of total count	1	21.2	4	1	1	15.2	7.1	3	3	2	58.6
	% with site scars	50	91[a]	80	50	7.1	62	41	75	75	50	58.6
	Count	1	21	4	1	1	15	7	3	3	2	58
	Total	2	23	5	2	14	24	17	4	4	4	99

[a] High percent

Table 4 Rate of cutaneous leishmaniasis infection in relation to certain social factors

Parameter	No. examined	Overall infection		Odds ratio	(95% CI)	P value
		No.	%			
Primary	86	18	18.2	3.955	0.443–0.424	0.412[n]
Secondary	81	18	18.2			
Diploma	22	4	4.0			
Bachelor	14	5	5.1			
Total	322	54	54.6			

[n] no significant P > 0.05

Table 5 Effect of certain environmental and others social factors on infection with CL

Parameter	No. examined	Over all infection		Odds ratio	(95% CI)	P value
		No.	%			
Residents type						
Populist	346	65	12.38	0.035	0.985–0.456	0.040*
New	179	34	6.47			
Floor type						
First floor	270	61	51.42	5.50	0.778–0.066	0.030*
Second floor	237	34	45.14			
Third floor	18	4	3.43			
House protection						
Found protection	294	55	10.4	0.010	1.00–0.922	0.040*
Not found	231	44	8.38			
Animals found						
Found	314	59	11.23	0.002	1.00–0.524	0.023*
Not found	211	40	7.6			

* Significant P < 0.05

Table 6 Levels of maloniadealdhyde (MDA), catalase (Cat.) and uric acid (UA) of patients and healthy control

Test	Number	Mean ± SEM	P value
UA mg/l	Patient (99) Control (51)	Patient 8.5 ± 0.27 Control 5.6 ± 0.17	<0.001*
Cat. kU/l	Patient (99) Control (51)	Patients 72.5 ± 4.5 Control 83.1 ± 4.9	0.115[n]
MDA nM/ml	Patient (99) Control (51)	Patients 3.40 ± 0.06 Control 1.38 ± 0.07	<0.001*

[n] no significant P > 0.05

* Significant P < 0.05

dampness which makes suitable environmental for sand flies colonies. Also, this result was the same by Alkhavan et al. [30]. The present study shows a significant correlation (OR = 5.50, P < 0.05) between infection and sitting in the floor house. The same results were found by Surendrana et al. [26]. They found that floors and plinths of houses, soil at the edges of heaps of refuse, and soil at the bases of stone walls are good breeding sites for the sand flies.

The results of this study show that the sites of CL distribution among the infected cases are related to age. The highest percent of lesions among adults were present in hand, leg, cheek and nose respectively, but the highest lesions of children lesions were present in ears, nose, and legs respectively. These results were in agreement with the results of AL-Jawabreh et al. [20] who found that in children the head was a more frequently infected area (61.3%) than other body sites of children, whereas the limbs were more involved in adults (78.3%). The distribution of lesions in the head area had a certain pattern with lesions more often appearing on the cheek (29.6% of 115 lesions) than on the nose (23.5%), the forehead (14.8%) or the chin (13.0%). Our results show that the infection of hands is the highest with (36%). The lesions were increased in hand than in the others parts because hands are for the most part that might be exposed to the bites. Similar results were observed by Ullah et al. [31].

In the present study, the single lesions are observed in most of the patients, which is supported by Parks [32]. The cause of differences of scars type maybe due to the

Table 7 Serum levels of maloniadealdhyde (MDA), catalase (Cat.) and uric acid (UA) in relation to age groups of patients infected with CL

Groups	N	Mean ± SEM	P value
UA mg/l			
1–15	28	8.62 ± 0.42	0.402[n]
16–30	38	8.93 ± 0.50	
31–45	28	7.77 ± 0.50	
45–60	5	8.28 ± 1.49	
Total	99	8.4892 ± 0.27	
Cat. kU/l			
1–15	28	81.96 ± 9.7	0.828[n]
16–30	38	85.34 ± 7.9	
31–45	28	79.49 ± 8.9	
45–60	5	103.11 ± 27.5	
Total	99	83.43 ± 4.9	
MDA nM/ml			
1–15	28	3.49 ± 0.13	0.139[n]
16–30	38	3.49 ± 0.09	
31–45	28	3.23 ± 0.12	
45–60	5	2.92 ± 0.30	
Total	99	3.39 ± 0.06	

n no significant P > 0.05

Table 8 Effect of sex on catalase among patients and control groups

Sex	Catalase				
	No.	Mean ± SEM	CI 95%	x^2	P value
Males patients	47	73.100 ± 0.021	0.439	39.0	0.561[n]
Females patients	52	72.29 ± 0.014	0.539	44.0	0.461[n]
Males control	27	83.1 ± 0.49	0.0477	138	0.523[n]
Females control	24	80.1 ± 0.32	0.677	140	0.323[n]

n no significant P > 0.05

Table 9 Effect of age on uric acid levels among patients and control

Age group	Uric acid		
	x^2	OR	P value
Patients	3900.187	692.471	0.363[n]
Control	1063.91	293.908	0.182[n]

n no SIGNIFICANT P value >0.05

Table 10 Effect of age on catalase levels among patient and control groups

Age group	Catalase		
	x^2	OR	P value
Patients	40.5	0.0512	0.213[n]
Control	63.48	0.033	0.588[n]

n no significant P > 0.05

Table 11 Effect of sex on uric acid level among infected group with CL and control group

Test group	Sex	Number	Mean and SEM	P value
Uric acid	Patients males	47	9.70 ± 0.35	0.050*
	Control males	27	6.62 ± 0.40	0.527[n]
	Patients females	52	8.10 ± 0.44	0.511[n]
	Control females	24	6.91 ± 0.41	0.492[n]

n no significant P > 0.05
* Significant P < 0.05

there was not study made about the species that cause the disease. The incubation period ranges from weeks to months. Present study shows some lesions appeared typically on exposed areas of the body where inoculation occurs. The same scars have been founded by Mandel et al. [33]; Mings et al. [34]. Lesions appear as small nodules, or round with raised margins and a granulating center with yellowish exudates which increase in size and eventually ulcerate, that depend on parasite, host, and sand fly factors; dose or route of inoculation; and the maintenance of macrophages in an inert, deactivated state [35]. The morphologic characteristics depend on the complex interactions between the virulent characteristics of the infecting *Leishmania* sp. and T-cell mediated immune responses of its human host [36].

Changes in lipid peroxidation and some free radicals scavengers in patients and control

Serum lipid peroxidation malondialdehyde (MDA) levels

Highly reactive oxygen species free radicals (ROS) have been indicated in the pathogenesis of various parasitic infections including *Leishmania* [37], *Plasmodium falciparum* (Kumar and Das 1999). *Ascaris lumbricoides* (Kilic et al. 2003), *Toxoplasma gondii* [38] *Trypanosoma cruzi* [39]. Lipid peroxidation is an ongoing physiological process, but several lines of evidence have suggested an important role for peroxidation in the pathogenesis of several parasitic diseases [40]. Lipid peroxidation is caused by ROS results in the disarrangement and ultimately, disruption of cell membranes, which leads to necrotic and cell death. The significant higher increased of serum MDA

variation of the vectors. The same discussion explained by Kharfi [25], present study does not cover the vector. Cutaneous leishmaniasis in Shara'b is caused by *Leishmania*. The vectors are sand flies of the genus *Phlebotomies*,

(P < 0.001) in CL patients, as comparing to control level of MDA, may suggest that the overproduction of ROS and RNS results in oxidative stress, and the acceleration of lipid peroxidation in CL patients, resulting from altered enzymatic antioxidant activities may be considered as an indication of cell injury caused by *Leishmania*.

Increased levels of MDA in serum of infected animals is related to the host defense against parasitic infections. The similar results were observed by Kocyigit et al. [4] and Serarslan et al. [41]. They found significant increase of serum MDA and NO⁻ in CL patients, as compared to their control and by Ozbilge et al. [42] who showed significant increase in LPO, superoxide dismutase peroxidation (SOP), glutathione and decrease catalase activity levels in patients with active CL than those of healthy control. Our result reveals that no effect of age and sex on the mean MDA levels in patients groups with CL and controls groups. Similar findings were reported by Quassim [43] and AL-Shamiri [44] as they found no significant changing in MDA levels among age groups of control and patients groups which disagree with the results of Hassan [45] who observed a significant increase in plasma MDA in the age of control group of (27–44 years) as compared to older age groups (45–58 years) and she suggested that this increased in MDA level to decreased SOD scavenger. From the previous speculation and the present observation, it might be postulated that the high serum MDA values in CL reflects an increased lipid peroxidation initiated by reaction of free radicals with poly unsaturated fatty acids in biological membranes. More over rapid production of oxygen free radicals depletes the protective antioxidant and enzymes.

Free radical scavengers

Enzymatic scavenger's catalase In the present study there was no significant decrease of catalase activity in patient as comparing to control and these result was in disagreement with result of Erel et al. [46]; Kocyigit et al. [4] they found that there was a significant decrease of mean catalase activity which level and increased MDA levels in patient with cutaneous leishmaniasis as compared to control. The mechanism of decrease catalase activity was due to that serum catalase activity can alter H_2O_2-dependent reactions and in the other site resistant the parasite to H_2O_2 which causes a consumed catalase serum.

The non-significant decrease of catalase activity in our study may happen due to the fact that the parasite itself is protected to some extent against toxic oxygen metabolites. As discussed earlier, by Murray [47]. Amastigotes appear to contain catalase and superoxide dismutase although leishmania is poorly endowed in glutathione peroxidase [47] a novel reducing agent specific to trypanosomes has been described, which may serve to mop up

hydrogen peroxide evolved during the respiratory burst [48]. This happens, maybe due to the method that we used in the present study, as well.

The large variation in age groups of patients in the present study may explain a decrease of catalase activity. Different result in catalase activates was recorded by Niwa et al. [49]. They found that catalase, glutathione peroxidase and D-glucose-6-phosphate dehydrogenase, was significantly higher in younger adults than in elderly individuals. The basic levels of three other H_2O_2 scavenging enzyme activities were found to be decreased in leukocytes of elderly adults in comparing with young adults. This results shows that there is any significant effect of age and sex on catalase levels among controls and patients groups. Our study of Yemeni individual has not been studied yet and there were not a number of normal values of serum catalase activity.

Non enzymatic scavengers Uric acid: Uric acid is an important contributor to total antioxidant capacity; it provides a significant antioxidant defense against nitration by proxy nitrite. It has an important role as an oxidative stress marker and a potential therapeutic role as an antioxidant [50].

This study shows that there is a high significant (P < 0.001) increase of the uric acid level in patients groups than those of controls. The same result was reported by Frederico et al. [51]. This increase in uric acid level which may refer to the physiological activity and the influence of destroyed or catabolism [52, 53]. Increased level of uric acid may contribute much more to scavenging of free radicals. This may support the powerful antioxidant role of uric acid in scavenging singlet oxygen and other free radicals [54] and [55]. Uric acid may act as a defense mechanism against oxidative stress, or uric acid acting as a pro-oxidant and contributing to the damage caused in these diseases [56, 57]. Uric acid is released from tissues that are short of oxygen and elevated uric acid levels may an important part of acclimatization to high altitude [58, 59]. There is a significant increase due to the effect of sex on uric acid in male than female this may due to its scavenger activities.

Conclusions

We conclude from this study that there was a high spread of CL and there were high prevalence rates of cutaneous leishmaniasis in Shara'b District, Taiz, Yemen, The prevalence of CL was highly positive in Nakhla village. The rate of infection among males was higher than females. There was an association between the infection and age group. The patient who had cutaneous leishmaniasis has many changes in some biochemical levels. This study provides a clear indication of the role of MDA as an early biochemical marker of peroxidation damage occurring during cutaneous leishmaniasis. Increased uric acid, and catalase activity was provided of free radical scavengers.

Authors' contributions

QA, carried out the prevalence with stuff of nurses and experimental chemical parasitological diagnosis in lab. ASS, Oversees the biochemical analysis and participated. ATM, carried out the diagnosis and Supervises on it. ASA participated during our responses. BHO and YL conceived the study and participated on its design, evaluation of the results and writing of the manuscript. All authors read and approved the final manuscript.

Author details

[1] College of Environment, Hohai University, Nanjing 210098, China. [2] Faculty of Medical Science, Taiz University, Taiz, Yemen. [3] Department of Applied Microbiology, Taiz University, Taiz, Yemen. [4] Faculty of Applied Science, Direction of Scientific Research, Taiz University, Taiz, Yemen. [5] College of Engineering, Sinnar University, Sinnar, Sudan.

Acknowledgements

My deep appreciation goes to Banny Ziad center in Shara'b, the Microbiology laboratories, villagers and Yemeni clinical laboratory Specialized Alborehee hospital, Palestine hospital and Specialized Almadaen laboratories for their assistance with samples examination. Tiaz University.

Competing interests

The authors declare that they have no competing interests.

Funding

The research was supported by the Chinese National Science Foundation (51579071, 51379061), Fok Ying Tong Education Foundation (141073), the Fundamental Research Funds for the Central Universities (2014B07314), and National Science Funds for Creative Research Groups of China (No. 51421006); the Priority Academic Program Development of Jiangsu Higher Education Institutions; the program of Dual Innovative Talents Plan and Innovative Research Team in Jiangsu Province, and the Special Fund of State Key Laboratory of Hydrology-Water Resources and Hydraulic Engineering.

References

1. Svobodová M, Alten B, Zídková L, Dvořák V, Hlavačková J, Myšková J. Cutaneous leishmaniasis caused by *Leishmania infantum* transmitted by *Phlebotomus tobbi*. Int J Parasitol. 2009;39:251–6.
2. World Health Organization, 2014. Framework for action on cutaneous leishmaniasis in the Eastern Mediterranean Region 2014–2018.
3. Abd Al-Warith Y, Mukhtar M. Leishmaniasis in Yemeni children: seroepidemiological study in Taiz and Lahj Governorates Ph.D. thesis, uofk. 2009.
4. Kocyigit A, Keles H, Selek S, Guzel S, Celik H, Erel O. Increased DNA damage and oxidative stress in patients with cutaneous leishmaniasis. Mutat Res. 2005;585(1):71–8.
5. Djaldetti M, Salman H, Bergman M. Phagocytosis-the mighty weapon of the silent warriors. Microsc Res Tech. 2002;57:421–31.
6. Magni F, Panduri G, Paolocci N. Hypothermia triggers iron-dependent lipoperoxidative damage in the isolated rat heart. Free Radic Biol Med. 1994;16:465–76.
7. Khovidhunkit W, Memon RA, Feingold KR, Grunfeld C. Infection and inflammation-induced proatherogenic changes of lipoproteins. J Infect Dis. 2000;181(Supplement 3):S462–72.
8. Neupane DP, Majhi S, Chandra L, Rijal S, Baral N. Erythrocyte glutathione status in human visceral leishmaniasis. Indian J Clin Biochem. 2008;23(1):95–7.
9. Kilic E, Yazar S, Saraymen R, Ozbilge H. Serum malondialdehyde level in patients infected with *Ascaris lumbricoides*. World J Gastroenterol. 2003;9(10):2332–4.
10. Maco V, Marcos L, Terashima A, Samalvides F, Miranda E, Espinoza JR, Gotuzzo E. ELISA Technical de Sedimentation Rapid Modificad por Lumbreras en el diagnostic de la infection por *Fasciola hepatica*. Rev Med Hered. 2002;13:49–57.
11. Aydemir T, Ozturk R, Bozkaya L, Tarhan L. Effect of antioxidant vitamins A, C, E and trace elements Cu, Se on Cu Zn SOD, GSHPx, CAT and LPO levels in chicken erythrocytes. Cell Biochem Funct. 2000;18:109–15.
12. Simons K, Toomre D. Lipid rafts and signal transduction. Nat Rev Mol Cell Biol. 2000;1(1):31–9.
13. Escobar MA, Martinez F, Scott S, Palma GI. American cutaneous and mucocutaneous leishmaniasis (tegumentary): a diagnostic challenge. Trop Dr. 1992;22:69–78.
14. Van Kampan EJ, Zijlstra WG. Standardization of hemoglobin cyanide method. Clin Chim Acta. 1961;22(6):538–44.
15. Goth L, Nometh H, Mészáros I. Clinical study of the determination of serum catalase enzyme activity. Hung Sci Inst. 1986;57:7–12.
16. Fong KL, McCay PB, Poyer JL, Keele BB, Misra H. Evidence that peroxidation of lysosomal membranes is initiated by hydroxyl free radicals produced during flavin enzyme activity. J Biol Chem. 1973;248(22):7792–7.
17. Caraway WT. Uric acid in stander methods of clinical chemistry. In: Seligson D, editor. vol. 4. New York: Academic Press, Inc; 1965. p. 239–47.
18. Khatri ML, Haider N. Cutaneous leishmaniasis in Yemen. Int J Dermatol. 1999;38(8):587–90.
19. Green SJ, Meltzer MS, Hibbs JB, Nacy CA. Activated macrophages destroy intracellular Leishmania major amastigotes by an L-arginine-dependent killing mechanism. J Immunol. 1990;144(1):278–83.
20. Al Jawabreh A, Barghuthy F, Schnur LF, Jacobson RL, Schonian G, Abdeen Z. Epidemiology of cutaneous leishmaniasis in the endemic area of Jericho, Palestine. 2003.
21. de Oliveira Silva S, Wu AA, Evans DA, Vieira LQ, Melo MN. *Leishmania* sp. isolated from human cases of cutaneous leishmaniasis in Brazil characterized as Leishmania major-like. Acta Trop. 2009;112(3):239–48.
22. Khatami A. Development of a disease-specific instrument for evaluation of quality of life in patients with acute old world cutaneous leishmaniasis in adult iranian patients. A Study Protocol Ph.D. thesis, Centre for the Public Health; 2007.
23. Khatri ML, Muccio T, Gramiccia M. Cutaneous leishmaniasis in North-Western Yemen: a clinic epidemiologic study and Leishmania species identification by polymerase chain reaction-restriction fragment length polymorphism. J Am Acad Dermatol. 2009;61(4):15–21.
24. Haidar NA, Diab AB, El-Sheik AM. Visceral leishmaniasis in children in the Yemen. Saudi Med J. 2001;22(6):516–9.
25. Kharfi M, Benmously R, Fekih NE, Daoud M, Fitouri Z, Mokhtar I, Becher SB, Kamoun MR. Childhood leishmaniasis: report of 106 cases. Dermatol Online J. 2004;10(2).
26. Surendran SN, Kajatheepan A, Ramasamy R. Socio-environmental factors and sandfly prevalence in Delft Island, Sri Lanka: implications for leishmaniasis vector control. J Vector Borne Dis. 2007;44(1):65.
27. Ahmed AA. The water resources in Yemen, Ministry of Oil and Mineral Resources, Mine. Explo. Report WRAY-35. 1995. (Arabic Reference).
28. Banuls AL, Hide M, Prugnolle F. Leishmania and the leishmaniases: a parasite genetic update and advances in taxonomy, epidemiology and pathogenicity in humans. Adv Parasitol. 2007;64:1–458.
29. Guerin PJ, Olliaro P, Sundar S. Visceral leishmaniasis: current status of control, diagnosis, and treatment, and a proposed research and development agenda. Lancet Infect Dis. 2002;2:494–501.

30. Akhavan AA, Yaghoobi-Ershadi MR, Mehdipour D, Abdoli H, Farzinnia B, Mohebali M, Hajjaran H. Epidemic outbreak of cutaneous leishmaniasis due to Leishmania major in Ghanavat rural district, Qom Province, Central Iran. Iranian J Publ Health. 2003;32(4):35–41.

31. Ullah S, Jan AH, Wazir SM, Ali N. Prevalence of cutaneous leishmaniasis in lower Dir District (NWFP), Pakistan. J Pak Assoc Dermatol. 2009;19:212–5.

32. Parks K. Epidemiology of communicable diseases In: Text book of preventive and social medicine Jabalpur India, vol. 24. M/S Banarsidas Bhanot; 2004. p. 325–35.

33. Mandel GL, Bennett JE, Dolin R. New York, Churchill-Livingstone; 5th sporotrichoid cutaneous leishmaniasis Iran. J Med Sci. 2006;31(3–175):2831–41.

34. Mings S, Beck JC, Davidson C, Ondo AL, Shanler SD, Berman J. Cutaneous leishmaniasis with boggy induration and simultaneous mucosal disease. Am J Trop Med Hyg. 2009;80(1):3–5.

35. Basu MK, Ray M. Macrophage and Leishmania: an unacceptable coexistence. Crit Rev Microbiol. 2005;31(3):145–54.

36. Reed SG, Scott P. T cell and cytokine responses in leishmaniasis. Curr Opin Immunol. 1993;5:524–31.

37. Oliveira FJA, Cechini R. Oxidative stress of liver in hamsters infected with *Leishmania* (L.) *chagasi*. J Parasitol. 2002;86:1067–72.

38. Kilic E, Saraymen R, Sahin I. Serum malondialdehyde levels in toxoplasma seropositive patients. Ann Saudi Med. 2003;23(6):413.

39. Finzi JK, Chiavegatto WMC, Lopez JA, Cabrera OG, Mielniczki-Pereira AA, Colli W, Alves MJM, Gadelha FR. *Trypanosoma cruzi* response to the oxidative stress generated by hydrogen peroxide. Mol Biochem Parasitol. 2004;133(1):37–43.

40. Bagchi M, Mukherjee S, Basu MK. Lipid peroxidation in hepatic microsomal membranes isolated from mice in health and in experimental leishmaniasis. Indian J Biochem Biophys. 1993;30(5):277–81.

41. Serarslan G, Yılmaz HR, Söğüt S. Serum antioxidant activities, malondialdehyde and nitric oxide levels in human cutaneous leishmaniasis. Clin Exp Dermatol. 2005;30(3):267–71.

42. Ozbilge H, Aksoy N, Kilic E, Saraymen R, Vural H. Evaluation of oxidative stress in cutaneous leishmaniasis. J Dermatol. 2005;32(1):7–11.

43. Quassim MM. Oxidative stress in hypertensive patients on different types of treatment. M. Sc thesis. 2001. AL-Mustansirriyah University. Iraq. (Arabic reference).

44. Al-Shamiri SAA. Evaluation of some biochemical markers of the oxidative damage and myocardial injury, Ph. D. Thesis Medical College, University of Baghdad, Iraq. 2003. p. 95–102 (Arabic reference).

45. Hassan, N. A. R., Antioxidant Activities of free radical scavengers in ischemic heart disease, doctors of philosophy in biochemistry, University of Baghdad, Iraq. 1996. A thesis. p. 34–56 (Arabic reference).

46. Erel O, Kocyigit A, Bulut V, Gurel MS. Reactive nitrogen and oxygen intermediates in patients with cutaneous leishmaniasis. Memórias do Instituto Oswaldo Cruz. 1999;94(2):179–83.

47. Murray HW. Susceptibility of Leishmania to oxygen intermediates and killing by normal macrophages. J Exp Med. 1981;153:1302.

48. Fairlamb AH. Trypanothione: a novel bias-(glutathione) spermidine cofactor for glutathione reductase in trypanosomatids. Sci J. 1985;227:1485–7.

49. Niwa Y, Iizawa O, Ishimoto K, Akamatsu H, Kanoh T. Age-dependent basal level and induction capacity of copper–zinc and manganese superoxide dismutase and other scavenging enzyme activities in leukocytes from young and elderly adults. Am J Pathol. 1993;143(1):312.

50. Teng RJ, Ye YZ, Parks DA, Beckman JS. Urate produced during hypoxia protects heart proteins from peroxynitrite-mediated protein nitration. Free Radic Biol Med. 2002;33:1243–9.

51. Glantzounis GK, Tsimoyiannis EC, Kappas AM, Galaris DA. Uric acid and oxidative stress. Curr Pharm Des. 2005;11:4145–51.

52. Mahajan M, Kaur S, Mahajan S, Kant R. Uric acid a better scavenger of free radicals than vitamin C in rheumatoid arthritis. Indian J Clin Biochem. 2009;24(2):205–7.

53. Verde FA, Verde FA, Veronese FJ, Neto AS, Fuc G, Verde EM. Hyponatremia in visceral leishmaniasis. Rev Inst Med Trop Sao Paulo. 2010;52(5):253–8.

54. Chuang CC, Shiesh SC, Chi CH, Tu YF, Hor LI, Shieh CC, Chen MF. Serum total antioxidant capacity reflects severity of illness in patients with severe sepsis. Crit Care. 2006;10(1):R36.

55. Bayiroğlu F, Cemek M, Çaksen H, Cemek F, Dede S. Altered antioxidant status and increased lipid peroxidation in children with acute gastroenteritis admitted to a pediatric emergency service. J Emerg Med. 2009;36(3):227–31.

56. Strazzullo P, Puig JG. Uric acid and oxidative stress relative impact on cardiovascular risk? Nutr Metab Cardiovasc Dis. 2007;17(6):409–14.

57. Dimitroula HV, Hatzitolios AI, Karvounis HI. The role of uric acid in stroke: the issue remains unresolved. Neurologist. 2008;14(4):238–42.

58. Baillie JK, Bates MG, Thompson AR, Waring WS, Partridge RW, Schnopp MF, Simpson A, Gulliver-Sloan F, Maxwell SR, Webb DJ. Endogenous urate production augments plasma antioxidant capacity in healthy lowland subjects exposed to high altitude. CHEST J. 2007;131(5):1473–8.

59. Araujo CF, Lacerda MV, Abdalla DS, Lima ES. The role of platelet and plasma markers of antioxidant status and oxidative stress in thrombocytopenia among patients with vivax malaria. Mem Inst Oswaldo Cruz. 2008;103(6):517–21.

A pre-therapeutic coating for medical devices that prevents the attachment of *Candida albicans*

Diego Vargas-Blanco, Aung Lynn, Jonah Rosch, Rony Noreldin, Anthony Salerni, Christopher Lambert and Reeta P. Rao*⬤

Abstract

Background: Hospital acquired fungal infections are defined as "never events"—medical errors that should never have happened. Systemic *Candida albicans* infections results in 30–50% mortality rates. Typically, adhesion to abiotic medical devices and implants initiates such infections. Efficient adhesion initiates formation of aggressive biofilms that are difficult to treat. Therefore, inhibitors of adhesion are important for drug development and likely to have a broad spectrum efficacy against many fungal pathogens. In this study we further the development of a small molecule, Filastatin, capable of preventing *C. albicans* adhesion. We explored the potential of Filastatin as a pre-therapeutic coating of a diverse range of biomaterials.

Methods: Filastatin was applied on various biomaterials, specifically bioactive glass (cochlear implants, subcutaneous drug delivery devices and prosthetics); silicone (catheters and other implanted devices) and dental resin (dentures and dental implants). Adhesion to biomaterials was evaluated by direct visualization of wild type *C. albicans* or a non-adherent mutant $edt1^{-/-}$ that were stained or fluorescently tagged. Strains grown overnight at 30 °C were harvested, allowed to attach to surfaces for 4 h and washed prior to visualization. The adhesion force of *C. albicans* cells attached to surfaces treated with Filastatin was measured using Atomic Force Microscopy. Effectiveness of Filastatin was also demonstrated under dynamic conditions using a flow cell bioreactor. The effect of Filastatin under microfluidic flow conditions was quantified using electrochemical impedance spectroscopy. Experiments were typically performed in triplicate.

Results: Treatment with Filastatin significantly inhibited the ability of *C. albicans* to adhere to bioactive glass (by 99.06%), silicone (by 77.27%), and dental resin (by 60.43%). Atomic force microcopy indicated that treatment with Filastatin decreased the adhesion force of *C. albicans* from 0.23 to 0.017 nN. Electrochemical Impedance Spectroscopy in a microfluidic device that mimic physiological flow conditions in vivo showed lower impedance for *C. albicans* when treated with Filastatin as compared to untreated control cells, suggesting decreased attachment. The anti-adhesive properties were maintained when Filastatin was included in the preparation of silicone materials.

Conclusion: We demonstrate that Filastatin treated medical devices prevented adhesion of Candida, thereby reducing nosocomial infections.

Keywords: *C. albicans*, Filastatin, Fungal pathogens, Inhibition of attachment, Biomaterials

Background

Hospital acquired infections are described as "never events"—medical errors that should never have

happened. These are largely preventable, serious events that have an adverse effect on public health. The CDC estimates that there are 1.7 million hospital acquired infections each year causing nearly 100,000 deaths, which costs the US healthcare system between 28 billion and 33 billion dollars each year [1]. *Candida albicans*, a normally human commensal organism, has become a significant

*Correspondence: rpr@wpi.edu
Life Science and Bioengineering Center, Worcester Polytechnic Institute, 60 Prescott Street, Worcester, MA 01609, USA

cause of most nosocomial diseases of fungal origin [2–4]. The number of immunocompromised patients, the population "at risk" and susceptible to fungal diseases [5, 6], steadily increased worldwide at the beginning of the century due to better medical facilities and changes in life style. As expected, this had serious repercussions in the number of reported cases of *C. albicans* infections [7, 8]. In the United States alone, the estimated healthcare cost to treat *C. albicans* systemic infections is between \$1.5 and \$2 billion per year, which accounts for ~70% of the total amount spent on systemic fungal infections [9–11]. This is in part due to a reduced number of antifungal drugs, a consequence of the fact that it is difficult to find fungi-specific drug targets that are not also present on host cells. Among the commercially available antifungals, azoles, polyenes and echinocandins are the most effective [12]. In the last few years strains resistant to fluconazole have been reported, and with it a new threat to public health [13–16]. Therefore, new methods to prevent hospital-acquired infections by this opportunistic fungus are becoming more important than ever.

Candida albicans is commonly found in the skin and urogenital tract of humans. However, it can become pathogenic causing localized infections such as thrush and vaginitis, the latter being suffered by 75% of females at least once in their lifetime [17, 18]. Furthermore, *C. albicans* can reach the bloodstream and cause systemic infections where the mortality rate can be as high as 50%, even with treatment [19, 20]. Individuals who contract systemic infections caused by this pathogen are typically immunocompromised, such as HIV-infected persons, transplant recipients, patients receiving chemotherapeutic agents, patients receiving large amounts of antibiotics for bacterial infection treatment, and low-birth weight infants [7, 8, 21–24], who are now at an increased risk due to drug resistant *C. albicans* [12, 25–27]. Treating such drug-resistant strains involves long term combination therapy that is often cost prohibitive.

Filastatin was recently identified as a potential agent to prevent *C. albicans* filamentation and adhesion to abiotic and biotic surfaces [10], both of which contribute to biofilm formation and virulence [25, 28–30]. We have previously reported that Filastatin also inhibits the adhesion of *C. dubliniensis*, *C. tropicalis* and *C. parapsilosis* to polystyrene surfaces [10]. Here, we specifically focus on the antiadhesive properties of Filastatin, and propose its use as a pre-therapeutic coating for biomaterials, specifically, dental resin used in dentures and dental implants; silicone elastomers which is widely used as a biomaterial in catheters or as a component of implanted devices that contact the body; bioactive glass which is a component of some medical devices, such as cochlear implants or subcutaneous drug delivery devices that have embedded

electronics, and used in prosthetic devices along with titanium to repair and replace diseased or damaged bone [31, 32]. These materials are at high risk of being contaminated with *C. albicans* due to their composition and physical properties [33, 34]. Even more, their common use in clinical settings makes them a suitable reservoir for nosocomial infections [35, 36]. Previous studies have demonstrated, to different extents, the efficiency of coating agents, such as chitosan [37], curcumin on dental resins [38], or the covalent immobilization of the antimicrobials vancomycin and caspofungin on titanium [39] preventing *C. albicans* adhesion and biofilm formation. Thus, we tested various biomaterials under steady-state laboratory conditions as well as physiological flow conditions where the abiotic surfaces were co-incubated or pre-treated with Filastatin. We used analytical techniques such as atomic force microscopy (AFM) to measure the force of adhesion to abiotic surfaces and electrochemical impedance spectroscopy (EIS) to measure the anti-adhesive properties of Filastatin on *C. albicans* under conditions that mimics physiological flow conditions. Finally, we tested silicone material where Filastatin was incorporated into its composition.

Methods

Strains and culture conditions

Candida albicans isolate, SC5314, obtained from a patient with disseminated candidiasis [40], an mCherry-tagged derivative [41], and the non-adherent mutant *edt1*$^{-/-}$ [42] were used in this study. *C. albicans* cultures were stored at −80 °C and were propagated on synthetic complete media (SC) agar plates at 30 °C. A single colony obtained from the plates was used to prepare the inoculum in conical tubes containing 10 mL of tryptic soy broth (TSB) that allows cells to grow as planktonic cells. *C. albicans* cells were growth overnight (12–15 h) at 30 °C in a roller drum incubator (64 rpm).

Preparation of biomaterials

96 well polystyrene plates were used for assay development to test *C. albicans* adhesion. To measure the effect Filastatin wells were pre-treated with Filastatin using 198 μL of diH$_2$O + 2 μL of DMSO, or 2 μL of 50 μM Filastatin in DMSO. The wells were washed 10 times in diH$_2$O and dried using N$_2$ gas. Treated surfaces were visually monitored since the nitrophenyl group on Filastatin absorbs in the visible spectrum (400 ηm).

Glass coupons (1.2 cm diameter) were cleaned using Piranha solution (30 of 35% H$_2$O$_2$ + 70% H$_2$SO$_4$) for 1 h, then washed with deionized water for at least 10 min, rinsed with ethanol wash and dried with N$_2$ gas. Once dried, the coupons were oxygen plasma cleaned for 2 min, and then silane-coated using 1% APTMS

(3-aminopropyltrimethoxysilane) in 96% ethanol (aqueous) for at least 6 h at room temperature and agitated at 60 rpm. The bioactive coupons were finally washed with ethanol, dried with N_2 gas, and stored at 4 °C until use.

Dental implants resin coupons, made from a fast self-curing acrylic methacrylate resin using the Lang dental Jet Tooth Shade kit, were obtained from Dr. M. Noverr (LSUHSC, New Orleans, LA 70112).

Silicone coupons were made using a mix of polydimethylsiloxane elastomer (PDMS, a silicone elastomer). Briefly, 6 mL of polydimethylsiloxane elastomer were combined with 600 μL of silicone curing agent. After degassing the mix using vacuum for 2 h, the mix was poured on a plane surface and compressed into a fine pellicle of approx. 2 mm of height. Polymerization of the mix took place at 72 °C for 3 h. Coupons of 1.2 cm diameter were then cut from the PDMS pellicle. PDMS coupons including Filastatin were made adding 60 μL of 2.5 mM Filastatin in DMSO to the polydimethylsiloxane elastomer and curing agent mix. PDMS control coupons were made adding 60 μL of DMSO.

Dental resin and PDMS coupons treated with Filastatin prior exposure to cells were placed in a 1.5 mL of diH_2O containing 50 μM Filastatin in 1% DMSO for 30 min at 37 °C. The coupons were vigorously washed with abundant diH_2O, dried using N_2 gas, and stored at 4 °C until use. The presence of Filastatin on the surface of the coupon was confirmed by the evident change of color to yellow.

Assay development for surface adhesion of C. albicans on polystyrene

SC5314 grown overnight were recovered by centrifugation at 1000g, 18 °C; washed twice with SC + 0.15%; and adjusted to 0.3 OD_{600} (equivalent to $9 \cdot 10^6$ cells mL^{-1}). Cells were incubated in a polystyrene 96 well plate (198 μL per well) including 2 μL of DMSO (control) or 5, 2.5, or 1.25 mM Filastatin in DMSO for 2.5 h at 37 °C. The wells were emptied and 50 μL of crystal violet 0.5% aqueous solution was added to each well. After 45 min of incubation under static conditions the 96 well plate was washed 10 times with diH_2O. 200 μL of 75% methanol were added to each well, and the absorbance was read at 590 nm in a plate reader (PerkinElmer, VICTOR^3) [10]. The absorbance values obtained were used to calculate a relative absorbance. Typically, the relative absorbance was calculated per biological replicate by dividing each sample's absorbance by the average of the DMSO control absorbance.

For the time-dependent assay, cells were co-incubated with Filastatin following the protocol previously described in 96 well polystyrene plates for varying lengths of time: 5, 15, 30 min, and then every 30 min until 240 min. For Filastatin pre-treated polystyrene, 200 μL of the cell suspension was added to each well. Controls including 1% DMSO or 50 μM Filastatin in 1% DMSO in non-treated wells were also included, as well as a negative control of $edt1^{-/-}$. The 96 well plate was incubated for 4 h at 37 °C, without agitation and light exposure. Adherent cells were also quantified using crystal violet staining following extensive washing. Absorbance was normalized as described above.

Measurement of surface adhesion of C. albicans on various biomaterials

Adhesion was measured using direct cell counts. SC5314 or SC5314 mCherry grown overnight were washed with SC + 0.15% dextrose and adjusted to 0.3 OD_{600}. APTMS-treated glass were incubated in a 24 well plates, each well containing 1.5 mL of the cell suspension and 15 μL of 5 mM Filastatin in DMSO, or an equal volume of the solvent as control. Cells were incubated for 2.5 h at 37 °C under static conditions (no agitation). Coupons were then recovered and washed twice with diH_2O, 10 min each time. Fluorescent images were taken with an Axio Imager Z1 with ApoTome (Zeiss). Twenty images were obtained per coupon, and the cells per imaged field (0.15 mm^2) were counted using ImageJ v1.49 m [43] and averaged. To visualize the non-tagged SC5314, after washing the coupons the cells were stained with Syto®9 and propidium iodide (PI) for 15 min (live/dead assay).

A similar protocol was used for other biomaterials. Briefly, a 24 well plate containing a 1.5 mL of a C. albicans cell suspension (0.3 OD_{600}) per well was incubated at 37 °C using either APTMS-treated glass coupons, acrylic dental implants coupons, or PDMS coupons in presence and absence of 50 μM Filastatin in 1% DMSO. Acrylic dental coupons and PDMS treated with Filastatin; and PDMS coupons including Filastatin were only incubated with 1.5 mL of C. albicans (0.3 OD_{600}). The coupons were recovered after 2.5 h, and were gently rinsed with diH_2O. Then, the coupons were placed in a new plate containing 500 μL of crystal violet per well for a 45 min incubation. Subsequently, the coupons were rinsed in situ using 1000 μL of diH_2O, three times. The crystal violet stain was recovered from the cells using 500 μL of an aqueous solution of 75% methanol, and the absorbance read at 590 nm.

Atomic Force Microscopy to measure adhesion force of C. albicans

AFM was used to quantify the adhesion force of single C. albicans cells to bioactive glass coupons. A 0.3 OD_{600} suspension of SC5314 cells was prepared using SC + 2% dextrose. Two tubes were filled with 2475 μL of cells and 25 μL of DMSO or 5 mM Filastatin in DMSO and incubated at 30 °C in a roller drum incubator. After 30 min the cells were centrifuged at 1000*g* for 5 min and 18 °C, and washed with PBS. A small volume of the cell suspension was pipetted on an agar plate, and using a cantilever coated with Concanavalin A (ConA) a single cell was picked up. This *C. albicans* cell was used for a series of ≥39 adhesion force measurements against a bioactive glass surface, with readings every 5 s using AFM (Asylum MFP-3D-BIO). As an additional control, the non-adherent *edt1*$^{-/-}$ mutant was also tested for adhesion.

Electrochemical impedance spectroscopy of *C. albicans* under physiological microfluidic conditions

A microfluidic chamber of 4 mm × 6 mm × 1 mm was fabricated by casting PDMS into an aluminum chamber. Interdigitated micro electrodes (IDE) were fabricated from gold coated glass slides, with the electrode pattern carved using a VersaLaser VLS 2.30 CO2 laser cutter. Each sensor is comprised of a 4 × 6 mm active sensitive surface made of 4 pairs of microelectrodes (400 μm wide with 7.2 mm-long fingers, each finger separated by 400 μm). Before use, the IDE sensors were cleaned with piranha solution, washed for 10 min with abundant diH$_2$O, sonicated for 5 min in 96% ethanol, and dried in a stream of N$_2$ gas. IDEs were then activated with O$_2$ plasma for 2 min and immersed overnight in a 1 mM cysteamine hydrochloride 3% triethylamine ethanoic solution at room temperature. The IDEs were then rinsed with 96% ethanol, submerged in 10% acetic acid in ethanoic solution, and rinsed with 96% ethanol before being dried with N$_2$ gas.

A 0.3 OD$_{600}$ suspension of SC5314 in SC + 0.15% dextrose with 50 μM Filastatin in 1% DMSO or 1% DMSO was pumped through the IDEs assembled microfluidic channels (each of 6 mm × 4 mm × 1 mm) at 120 μL min^{-1} for 3 h, and at 37 °C. A syringe pump (KD Scientific) and silicone tubing were used to maintain the continuous flow. EIS measurements were performed every 5 min over a frequency range of 4–100 kHz, 0 V DC bias and a 20 mV p–p sinusoidal excitation signal. Adhesion of *C. albicans* cells over time was measured indirectly by using impedance changes (Zreal at 4 kHz). The experiment was also performed for the non-adherent mutant *edt1*$^{-/-}$ in presence of the DMSO vehicle (negative control). Each experiment consists of at least three biological replicates. Moreover, a single *C. albicans* cell is regarded as a dielectric component since it consists of biomaterials that have double-layer capacitance [44]. At higher frequencies, the electric current can penetrate the cell body and the impedance is independent of the frequency. At lower frequencies, the double layer capacitance of the cell body and EPS results in

a high impedance. The EIS frequency used in biosensing research is usually below 1 MHz, at which there is greater sensitivity to biological bodies, such as cells [45]. In this microfluidic physiological flow [46] experiment, *C. albicans* cells flowing through the IDE were attached and detached from its surface over time due to the nature of the surface, flow shear stress and hydrodynamic forces [47, 48]. As expected, the attachment of cells on the IDE covered the IDE conductive surface and increased the impedance, while the detachment exposed the IDE conductive surface and thus decreased the impedance.

Results

Filastatin inhibits *C. albicans* adhesion in a time and concentration dependent manner

We have previously demonstrated that Filastatin inhibits adhesion of many fungal pathogens of the *Candida* spp. to polystyrene surfaces [10]. To further study its anti-adhesion properties we exposed *C. albicans* to increasing concentrations of Filastatin (Fig. 1a). Unbound cells were washed and attached cells were stained with crystal violet to measured absorbance at 590 nm and quantify adhesion. We measured the effect of 12.5, 25 and 50 μM Filastatin compared to the solvent (DMSO) control. Our results indicate that treatment with Filastatin significantly decreases adhesion by 58.7, 68.1 and 70.8%, respectively ($p < 0.0001$, one-way ANOVA) for *C. albicans*, as compared to the control (Fig. 1a).

In order to determine the exposure time required for Filastatin to trigger an anti-adhesion response in *C. albicans*, we performed a time course experiment from 5 to 240 min using 50 μM Filastatin. Our results showed that the anti-adhesion effect of Filastatin increases overtime (Fig. 1b). Significant reduction of *C. albicans* attachment was observed 15 min post Filastatin treatment as compared to control (DMSO solvent). The effect of Filastatin was exaggerated with increased exposure time: at 15 min post exposure 29.6% of cells were attached, 19.4% after 60 min, and less than a 6% after 240 min. Together these results indicate that effects of Filastatin are concentration and time dependent, and measurable as early as 15 min.

Filastatin decreases the force of attachment between *C. albicans* and abiotic surfaces

To measure the direct force of attachment of *C. albicans* to an abiotic surface we used AFM. Briefly, cells attached to a surface are probed to measure the force necessary to "pluck" them off the surface [49]. Wild type *C. albicans* was exposed to 50 μM Filastatin and control population was exposed to the solvent (DMSO) for 30 min. The force of attachment for wild type *C. albicans* was recorded at 0.23 nN compared to 0.017 nN when cells were treated with Filastatin (Fig. 2, $p < 0.001$, one-way ANOVA). This

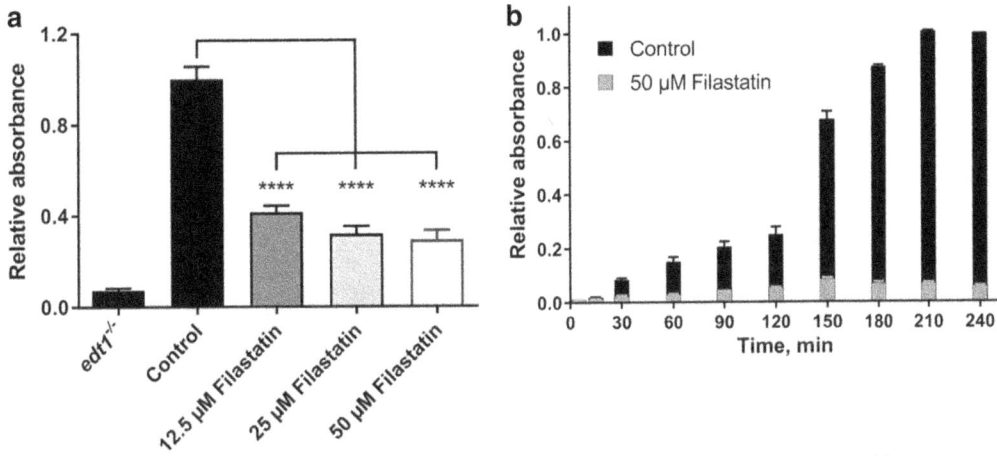

Fig. 1 Filastatin-mediated inhibition of *C. albicans* adhesion to abiotic surfaces is **a** dependent on its concentration and **b** increases over time. *C. albicans* were incubated in the presence of Filastatin. Adherent cells were stained with crystal violet and absorbance was measured. Relative absorbance values for each of the three biological replicates and standard error bars displayed, $p < 0.0001$. The $edt1^{-/-}$ mutant lacking an adhesion protein is used as a negative control

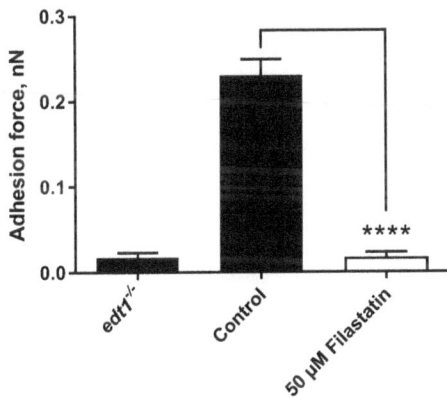

Fig. 2 Atomic force microscopy (AFM) to measure adhesion force on *C. albicans* to abiotic surfaces. *C. albicans* cells were lifted with an AFM cantilever and probed against an abiotic surface to measure the adhesion force. The adhesion force of cells treated with Filastatin (*white bar*) is shown in contrast to untreated cells and the $edt1^{-/-}$ non-adherent mutant (*black bars*). Each force measurement is calculated from 35–50 trials, standard error bars displayed, $p < 0.001$. The *graphic* shows one representative experiment

decreased force was comparable to the non-adherent $edt1^{-/-}$ mutant cell attachment to surfaces. These physical measurements further support our previous observations that Filastatin decreases the force of attachment between *C. albicans* and an abiotic surface.

Filastatin inhibits adhesion of *C. albicans* to a variety of biomaterials

To establish the utility of Filastatin in preventing adhesion of *C. albicans* we tested biomaterials such as dental resin, bioactive glass, and silicone. We used 1.2 cm coupons composed of these biomaterials that fit at the bottom of 24 well plates. We standardized the protocol using bioactive glass where we measured adhesion by direct counting of cells attached to the surfaces (Fig. 3a), and spectroscopic measurement of crystal violet stained cells attached to the surface (Fig. 3b). As described earlier we exposed *C. albicans* to varying concentration of Filastatin (12.5, 25 and 50 μM) and allowed cells to attach to bioactive glass coupons. Our results indicate that there was a significant decrease ($p < 0.0001$) in the number of *C. albicans* cells attached to bioactive glass after treatment with Filastatin as compared to the untreated control (Fig. 3a). Similar results were obtained when adherent cells were stained and the absorbance at A_{590} was measured (Fig. 3b).

To determine whether Filastatin affects viability of the cells, we used a live-dead assay (Syto9® and PI) where metabolically active and live cells fluoresce green (Syto9®) and dead cells fluoresce red (PI). These studies indicate that adherent *C. albicans* cells treated with Filastatin or those removed from the media containing Filastatin are viable. A representative microscopy image of a coupon surface with fluorescent stained cells is shown in Fig. 4a. To test whether the continuous exposure to Filastatin is needed to disrupt adhesion, we exposed *C. albicans* to 50 μM Filastatin, washed them, and then tested cell adhesion on bioactive glass. The experimental design is outlined in Fig. 4b. Briefly, surface adhesion of *C. albicans* cells was measured after continuous exposure to Filastatin or DMSO compared to that of cells that were washed and recovered in fresh media after Filastatin

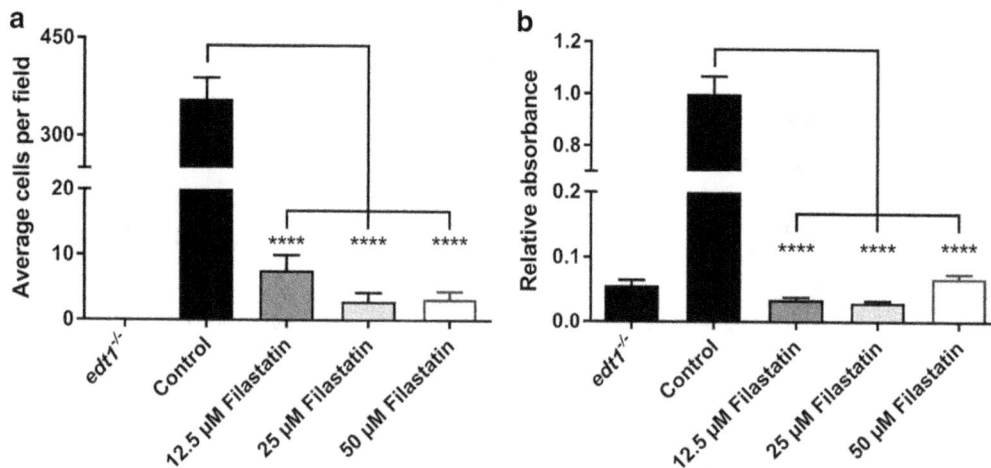

Fig. 3 Filastatin inhibits attachment of *C. albicans* to bioactive glass. *C. albicans* was incubated in varying concentrations of Filastatin in 24 well plates containing bioactive glass coupons. **a** Direct cell counts were obtained by propidium iodide and Syto9® staining. *Black bars* represent the number of wild type cells (control) or non-adherent cells (*edt1−/−*) that attach to untreated bioactive glass. *Grey and white bars* represent wild-type cells treated with varying concentrations of Filastatin. Standard error bars displayed, *p* < 0.0001. **b** Crystal violet staining to determine adhered cells to the surface of bioactive glass coupons

treatment. Our results (Fig. 4c) indicated that continuous exposure to Filastin decreased surface adhesion by 78% as compared to short exposure to Filastatin where adhesion was decreased by 24%. These results suggest that Filastatin is more effective when present continuously. This prompted us to consider Filastatin as a pre-therapeutic coating for biomaterials.

Filastatin, can serve as a pre-therapeutic coating for various biomaterials

Since Filastatin is most effective when present continuously we wanted to test whether it can be used as pre-therapeutic for biomaterials that pose a high risk of contamination with *C. albicans*. *C. albicans* cells incubated on 50 µM Filastatin-treated polystyrene wells showed 24.5% of cell adhesion when compared to the DMSO solvent control. A similar result was obtained when Filastatin was co-incubated (25.37% of cells adhered) with cells. 74% of cells adhered to DMSO solvent treated polystyrene wells, while the positive control *edt1−/−* mutant strain, registered a 6.77% of cell adhesion (Fig. 5).

Similar decrease in adhesion was observed when silicone surfaces and dental resin were incubated with *C. albicans* cells in presence of 50 µM Filastatin. Cell attachment was decreased by 87.27 and 60.43% as compared to DMSO solvent controls, respectively (Fig. 6a, b).

Silicone and dental resin coupons were also pretreated with 50 µM Filastatin for 30 min prior to exposure to *C. albicans*. Silicone surfaces where Filastatin was chemisorbed showed a 62.7% of reduction of adhesion of *C. albicans*, while similarly treated dental resin showed a

79.7% (Fig. 6c, d). Together these results indicate that biomaterials such as silicone and dental resin when superficially treated with Filastatin prevent attachment of *C. albicans*. These results further establish the utility of Filastatin as a pre-therapeutic for biomaterials. The anti-adhesion effect of Filastatin is lost after treatment with harsh chemicals such as methanol. Binding of *C. albicans* to methanol-treated coupons was similar when compared to untreated resin surfaces. These observations informed our next experiments to incorporate Filastatin into the matrix of biomaterials.

The anti-adhesive properties of Filastatin persists when incorporated into the chemical composition

To be used as a pre-therapeutic Filastatin may also be incorporated into the composition of the biomaterial. For this purpose, we choose to test silicone since it is a versatile biomaterial specifically used in catheters, a surface that often initiates a candida infection. Our results indicate that incorporation of 25 µM filastatin into the composition of silicone coupons decreased adhesion of *C. albicans* by 6.5-fold when compared to untreated silicone coupons (Fig. 7, *p* < 0.001). These results demonstrate that Filastatin retains its biological activity when it is incorporated into the silicone material, despite of being exposed at 72 °C for 3 h.

The anti-adhesive properties of Filastatin persist in physiological flow conditions

The effectiveness of Filastatin in a dynamic flow system that mimics physiological conditions was assessed using EIS to measure surface impedance. Higher impedance

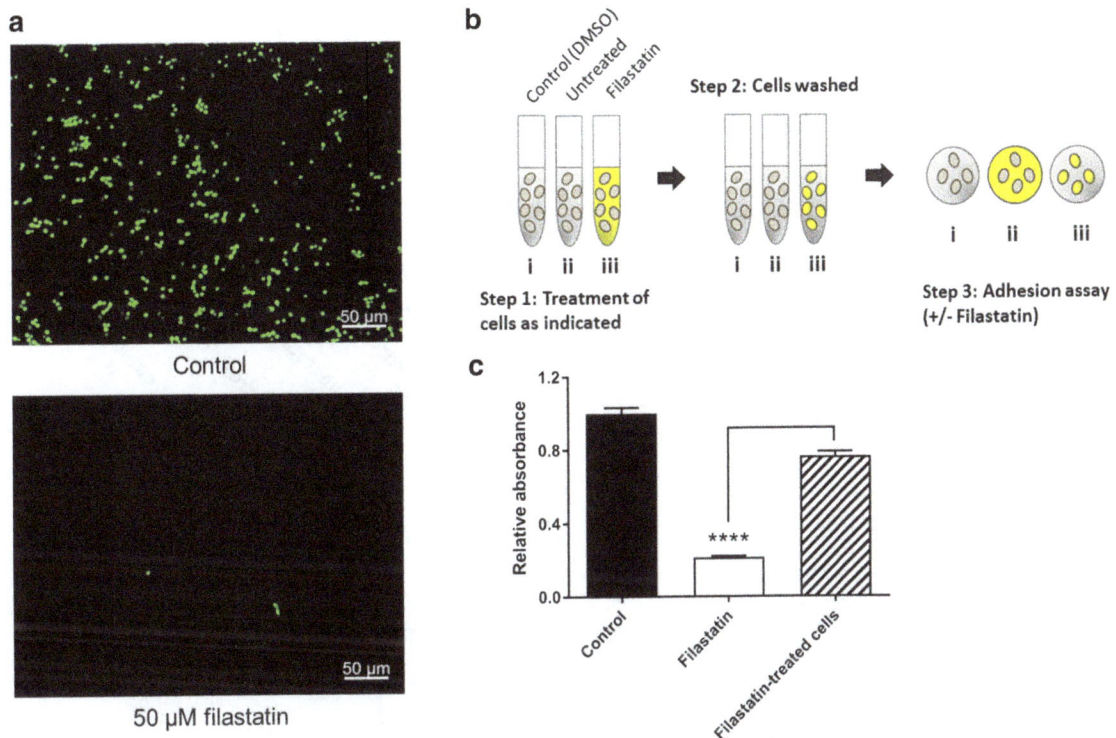

Fig. 4 The anti-adhesion effect of Filastatin depends on a continuous exposure to the drug and does not affect *C. albicans* viability. **a** *C. albicans* cells are viable upon exposure to Filastatin. Microscopic imaging of untreated cells attached to bioactive glass (*top panel*, labeled control) indicate that cells were viable but were unable to attach when treated with Filastatin (*bottom panel*). Filastatin treated cells were removed from the incubation media and stained for viability to ascertain that 100% of the cells were accounted for. **b** Experimental design to compare SC5314 cells pretreated with Filastatin vs those under continuous exposure to Filastatin. *Step 1* Cells were incubated with 1% DMSO (*i*), untreated (*ii*), or 50 μM Filastatin in 1% DMSO (*iii*). *Step 2* After 15 min, all the cells were washed three times. *Step 3* Adhesion assay using cell suspensions (*i* control, *ii* continuous exposure to Filastatin, or *iii* pre-treated with Filastatin). *Yellow* represents Filastatin in the media, or cells that were exposed to Filastatin. **c** *C. albicans* cells exposed to Filastatin either as a pre-treatment (*hatched*) or continuously (*white*) were unable to attach to bioactive glass as compared to the untreated cells (*black*). The decrease in adhesion is more dramatic when Filastatin is present continuously. Standard error bars displayed, $p < 0.0001$. Cell adhesion was measured using the crystal violet assay

is indicative of more *C. albicans* cells being attached to surfaces. EIS is widely used in biosensing [50] to measure impedance on amine-terminated IDE (a schematic of the IDE is shown in Fig. 8a, b). Through the course of this microfluidic experiment, the cells experience a continuous flow rate of 120 μL min^{-1} for 3 h, mimicking the conditions in the circulatory system of the mammalian host [46]. *C. albicans* cells continually attached and detached from the surface of the electrode during the experiment. Due to the double-layer capacitance nature of the cells at low frequency range, attachment of the cells on IDE surface is recorded as an increase in impedance changes and detachment of the cells exposes the electrode's conductive surface and is recorded as a decrease in the impedance [44, 45]. This allows us to measure the impedance as a readout for cell attachment and to determine the effects of Filastatin. *C. albicans* cells treated with Filastatin showed lower impedance as compared to untreated cells.

The impedance of the non-adherent mutant *edt1*$^{-/-}$ was measured as a positive control (Fig. 8c). Indeed, these results indicate that Filastatin is effective under dynamic flow conditions and supports the finding that Filastatin reduces attachment of *C. albicans* to abiotic surfaces.

Discussion

Over the last few decades the number of cases of systemic candidiasis has increased, outpacing the development of antifungal drugs to fight it. As an opportunistic pathogen, *C. albicans* is responsible for common clinical problems including oral thrush and vaginitis, but can also lead to life-threatening systemic infections in immunocompromised individuals [51], resulting in 30–50% mortality rates [52, 53]. A contributing factor to these statistics is the ability of *C. albicans* to develop resistance to antifungal drugs. In fact, fluconazole-resistant *Candida* strains were more frequently reported [27] and

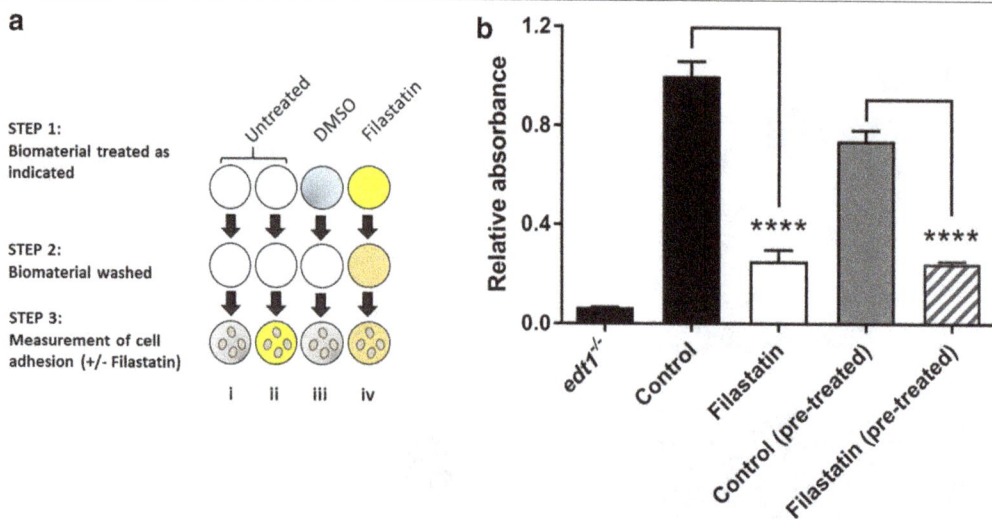

Fig. 5 Filastatin-treatment of polystyrene prevents *C. albicans* attachment. **a** Diagram representing the experimental setup. *Step 1* Polystyrene surfaces were untreated (*i*, *ii*), treated with the DMSO solvent (*iii*), or treated with Filastatin (*iv*). *Step 2* Washing. *Step 3* Incubation with *C. albicans* in the presence of solvent (*i*), Filastatin (*ii*), or none (*iii*, *iv*). **b** Crystal violet staining to determine *C. albicans* attachment to Filastatin-treated polystyrene. The *black bars* (control and *edt1*$^{-/-}$) represent *C. albicans* attachment to untreated polystyrene. The *white bar* represents Filastatin treated *C. albicans* attachment to untreated polystyrene. The *grey bar* represents adhesion of *C. albicans* to polystyrene exposed to the solvent only, and the *grey hatched bar* represents *C. albicans* adhesion to Filastatin-treated polystyrene

with it the fear of a new threat. The Center for Disease Control (CDC) recently declared drug-resistant *C. albicans* as a major public health threat [13–16, 54]. With the Pharmaceutical industry reporting a low inventory of antimicrobials [55], the search for non-traditional methods to prevent and manage nosocomial fungal infections is becoming more important than ever.

Inhibitors of adhesion are excellent lead compounds for pre-therapeutic and therapeutic drug development because (1) adhesion is the first step of an infection, and (2) inhibition of a general property such as fungal adhesion are likely to have a broad spectrum and affect other fungal pathogens. Efficient adhesion is required for formation of aggressive biofilms, which in turn make *Candida* a successful pathogen [56]. Therefore, adhesion is a pivotal step in fungal pathogenesis, but to our knowledge, one that has not yet been targeted by small molecules.

The discovery of Filastatin and other small molecules with attachment and biofilm disrupting properties [57] can lead to new alternatives for the prevention of nosocomial infections. Here, we further tested the effects of Filastatin on *C. albicans*, showing promising uses as a pre-therapeutic material and even as a composition additive for silicone-based devices.

AFM measurements revealed that Filastatin-exposed *C. albicans* cells were unable to attach to abiotic surfaces and resembled those of the non-adherent *edt1*$^{-/-}$ mutant cells. The effect of Filastatin is most dramatic when it is continuously present, because cells that were washed to

remove Filastatin were capable of binding abiotic surfaces again, albeit with reduced efficiency. These results led us to explore surface-treatment with Filastatin. For this purpose, three biomaterials were tested for co-incubations with Filastatin, and surface-treatment experiments: polystyrene, silicone and acrylic dental resin. In each case, materials treated with Filastatin showed a dramatic decrease in the number of cells adhered and correlated well with results of experiments where cells were co-incubated with Filastatin. The extent of adhesion of cells co-incubated with Filastatin was greater in polystyrene and silicone compared to acrylic dental resin. These results might be caused by DMSO, due to its moderate compatibility/solubility with PDMS and polystyrene [58]. In this present report, the nature of Filastatin attachment to surfaces is ill understood. We conducted preliminary studies using Quartz Crystal Microbalance with Dissipation monitoring technology (QCM-D), which showed Filastatin covering the surface of an APTMS-treated crystal. Future studies will focus on better methods to tether Filastatin to biomaterials.

Our results involving bioactive glass surfaces and plastics confirmed the efficacy of Filastatin as a potent anti-adhesion molecule for *C. albicans* in concentrations as low as 12.5 μM while in co-incubation. Moreover, this effect also extents to *C. dubliniensis*, *C. parapsilosis* and *C. tropicalis* [10]. Due to its potential use as a pre-therapeutic drug, IES and a microfluidics bioreactor were used to determine the effect of Filastatin under a

A pre-therapeutic coating for medical devices that prevents the attachment...

193

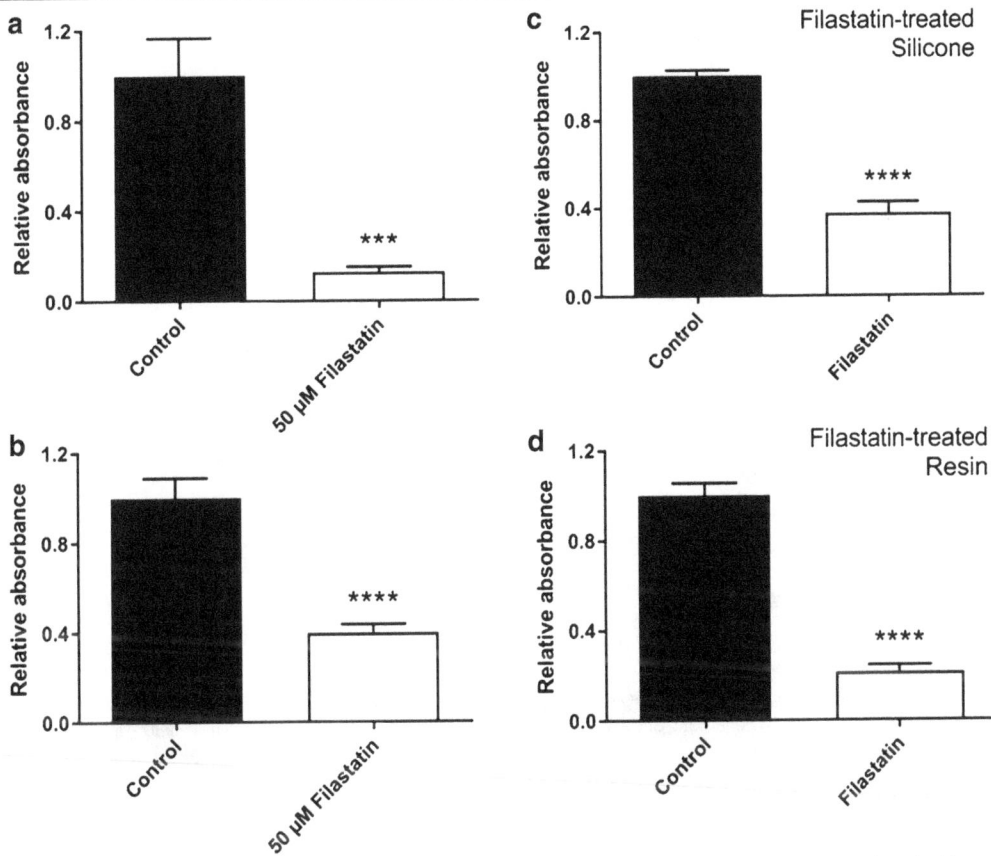

Fig. 6 Biomaterials treated with Filastatin prevent *C. albicans* attachment. **a** Adhesion of wild type *C. albicans* cells incubated with or without Filastatin on silicone coupons; or **b** on acrylic dental resin coupons. **c** *C. albicans* incubated on Filastatin-treated silicone coupons, or DMSO-exposed silicone coupons (control); or **d** on Filastatin-treated acrylic dental resin coupons. *C. albicans* adhesion measured using the crystal violet assay. Standard error bars displayed. ***$p < 0.001$, ****$p < 0.0001$

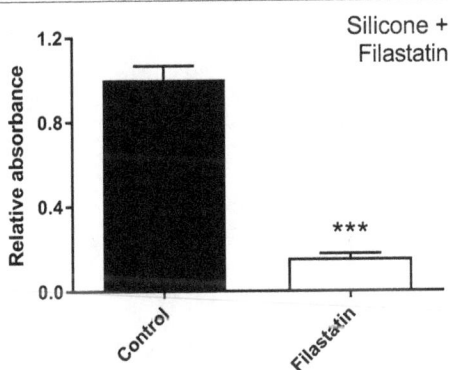

Fig. 7 Filastatin incorporated into silicone during formulation confers anti-adhesive properties against *C. albicans*. Crystal violet assay results for *C. albicans* attached to silicone surfaces prepared with Filastatin (*white bar*) or including the DMSO solvent (*black bar*). Standard error bars displayed, $p < 0.001$

microenvironment that mimics physiological flow conditions of bodily fluids. The impedance readings can be interpreted as a disruption on the adhesive properties of *C. albicans* cells in the presence of Filastatin, reinstating not only the efficacy of this molecule under steady conditions but also under flow conditions.

It is known that *C. albicans* cell surface interacts directly with host cells and is highly dynamic [59]. Its protein composition changes in the presence of environmental stresses, during switching between budded and hyphal morphologies and also when treated with antifungal agents [59, 60]. Notably, cell surface proteins, nutrient sensing and uptake, morphological switching, and biofilm formation are interrelated factors that contribute directly to the virulence and fitness of *C. albicans* within the host environment [59, 61–63]. Therefore, discovery of compounds that block adhesion, perturb

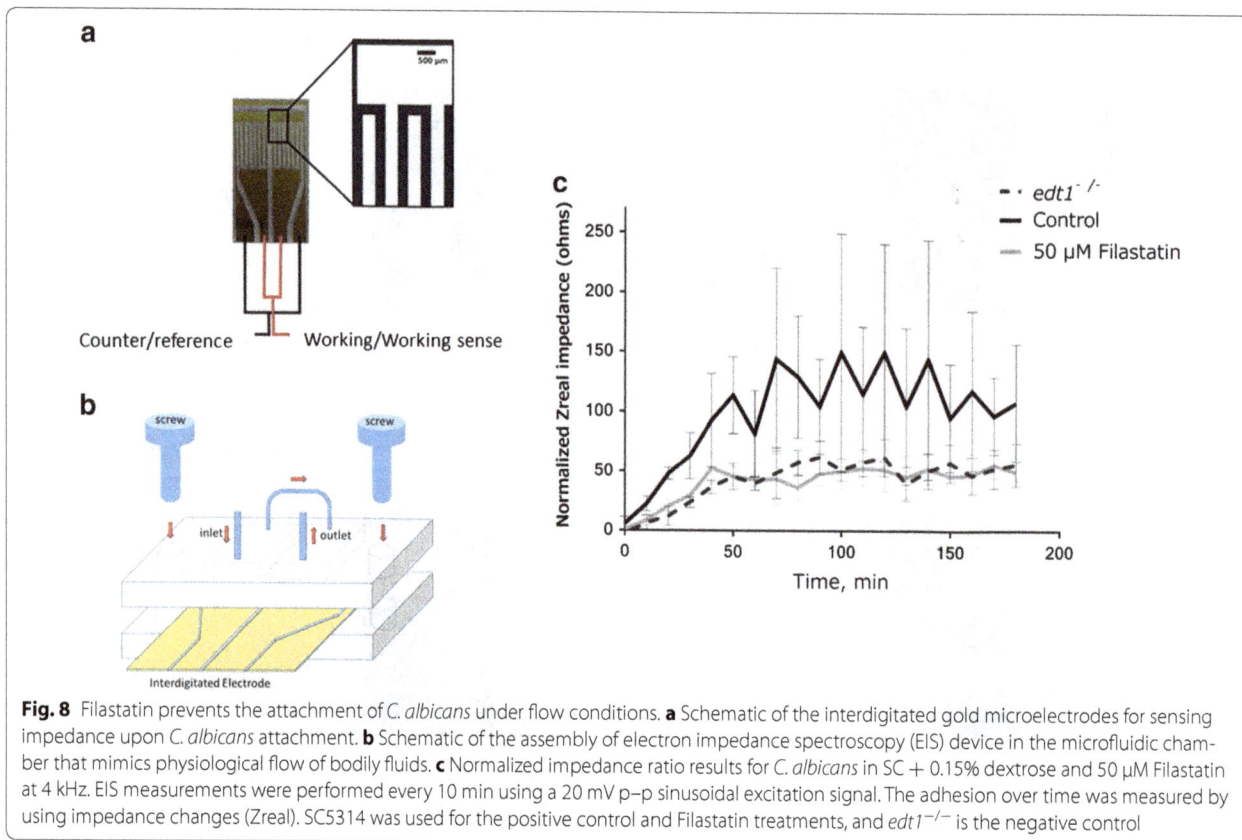

Fig. 8 Filastatin prevents the attachment of *C. albicans* under flow conditions. **a** Schematic of the interdigitated gold microelectrodes for sensing impedance upon *C. albicans* attachment. **b** Schematic of the assembly of electron impedance spectroscopy (EIS) device in the microfluidic chamber that mimics physiological flow of bodily fluids. **c** Normalized impedance ratio results for *C. albicans* in SC + 0.15% dextrose and 50 μM Filastatin at 4 kHz. EIS measurements were performed every 10 min using a 20 mV p–p sinusoidal excitation signal. The adhesion over time was measured by using impedance changes (Zreal). SC5314 was used for the positive control and Filastatin treatments, and *edt1*$^{-/-}$ is the negative control

morphological switching and reduce biofilm formation or limit uptake of essential nutrients by *C. albicans* would be an important first step towards developing new antifungal therapeutics.

Conclusion

We have shown that Filastatin is an effective agent against *C. albicans* adhesion to multiple surfaces under steady and dynamic conditions. Furthermore, *C. albicans* was unable to attach to biomaterials treated with Filastatin. Future studies will focus on the molecular targets of Filastatin and tethering to biomaterials, as well as in safety and of Filastatin as a pre-therapeutic coating.

Abbreviations

AFM: atomic force microscopy/microscope; APTMS: (3-aminopropyl) trimethoxysilane; CDC: Center for Disease Control; diH$_2$O: deionized water; DMSO: dimethyl sulfoxide; EIS: electrochemical impedance spectroscopy; HIV: human immunodeficiency virus; IDE: interdigitated electrode; PDMS: polydimethylsiloxane; PI: propidium iodide; QCM-D: quartz crystal microbalance with dissipation monitoring; SC: synthetic complete (media); TSB: tryptic soy broth.

Authors' contributions

DVB, RPR, CL and AL contributed to the intellectual content, experimental design of the study. DVB and RPR drafted the manuscript. DVB and AL carried out the laboratory studies, JR and RN performed the AFM studies, AS designed and prepared the microfluidics device used in this study. CL was involved with critically evaluation and constructive discussions during all stages of this study. All authors read and approved the final manuscript.

Acknowledgements

The authors thank Dr. Mairi Noverr (LSU Health Science Center) for generously providing the dental resins used in this study. We would like to acknowledge, T. Gawain for his help in the acquisition of the AFM data.

Competing interests

The authors declare that they have no competing interests.

Funding

This work was partially supported by a WPI, Pilot Project Initiative Grant to RPR. DVB was partially supported by the LASPAU, Fulbright Foreign Student Program.

References

1. Scott RD. The direct medical costs of healthcare-associated infections in US hospitals and the benefits of prevention: Division of Healthcare Quality Promotion National Center for Preparedness, Detection, and Control of Infectious Diseases, Centers for Disease Control and Prevention; 2009.

2. Pfaller MA. Nosocomial candidiasis: emerging species, reservoirs, and modes of transmission. Clin Infect Dis. 1996;22(Suppl 2):S89–94.

3. Kabir MA, Hussain MA, Ahmad Z. *Candida albicans*: a model organism for studying fungal pathogens. ISRN Microbiol. 2012;2012:538694.

4. Wisplinghoff H, Bischoff T, Tallent SM, Seifert H, Wenzel RP, Edmond MB. Nosocomial bloodstream infections in US hospitals: analysis of 24,179 cases from a prospective nationwide surveillance study. Clin Infect Dis. 2004;39(3):309–17.

5. Low CY, Rotstein C. Emerging fungal infections in immunocompromised patients. F1000 Med Rep. 2011;3:14.

6. Barnes RA. Early diagnosis of fungal infection in immunocompromised patients. J Antimicrob Chemother. 2008;61(Suppl 1):i3–6.

7. Pfaller MA, Diekema DJ. Epidemiology of invasive candidiasis: a persistent public health problem. Clin Microbiol Rev. 2007;20(1):133–63.

8. Schelenz S. Management of candidiasis in the intensive care unit. J Antimicrob Chemother. 2008;61(Suppl 1):i31–4.

9. Miceli MH, Diaz JA, Lee SA. Emerging opportunistic yeast infections. Lancet Infect Dis. 2011;11(2):142–51.

10. Fazly A, Jain C, Dehner AC, Issi L, Lilly EA, Ali A, Cao H, Fidel PL Jr, Rao RP, Kaufman PD. Chemical screening identifies filastatin, a small molecule inhibitor of *Candida albicans* adhesion, morphogenesis, and pathogenesis. Proc Natl Acad Sci USA. 2013;110(33):13594–9.

11. Wilson LS, Reyes CM, Stolpman M, Speckman J, Allen K, Beney J. The direct cost and incidence of systemic fungal infections. Value Health. 2002;5(1):26–34.

12. Spampinato C, Leonardi D. Candida infections, causes, targets, and resistance mechanisms: traditional and alternative antifungal agents. Biomed Res Int. 2013;2013:204237.

13. Giusiano G, Mangiaterra M, Garcia Saito V, Rojas F, Gomez V, Diaz MC. Fluconazole and itraconazole resistance of yeasts isolated from the bloodstream and catheters of hospitalized pediatric patients. Chemotherapy. 2006;52(5):254–9.

14. Wang Y, Liu JY, Shi C, Li WJ, Zhao Y, Yan L, Xiang MJ. Mutations in transcription factor Mrr2p contribute to fluconazole resistance in clinical isolates of *Candida albicans*. Int J Antimicrob Agents. 2015;46:552.

15. Rosana Y, Yasmon A, Lestari DC. Overexpression and mutation as a genetic mechanism of fluconazole resistance in *Candida albicans* isolated from human immunodeficiency virus patients in Indonesia. J Med Microbiol. 2015;64(9):1046–52.

16. Zhang SQ, Miao Q, Li LP, Zhang LL, Yan L, Jia Y, Cao YB, Jiang YY. Mutation of G234 amino acid residue in *Candida albicans* drug-resistance-related protein Rta2p is associated with fluconazole resistance and dihydrosphingosine transport. Virulence. 2015;6(6):611–9.

17. Sobel JD. Vaginitis. N Engl J Med. 1997;337(26):1896–903.

18. Ruhnke M, Maschmeyer G. Management of mycoses in patients with hematologic disease and cancer—review of the literature. Eur J Med Res. 2002;7(5):227–35.

19. Pappas PG, Rex JH, Lee J, Hamill RJ, Larsen RA, Powderly W, Kauffman CA, Hyslop N, Mangino JE, Chapman S, et al. A prospective observational study of candidemia: epidemiology, therapy, and influences on mortality in hospitalized adult and pediatric patients. Clin Infect Dis. 2003;37(5):634–43.

20. Sexton JA, Brown V, Johnston M. Regulation of sugar transport and metabolism by the *Candida albicans* Rgt1 transcriptional repressor. Yeast. 2007;24(10):847–60.

21. Pfaller MA. Epidemiology of nosocomial candidiasis: the importance of molecular typing. Braz J Infect Dis. 2000;4(4):161–7.

22. Jarvis WR. Epidemiology of nosocomial fungal infections, with emphasis on Candida species. Clin Infect Dis. 1995;20(6):1526–30.

23. Leroy O, Gangneux JP, Montravers P, Mira JP, Gouin F, Sollet JP, Carlet J, Reynes J, Rosenheim M, Regnier B, et al. Epidemiology, management, and risk factors for death of invasive Candida infections in critical care: a multicenter, prospective, observational study in France (2005–2006). Crit Care Med. 2009;37(5):1612–8.

24. Barberino MG, Silva N, Reboucas C, Barreiro K, Alcantara AP, Netto EM, Albuquerque L, Brites C. Evaluation of blood stream infections by Candida in three tertiary hospitals in Salvador, Brazil: a case-control study. Braz J Infect Dis. 2006;10(1):36–40.

25. Chandra J, Kuhn DM, Mukherjee PK, Hoyer LL, McCormick T, Ghannoum MA. Biofilm formation by the fungal pathogen *Candida albicans*: development, architecture, and drug resistance. J Bacteriol. 2001;183(18):5385–94.

26. Mathe L, Van Dijck P. Recent insights into *Candida albicans* biofilm resistance mechanisms. Curr Genet. 2013;59(4):251–64.

27. Antifungal Resistance. http://www.cdc.gov/fungal/antifungal-resistance.html.

28. Palanisamy SK, Ramirez MA, Lorenz M, Lee SA. *Candida albicans* PEP12 is required for biofilm integrity and in vivo virulence. Eukaryot Cell. 2010;9(2):266–77.

29. Samaranayake YH, Cheung BP, Yau JY, Yeung SK, Samaranayake LP. Human serum promotes *Candida albicans* biofilm growth and virulence gene expression on silicone biomaterial. PLoS ONE. 2013;8(5):e62902.

30. de Vasconcellos AA, Goncalves LM, Del Bel Cury AA, da Silva WJ. Environmental pH influences *Candida albicans* biofilms regarding its structure, virulence and susceptibility to fluconazole. Microb Pathog. 2014;69–70:39–44.

31. Bronzino JD. The biomedical engineering handbook 1. Berlin: Springer; 2000.

32. Srivatsan TS. Processing and fabrication of advanced materials, XVII: part 8: polymer-based composites and nano composites, vol. 2. New Delhi: I.K. International Publishing House; 2009.

33. Ellepola AN, Samaranayake LP. Adhesion of oral *Candida albicans* isolates to denture acrylic following limited exposure to antifungal agents. Arch Oral Biol. 1998;43(12):999–1007.

34. Nevzatoglu EU, Ozcan M, Kulak-Ozkan Y, Kadir T. Adherence of *Candida albicans* to denture base acrylics and silicone-based resilient liner materials with different surface finishes. Clin Oral Invest. 2007;11(3):231–6.

35. Ramage G, Martinez JP, Lopez-Ribot JL. Candida biofilms on implanted biomaterials: a clinically significant problem. FEMS Yeast Res. 2006;6(7):979–86.

36. O'Grady NP, Alexander M, Dellinger EP, Gerberding JL, Heard S, Maki D, Masur H, McCormick R, Mermel L, Pearson M. Draft guideline for the prevention of intravascular catheter-related infections. Atlanta: Centers for Disease Control; 2001.

37. Carlson RP, Taffs R, Davison WM, Stewart PS. Anti-biofilm properties of chitosan-coated surfaces. J Biomater Sci Polym Ed. 2008;19(8):1035–46.

38. Alalwan H, Rajendran R, Lappin DF, Combet E, Shahzad M, Robertson D, Nile CJ, Williams C, Ramage G. The anti-adhesive effect of curcumin on *Candida albicans* biofilms on denture materials. Front Microbiol. 2017;8:659.

39. Kucharikova S, Gerits E, De Brucker K, Braem A, Ceh K, Majdic G, Spanic T, Pogorevc E, Verstraeten N, Tournu H, et al. Covalent immobilization of antimicrobial agents on titanium prevents Staphylococcus aureus and *Candida albicans* colonization and biofilm formation. J Antimicrob Chemother. 2016;71(4):936–45.

40. Gillum AM, Tsay EY, Kirsch DR. Isolation of the *Candida albicans* gene for orotidine-5'-phosphate decarboxylase by complementation of S. cerevisiae ura3 and E. coli pyrF mutations. Mol General Genet MGG. 1984;198(2):179–82.

41. Brothers KM, Newman ZR, Wheeler RT. Live imaging of disseminated candidiasis in zebrafish reveals role of phagocyte oxidase in limiting filamentous growth. Eukaryot Cell. 2011;10(7):932–44.

42. Wheeler RT, Kombe D, Agarwala SD, Fink GR. Dynamic, morphotype-specific *Candida albicans* beta-glucan exposure during infection and drug treatment. PLoS Pathog. 2008;4(12):e1000227.

43. Schindelin J, Arganda-Carreras I, Frise E, Kaynig V, Longair M, Pietzsch T, Preibisch S, Rueden C, Saalfeld S, Schmid B, et al. Fiji: an open-source platform for biological-image analysis. Nat Methods. 2012;9(7):676–82.

44. Asami K, Hanai T, Koizumi N. Dielectric properties of yeast cells. J Membr Biol. 1976;28(2–3):169–80.

45. Benson K, Cramer S, Galla HJ. Impedance-based cell monitoring: barrier properties and beyond. Fluids Barriers CNS. 2013;10(1):5.

46. Bruchmann J, Sachsenheimer K, Rapp BE, Schwartz T. Multi-channel microfluidic biosensor platform applied for online monitoring and screening of biofilm formation and activity. PLoS ONE. 2015;10(2):e0117300.

47. Stone SD, Hollins BC. Modeling shear stress in microfluidic channels for cellular applications. In: Biomedical engineering conference (SBEC), 2013 29th Southern: 3–5 May 2013; 2013. p. 117–8.

48. Lu H, Koo LY, Wang WM, Lauffenburger DA, Griffith LG, Jensen KF. Microfluidic shear devices for quantitative analysis of cell adhesion. Anal Chem. 2004;76(18):5257–64.

49. De Oliveira R, Albuquerque D, Leite F, Yamaji F, Cruz T. Measurement of the nanoscale roughness by atomic force microscopy: basic principles and applications. Croatia: INTECH Open Access Publisher; 2012.

50. K'Owino IO, Sadik OA. Impedance spectroscopy: a powerful tool for rapid biomolecular screening and cell culture monitoring. Electroanalysis. 2005;17(23):2101–13.

51. Fidel PL Jr, Sobel JD. Immunopathogenesis of recurrent vulvovaginal candidiasis. Clin Microbiol Rev. 1996;9(3):335–48.

52. Gudlaugsson O, Gillespie S, Lee K, Vande Berg J, Hu J, Messer S, Herwaldt L, Pfaller M, Diekema D. Attributable mortality of nosocomial candidemia, revisited. Clin Infect Dis. 2003;37(9):1172–7.

53. Rangel-Frausto MS, Wiblin T, Blumberg HM, Saiman L, Patterson J, Rinaldi M, Pfaller M, Edwards JE Jr, Jarvis W, Dawson J, et al. National epidemiology of mycoses survey (NEMIS): variations in rates of bloodstream infections due to Candida species in seven surgical intensive care units and six neonatal intensive care units. Clin Infect Dis. 1999;29(2):253–8.

54. Centres for Disease Control and Prevention (CDC) Prevention: Antibiotic resistance threats in the United States, 2013. US Department of Health and Human Services; 2013.

55. Laxminarayan R, Duse A, Wattal C, Zaidi AK, Wertheim HF, Sumpradit N, Vlieghe E, Hara GL, Gould IM, Goossens H. Antibiotic resistance—the need for global solutions. Lancet Infect Dis. 2013;13(12):1057–98.

56. Finkel JS, Mitchell AP. Genetic control of *Candida albicans* biofilm development. Nat Rev Microbiol. 2011;9(2):109–18.

57. Pierce CG, Chaturvedi AK, Lazzell AL, Powell AT, Saville SP, McHardy SF, Lopez-Ribot JL. A novel small molecule inhibitor of Candida albicans biofilm formation, filamentation and virulence with low potential for the development of resistance. NPJ Biofilms Microb. 2015;1:15012.

58. Product information sheet for DMSO. https://www.sigmaaldrich.com/content/dam/sigma-aldrich/docs/Sigma/Product_Information_Sheet/d2650pis.pdf.

59. Chaffin WL. *Candida albicans* cell wall proteins. Microbiol Mol Biol Rev MMBR. 2008;72(3):495–544.

60. Dranginis AM, Rauceo JM, Coronado JE, Lipke PN. A biochemical guide to yeast adhesins: glycoproteins for social and antisocial occasions. Microbiol Mol Biol Rev MMBR. 2007;71(2):282–94.

61. Lo HJ, Kohler JR, DiDomenico B, Loebenberg D, Cacciapuoti A, Fink GR. Nonfilamentous *C. albicans* mutants are avirulent. Cell. 1997;90(5):939–49.

62. d'Enfert C. Hidden killers: persistence of opportunistic fungal pathogens in the human host. Curr Opin Microbiol. 2009;12(4):358–64.

63. Blankenship JR, Mitchell AP. How to build a biofilm: a fungal perspective. Curr Opin Microbiol. 2006;9(6):588–94.

Molecular characterization and genetic relatedness of clinically *Acinetobacter baumanii* isolates conferring increased resistance to the first and second generations of tetracyclines in Iran

Zahra Meshkat[1,2], Himen Salimizand[3], Yousef Amini[4], Mostafa Khakshoor[5], Davoud Mansouri[1,2,6], Hadi Farsiani[1,2], Kiarash Ghazvini[1,2] and Adel Najafi[1,2,6]*

Abstract

Background: The increasing resistance of *Acinetobacter baumannii* to antibiotics has recently been regarded as a notable therapeutic difficulty. Evaluating resistance rates of some *A. baumannii* isolates to tetracyclines had an impact on understanding the antibiotic resistance dissemination. By comparing genetic characteristics and relatedness of *A. baumannii* isolates, we are able to determine the transition dynamics of outbreak isolates.

Methods: A total of 72 non-duplicate isolates of *A. baumannii* were recovered in 2011 and 2015 and minimum inhibitory concentration (MIC) range distribution of the isolates to tetracyclines was performed by broth micro dilution (BMD) assay, and to determine the lineage relatedness of the outbreak isolates repetitive extragenic palindromic element based on polymerase chain reaction (rep-PCR) and international clonal (ICs) investigations were performed.

Results: Resistance rates to tetracycline, doxycycline and minocycline in 2011 were 73, 2 and 0%, while these rates in 2015 increased up to 90, 84 and 52%, respectively. The *tetB* existed in 100% of all the isolates of both years. *tetA* was not found in any of the isolates. According to the rep-PCR assays, up to 83% of all isolates clustered distinctly and only 6% of isolates had a common root. The percentage rates of IC1 decreased from 42% in 2011 to 22% in 2015, while those of IC2 increased from 28 to 36%, from 2011 to 2015.

Conclusions: Our data showed that resistance to the first and second generations of tetracyclines is on the rise and the clonal transition dynamics of isolates are in progress in our hospital.

Keywords: *Acinetobacter baumannii*, Tetracyclines, Molecular epidemiology, rep-PCR, IC clone

Background

Acinetobacter baumannii as an opportunistic pathogen has recently been known as a nosocomial pathogen which is associated with health care infections [1]. Due to the increasing antimicrobial resistance, *A. baumannii* has emerged as a life-threatening pathogen in the three past decades. The most important mechanisms of resistance to tetracyclines in *A. baumannii* isolates are efflux pumps followed by ribosomal protections and enzymatic inactivation. To date, tetracyclines were considered as a second-line therapy for *Acinetobacter* infections. However, due to the lack of any new under-development antibiotics and decreased effectiveness of the first-line antibiotics, older ones (e.g. tetracyclines) have been taken into consideration again [2]. Streptomyces species were the source of tetracycline, which is considered as the first

*Correspondence: najafia902@mums.ac.ir; adelnajafi1057@gmail.com
[2] Department of Microbiology and Virology, Ghaem hospital, Mashhad University of Medical Sciences, Ahmadabad Boulevard, Mashhad, Khorasan Razavi, PO Box: 91766-99199 (155), Iran
Full list of author information is available at the end of the article

generation of tetracyclines. Semisynthetic tetracyclines, doxycycline and minocycline, as the second generation of this group have wider spectrum. Tigecycline, a glycylcycline, has recently approved by US Food and Drug Administration (FDA) antibacterial agent. This minocycline structural analogue is indicated intravenously for the treatment of complicated infections [3].

Resistance to the first and second generations of tetracyclines in *A. baumannii* isolates mainly resulted from the acquired major facilitator superfamily (MFS) efflux pumps, including *tetA*, *tetB*, *tetG*, *tetH*, *tetL*, and *tet39*, resistance nodulation division family (RND) efflux pumps nominated as *adeABC*, *adeIJK*, *adeFGH*, *adeM*, *adeDE* [4], and finally ribosomal protections and enzymatic inactivation [5]. *tetA* is responsible for the resistance to tetracycline and doxycycline whereas *tetB* has been found in the isolates that were also resistant to minocycline [6]. Notably, the main resistance mechanisms of tetracyclines are *ade* efflux systems while coexistence with *tetA* and *tetB* determinants resulted in increasing MIC values [7].

Due to the lack of accuracy in disc diffusion method, determining susceptibility to doxycycline and minocycline was recommended to be carried out by Epsilometric test (E-test) or broth microdilution assays [8].

Regarding the impact of *A. baumannii* in healthcare—associated infections and rapid spreading of antibiotic-resistant strains, epidemiological investigation and determination of the clonal relationships among *A. baumannii* isolates should be considered. Some molecular techniques are currently at our disposal for typing and to clonal relatedness among clinically isolates of *A. baumannii*. The most common assay is the repetitive extragenic palindromic polymerase chain reaction-based (rep-PCR) that is simple, rapid and reliable compared to PFGE. Determining international clonal lineages (ICs) in *A. baumanii* is a useful tool for showing widespread distribution of global distributed clones [9]. Outbreak strains which are more resistant to antibiotics and might be associated with specific clinical syndromes, could be identified by such aforementioned studies [10]. The present study aimed to compare the resistance range of tetracycline, doxycycline and minocycline in the two periods of 2011 and 2015. Moreover, resistance determinants *tetA* and *tetB* were screened in clinical isolates of *A. baumannii*. Also, to determine the clonal transition dynamics and relatedness of isolates, international clonal lineage investigation and rep-PCR assays were performed in Ghaem Hospital, Mashhad, Iran.

Methods

Bacterial isolates and hospital setting

A total of 72 non-duplicate isolates of carbapenem resistant *A. baumannii* (CRAB) were collected from admitted patients at the Intensive Care Units (ICUs) of Ghaem Hospital (1000-bed referral university hospital, with NICU, PICU and adult's ICU wards). The ethics committee of hospital and institutional review boards approved this study, and recommendations by STROBE were considered to report the results [11]. Thirty-six isolates were collected in 2011, and the other 36 isolates were obtained in 2015. In the first stage, these isolates were identified by API20NE as *Acinetobacter baumannii-calcoaceticus* complex, and for confirming as *A. baumannii*, all of the isolates were investigated by OXA-51-like β-lactamase and *gyrB* multiplex PCR amplification according to previous studies [12]. The isolates were stored in 30% v/v glycerol/triptic soy broth medium at −70 °C.

Antibacterial susceptibility testing and efflux pump activity evaluation

In order to evaluate antimicrobial susceptibility to doxycycline, minocycline and tetracycline, broth micro dilution method was used according to CLSI M07-A9 instructions [13] and the results were interpreted according to CLSI M100-S25 guidelines [14]. In this study, the intermediate isolates were also considered as resistant. All antibiotic chemicals were purchased from Sigma Chemicals Co., Inc. (St. Louis, USA). *Escherichia coli* ATCC 25922 and *Pseudomonas aeruginosa* ATCC 27853 were used as reference strains.

For tetracyclines resistant isolates, MICs of the three aforementioned antibacterials were repeated in the presence of the following efflux pump inhibitors (EPIs) by broth microdilution method. Carbonyl cyanide 3-chlorophenylhydrazone (CCCP), phenyl-arginine-β-naphthylamide (PAβN), 1-(1-naphthylmethyl)-piperazine (NMP), reserpine and verapamil (Sigma), CCCP, PAβN, NMP, reserpine, and verapamil were added to the broth at the final concentrations of 5, 70, 100, 50, and 100 g/L, respectively [4]. A fourfold or greater decrease in the MIC values in the presence of EPIs was considered as significant inhibition.

PCR amplification of *tetA* and *tetB*

The existence of tetracycline resistant determinants, *tetA* and *tetB*, were detected by the PCR assay according to previous studies with some modifications [15]. Briefly, the template DNA for PCR reactions was obtained from heating 200 μL suspension of overnight bacterial cultures for 10 min at 95 °C and quickly refrigerating for 10 min followed by centrifugation at 15,000*g* for 5 min, and then discarding the supernatant. PCR products were analyzed by electrophoresis on agarose gels 2% using a 100plus DNA ladder Fermentase (Thermo Fisher Scientific, Germany) as a size marker.

Clonal and international lineage relatedness

To discover clonal relationships among the isolates of *A. baumannii*, we exploited two molecular typing methods. All the isolates were subjected to rep-PCR and international clonal lineage (IC) investigations.

A pair of primers with indication for REP sequences of *A. baumannii* were used as amplification primers, as described previously. The concentration of REP primers, REP1 and REP2, were 50 pmol/mL [16]. PCR products were detected by electrophoresis on 2% agarose using a 100 bp plus DNA ladder (Thermo Fisher Scientific, Germany), as a size marker. GelJ software (v. 1.3) was utilized in order to analyze the band patterns, considering dice tolerance 2.0 and UPGMA method to depict dendrogram. Isolates with at least 95% similarity were considered related and defined as the same rep-PCR cluster. IC lineages detection was done by a multiplex PCR assay of all the strains to find *csuE*, OXA-66/69 and *ompA* genes [9].

Statistical study

All statistical analyses were performed using SPSS v.16.0. A univariate analysis was carried out using Pearson's Chi square test for nominal variables in two independent groups. A P value of <0.05 was considered significant.

Results

Antimicrobial susceptibility and molecular detection of *tetA* and *tetB*

In two periods of 2011 and 2015, 72 CRAB isolates (36 isolates per year) were collected. The percentages of tetracyclines resistant isolates in 2015 were obviously higher than those in 2011. About 70% (26 of 36) of isolates in 2011 were resistant to tetracycline, while in 2015, the resistance rates were increased up to 90% (32 of 36). The increasing rates were also observed for doxycycline and minocycline. In 2011, 2.7% (1 of 36) of the isolates were resistant to doxycycline versus 84.2% (30 of 36) in 2015. None of the isolates were resistant to minocycline in 2011, but the resistance rate increased to 52.6% (19 of 36) after 4 years (Table 1).

MIC_{90} of minocycline, doxycycline and tetracycline were dramatically increased after passing 4 years (Fig. 1). $MICs_{90}$ for minocycline, doxycycline and tetracycline in 2011 were 2, 4 and 32 mg/L, respectively, whereas in 2015 they obviously increased to 16, 64 and 1024 mg/L, respectively. The MICs of resistant isolate for these antibacterials in the presence of EPIs were significantly changed. About 88% of tetracycline resistant isolates (51 out of 58) showed decreasing MIC when tetracycline was presented with EPIs. The effect of EPIs on the MICs of doxycycline and minocycline resistant isolates (31 and 19 out of 72, respectively), was reduced in 26% (8 of 31) and 47% (9 of 19) of doxycycline and minocycline, respectively. The tetracycline resistance determinant *tetB* was detected in all of the isolates of both years, however, tetA was not found in any of the isolates.

Epidemiological investigations and international clonal lineages

About 10 distinctive rep-PCR clusters (named A to J) and eight singleton isolates were inferred from the band patterns (Fig. 2). Clusters A–E and G consisted of

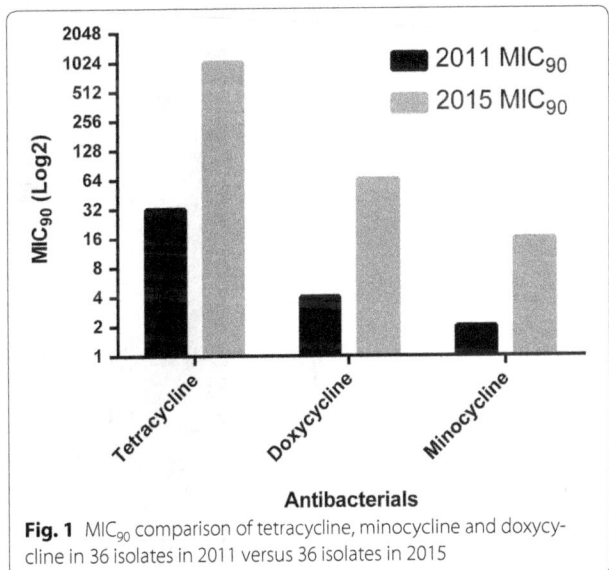

Fig. 1 MIC_{90} comparison of tetracycline, minocycline and doxycycline in 36 isolates in 2011 versus 36 isolates in 2015

Table 1 Broth microdilution susceptibilities and MIC range distribution of 72 *A. baumannii* isolates (results represented by %)

Agent/MIC$_{mg/L}$	2011			2015		
	≤4	8	≥16	≤4	8	≥16
TET	27	33	40	10	2.6	87.4
DOX	98	0	2	15.8	0	84.2
MIN	100	0	0	47.4	31.6	21

TET tetracycline, *DOX* doxycycline, *MIN* minocycline

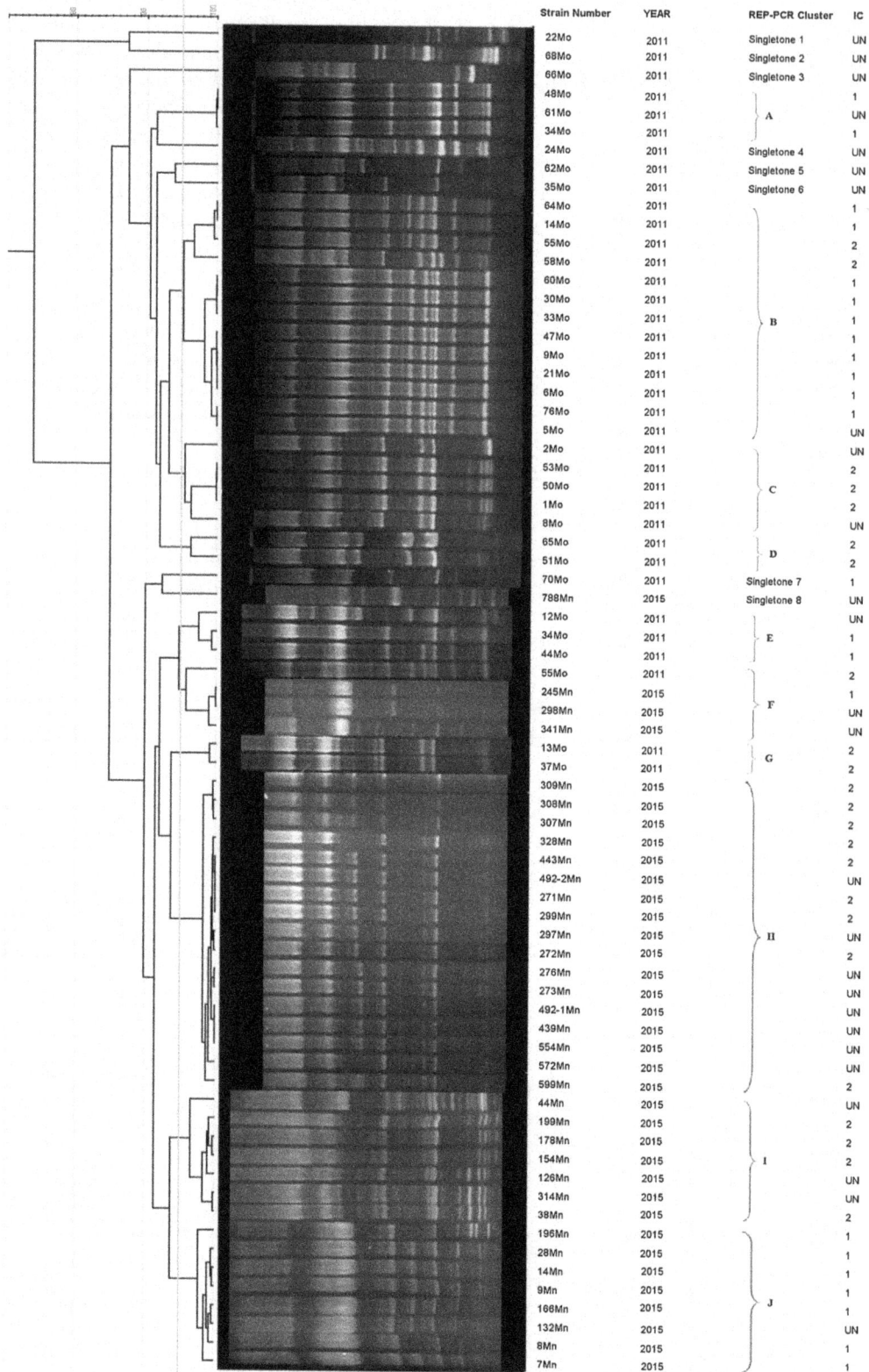

Strain Number	YEAR	REP-PCR Cluster	IC
22Mo	2011	Singletone 1	UN
68Mo	2011	Singletone 2	UN
66Mo	2011	Singletone 3	UN
48Mo	2011		1
61Mo	2011	A	UN
34Mo	2011		1
24Mo	2011	Singletone 4	UN
62Mo	2011	Singletone 5	UN
35Mo	2011	Singletone 6	UN
64Mo	2011		1
14Mo	2011		1
55Mo	2011		2
58Mo	2011		2
60Mo	2011		1
30Mo	2011		1
33Mo	2011	B	1
47Mo	2011		1
9Mo	2011		1
21Mo	2011		1
6Mo	2011		1
76Mo	2011		1
5Mo	2011		UN
2Mo	2011		UN
53Mo	2011		2
50Mo	2011	C	2
1Mo	2011		2
8Mo	2011		UN
65Mo	2011	D	2
51Mo	2011		2
70Mo	2011	Singletone 7	1
788Mn	2015	Singletone 8	UN
12Mo	2011		UN
34Mo	2011	E	1
44Mo	2011		1
55Mo	2011		2
245Mn	2015	F	1
298Mn	2015		UN
341Mn	2015		UN
13Mo	2011	G	2
37Mo	2011		2
309Mn	2015		2
308Mn	2015		2
307Mn	2015		2
328Mn	2015		2
443Mn	2015		2
492-2Mn	2015		UN
271Mn	2015		2
299Mn	2015		2
297Mn	2015	H	UN
272Mn	2015		2
276Mn	2015		UN
273Mn	2015		UN
492-1Mn	2015		UN
439Mn	2015		UN
554Mn	2015		UN
572Mn	2015		UN
599Mn	2015		2
44Mn	2015		UN
199Mn	2015		2
178Mn	2015		2
154Mn	2015	I	2
126Mn	2015		UN
314Mn	2015		UN
38Mn	2015		2
196Mn	2015		1
28Mn	2015		1
14Mn	2015		1
9Mn	2015		1
166Mn	2015	J	1
132Mn	2015		UN
8Mn	2015		1
7Mn	2015		1

Fig. 2 REP generated dendrogram of all isolates with considering more than 95% of similarity for clustering of isolates. *MN* Mashhad new, *Mo* Mashhad old, *UN* unknown

representatives of strains of 2011, and clusters H, I and J indicated strains of 2015. Cluster F consisted of strains of both years of 2011 and 2015. Our data showed that up to 94% of all the strains were included in nine distinct clusters and only 6% of them had common roots.

Results from Multiplex PCR revealed that 42% of strains in 2011 were IC1, 28% were IC2 and 30% were unknown, while only 22% of strains in 2015 were attributed to IC1, 36% to IC2 and 42% were unknown.

Discussion

This integrative study provides concerns about a formidable increase in drug resistance to *A. baumannii* concomitant with prospects to clonal transmission dynamics of outbreak isolates over a 4-year interval between 2011 and 2015.

Due to the increase in resistance to majority of antibiotics in *A. baumannii*, evaluating antimicrobial susceptibility of older agents that was not used in clinical practice is of interest to overcome the Acinetobacter infections. A previous study showed the satisfying effectiveness of tetracyclines against *A. baumannii* in vitro [15]. In this regard, our data showed that the resistance rates for tetracycline, doxycycline and minocycline in 2011 were 73, 2 and 0%, respectively. Meanwhile, these resistance rates increased to 90, 84.2 and 52.6% in the case of the noted antibiotics in 2015. Because of not using tetracyclines in clinical practice of *A. baumannii* infections in our hospitalized patients, the increased resistance to these three agents was not expected. Significant increasing resistance in our hospital setting is in correlation with another previous study in Iran [17]. Being consistent with our study, Maleki et al. reported that resistance rates of tetracycline, minocycline and doxycycline to *A. baumannii* isolates in Tehran in 2013 were 89, 35 and 25%, respectively.

The *tetA* and *tetB* determinants are common in tetracyclines resistant *A. baumannii* isolates [6]. Our results are also in agreement with a previous study by Farsiani et al. [18] in 2015 who reported that the *tetA* gene was not found in any of the strains whereas *tetB* was detected in 100% of the strains. In our study, the increased level of resistance to tetracyclines was observed in spite of any detectable differences in prevalence of *tetA* and *tetB* in all of the isolates. The effect of EPIs herein on most of the tetracycline resistant strains can explain that the increasing resistance is related to efflux pumps activity.

By using molecular typing methods, we are able to discriminates widespread clonal lineages of *A. baumannii* responsible for hospital clonal transition dynamics in outbreaks worldwide [19]. Amongst ten clusters obtained from evaluating all of the strains by rep-PCR, six clusters (A–E and G) included representatives of strains of 2011. The 2015 strains were classified in three clusters (H, I and

J), and one cluster (F) contained strains of both years. At a glance, it can be inferred that more than 94% of all the strains were classified in distinct clusters and less than 6% of the strains are in a common (F) cluster. Furthermore, up to 91% of the strains in 2015 were classified in three clusters. Considering the decrease in the number of clusters from 2011 to 2015, it certainly indicated that new lineages with different resistance patterns were replaced over 4 years.

In this study, the percentage rates of IC1 and IC2 in the strains of 2011 were 42 and 28%, whereas in the strains of 2015 they were 22 and 36%, respectively. Higher prevalence of IC2 strains in 2015 compared with 2011, is consistent with the previous reports which state that in the recent years IC2 was a more common lineage in antibiotic-rich environments of hospitals [20]. A pervious study by Turton et al. [9] showed that IC1 strains have been prevalent in the past years. Therefore, it can be concluded that the clonal transition dynamics of strains in our hospital is in progress. The increased prevalence of IC2 in our hospital concomitant with elevated resistance to the first and second generations of tetracycline strengthens the fact that the IC 2 strains have higher resistance genetic determinants than IC1 strains. This consequence is in accordance with the previous study where IC 2 strains were relatively older than the other ICs which have been undergoing extensive diversification [21].

Conclusions

With the best of our knowledge, this study is the first comparison of clinical strains of CRAB strains in the same location in two periods in Iran. Our data indicates that despite not using tetracyclines in treatment of Acinetobacter infections, the increased resistance to tetracyclines is likely duo to the clonal transition dynamics of strains with replacement of IC2 clones which contain higher prevalence of resistance determinants. Molecular detection of tetracycline resistance determinants in our hospital is due to the other efflux pumps rather than tetA and tetB efflux pumps. Eventually, to overcome the increasing resistance to antibiotics, some prerequisites should be considered e.g., improving antibiotic stewardship programs (ASPs), hygienic surveillance programs, epidemiological study of outbreak strains, and concrete infection control.

Authors' contributions

Concepts: ZM, YA, AN. Design: ZM, HS, YA, HF, KG, AN. Definition of intellectual content: ZM, HF, KG, AN. Literature search: HS, HF, AN. Clinical studies: HS, YA, KG. Experimental studies: HS, MK, DM, AN. Data acquisition: HS, YA, MK, AN. Data analysis: ZM, HS, DM, HF, AN. Statistical analysis: AN. Manuscript preparation: ZM, HS, YA, MK, DM, HF, KG, AN. Manuscript editing: ZM, HS, YA, MK, DM, HF, KG, AN. Manuscript review: ZM, HS, YA, MK, DM, HF, KG, AN. Guarantor: ZM. All authors read and approved the final manuscript.

Author details
[1] Antimicrobial Resistance Research Center, Bu Ali Research Institute, Mashhad, Iran. [2] Department of Microbiology and Virology, Ghaem hospital, Mashhad University of Medical Sciences, Ahmadabad Boulevard, Mashhad, Khorasan Razavi, PO Box: 91766-99199 (155), Iran. [3] Department of Microbiology, Faculty of Medicine, Kurdistan University of Medical Sciences, Sanandaj, Iran. [4] Department of Microbiology, Faculty of Medicine, Zahedan University of Medical Sciences, Zahedan, Iran. [5] Microbiology Department, Islamic Azad University, Tehran, Iran. [6] Student Research Committee, Faculty of Medicine, Mashhad University of Medical Sciences, Mashhad, Iran.

Acknowledgements
The authors appreciate the Ghaem laboratory staff for preparing the isolates.

Competing interests
The authors declare that they have no competing interests.

Funding
Financial support of Mashhad University of Medical Sciences are appreciated (Grant Number: Grant No. 931486).

References

1. Towner K. Acinetobacter: an old friend, but a new enemy. J Hosp Infect. 2009;73(4):355–63.
2. Viehman JA, Nguyen MH, Doi Y. Treatment options for carbapenem-resistant and extensively drug-resistant Acinetobacter baumannii infections. Drugs. 2014;74(12):1315–33.
3. Doan T-L, Fung HB, Mehta D, Riska PF. Tigecycline: a glycylcycline antimicrobial agent. Clin Ther. 2006;28(8):1079–106.
4. Deng M, Zhu MH, Li JJ, Bi S, Sheng ZK, Hu FS, et al. Molecular epidemiology and mechanisms of tigecycline resistance in clinical isolates of Acinetobacter baumannii from a Chinese University Hospital. Antimicrob Agents Chemother. 2014;58(1):297–303.
5. Chopra I, Roberts M. Tetracycline antibiotics: mode of action, applications, molecular biology, and epidemiology of bacterial resistance. Microbiol Mol Biol Rev. 2001;65(2):232–60.
6. Marti S, Fernandez-Cuenca F, Pascual A, Ribera A, Rodriguez-Bano J, Bou G, et al. Prevalence of the tetA and tetB genes as mechanisms of resistance to tetracycline and minocycline in Acinetobacter baumannii clinical isolates. Enfermedades infecciosas y microbiología clínica. 2006;24(2):77.
7. Huys G, Cnockaert M, Vaneechoutte M, Woodford N, Nemec A, Dijkshoorn L, et al. Distribution of tetracycline resistance genes in genotypically related and unrelated multiresistant Acinetobacter baumannii strains from different European hospitals. Res Microbiol. 2005;156(3):348–55.
8. Wang P, Bowler SL, Kantz SF, Mettus RT, Guo Y, McElheny CL, et al. Comparison of minocycline susceptibility testing methods for carbapenem-resistant Acinetobacter baumannii. J Clin Microbiol. 2016;54:2937–41.
9. Turton J, Gabriel S, Valderrey C, Kaufmann M, Pitt T. Use of sequence-based typing and multiplex PCR to identify clonal lineages of outbreak strains of Acinetobacter baumannii. Clin Microbiol Infect. 2007;13(8):807–15.
10. Dijkshoorn L, Aucken H, Gerner-Smidt P, Janssen P, Kaufmann M, Garaizar J, et al. Comparison of outbreak and nonoutbreak Acinetobacter baumannii strains by genotypic and phenotypic methods. J Clin Microbiol. 1996;34(6):1519–25.
11. Malmivaara A. Benchmarking controlled trial—a novel concept covering all observational effectiveness studies. Ann Med. 2015;47(4):332–40.
12. Higgins P, Wisplinghoff H, Krut O, Seifert H. A PCR-based method to differentiate between Acinetobacter baumannii and Acinetobacter genomic species 13TU. Clin Microbiol Infect. 2007;13(12):1199–201.
13. Standard A, Edition N. CLSI document M07-A9. Wayne: Clinical and Laboratory Standards Institute; 2012.
14. Clinical and Laboratory Standards Institute. Performance Standards for Antimicrobial Susceptibility Testing; Twenty-Fifth Informational Supplement. CLSI document M100-S25. Wayne: Clinical and Laboratory Standards Institute; 2015.
15. Miranda CD, Kehrenberg C, Ulep C, Schwarz S, Roberts MC. Diversity of tetracycline resistance genes in bacteria from Chilean salmon farms. Antimicrob Agents Chemother. 2003;47(3):883–8.
16. Snelling AM, Gerner-Smidt P, Hawkey PM, Heritage J, Parnell P, Porter C, et al. Validation of use of whole-cell repetitive extragenic palindromic sequence-based PCR (REP-PCR) for typing strains belonging to the Acinetobacter calcoaceticus-Acinetobacter baumannii complex and application of the method to the investigation of a hospital outbreak. J Clin Microbiol. 1996;34(5):1193–202.
17. Asadollahi P, Akbari M, Soroush S, Taherikalani M, Asadollahi K, Sayehmiri K, et al. Antimicrobial resistance patterns and their encoding genes among Acinetobacter baumannii strains isolated from burned patients. Burns. 2012;38(8):1198–203.
18. Farsiani H, Mosavat A, Soleimanpour S, Nasab MN, Salimizand H, Jamehdar SA, et al. Limited genetic diversity and extensive antimicrobial resistance in clinical isolates of Acinetobacter baumannii in north-east Iran. J Med Microbiol. 2015;64(7):767–73.
19. Ecker JA, Massire C, Hall TA, Ranken R, Pennella TTD, Ivy CA, et al. Identification of Acinetobacter species and genotyping of Acinetobacter baumannii by multilocus PCR and mass spectrometry. J Clin Microbiol. 2006;44(8):2921–32.
20. Higgins PG, Janßen K, Fresen MM, Wisplinghoff H, Seifert H. Molecular epidemiology of Acinetobacter baumannii bloodstream isolates from the United States 1995-2004 using rep-PCR and multilocus sequence typing. J Clin Microbiol. 2012:JCM. 01759-12.
21. Nemec A, Dolzani L, Brisse S, van den Broek P, Dijkshoorn L. Diversity of aminoglycoside-resistance genes and their association with class 1 integrons among strains of pan-European Acinetobacter baumannii clones. J Med Microbiol. 2004;53(12):1233–40.

Comparison of in-house and commercial real time-PCR based carbapenemase gene detection methods in *Enterobacteriaceae* and non-fermenting gram-negative bacterial isolates

M. Smiljanic[1], M. Kaase[2,3], P. Ahmad-Nejad[1] and B. Ghebremedhin[1*]

Abstract

Background: Carbapenemase-producing gram-negative bacteria are increasing globally and have been associated with outbreaks in hospital settings. Thus, the accurate detection of these bacteria in infections is mandatory for administering the adequate therapy and infection control measures. This study aimed to establish and evaluate a multiplex real-time PCR assay for the simultaneous detection of carbapenemase gene variants in gram-negative rods and to compare the performance with a commercial RT-PCR assay (Check-Direct CPE).

Methods: 116 carbapenem-resistant *Enterobacteriaceae*, *Pseudomonas aeruginosa* and *Acinetobacter baumannii* isolates were genotyped for carbapenemase genes by PCR and sequencing. The defined isolates were used for the validation of the in-house RT-PCR by use of designed primer pairs and probes.

Results: Among the carbapenem-resistant isolates the genes bla_{KPC}, bla_{VIM}, bla_{NDM} or bla_{OXA} were detected. Both RT-PCR assays detected all bla_{KPC}, bla_{VIM} and bla_{NDM} in the isolates. The in-house RT-PCR detected 53 of 67 (79.0%) whereas the commercial assay detected only 29 (43.3%) of the OXA genes. The in-house sufficiently distinguished the most prevalent OXA types (23-like and 48-like) in the melting curve analysis and direct detection of the genes from positive blood culture vials.

Conclusion: The Check-Direct CPE and the in-house RT-PCR assay detected the carbapenem resistance from solid culture isolates. Moreover, the in-house assay enabled the identification of carbapenemase genes directly from positive blood-culture vials. However, we observed insufficient detection of various OXA genes in both assays. Nevertheless, the in-house RT-PCR detected the majority of the OXA type genes in *Enterobacteriaceae* and *A. baumannii*.

Keywords: RT-PCR, Carbapenemases, *Acinetobacter baumannii*, MDR gram-negative bacteria

Background

An increase of infection triggered by multidrug-resistant gram-negative bacteria is a global problem because it is related to longer hospitalization, increased morbidity and mortality rates and to increased medical costs. The production of β-lactamase enzymes is the most common mechanism of bacterial resistance [1]. Carbapenemases are β-lactamases that have the ability to hydrolyse all β-lactam antibiotics, including carbapenem [2]. Rapid diagnostic tests for the identification and detection of specific resistance mechanism are necessary for therapy and prevent dissemination. Different techniques can be applied to identify carbapenem-resistant gram-negative bacteria. Phenotypic tests are used for detecting the carbapenemase activity while molecular based assays identify the resistance genes

*Correspondence: beniam.ghebremedhin@uni-wh.de
[1] Center for Clinical and Translational Research, Institute for Medical Laboratory Diagnostics, HELIOS University Clinic Wuppertal; Witten/Herdecke University, Heusnerstr. 40, 42283 Wuppertal, Germany
Full list of author information is available at the end of the article

[3]. Carbapenem-resistance can be detected by disc diffusion tests or Etest with imipenem, ertapenem or meropenem using agar plates or by automated systems (e.g. BD Phoenix, VITEK 2), selective chromogenic media for carbapenemase screening or the modified Hodge test (MHT) as additional phenotypic method [4]. The MHT is the only Clinical and Laboratory Standards Institute (CLSI)—recommended carbapenemase-screening method [4]. However, the gold standard for the detection of carbapenem-resistance are molecular based methods e.g. polymerase chain reaction (PCR)—either single- or multiplex PCR followed by a sequencing step if needed [3, 4]. However, these molecular methods are mainly implemented in reference laboratories. These diagnostic tools are necessary to administer the adequate therapeutic management for instance in septicaemia caused by carbapenemase-producing pathogens. Therefore, the distinction between carbapenem-resistance mediated by carbapenemases and those by other mechanisms is important for infection control in hospital setting. As the carbapenemase-producing gram-negative bacteria causing severe infections are generally multidrug-resistant, treatment options are compromised. Thus, the timely detection and monitoring of carbapenemases is important for therapeutic and prognostic means. Various carbapenemase genes may disseminate differently in the European countries, in the USA or the Asian countries. In the study region the predominance of the class D carbapenemase genes in *Enterobacteriaceae* and *Acinetobacter baumannii* is true [5].

In this study we established and evaluated a multiplex RT-PCR assay for the simultaneous detection of carbapenem resistance genes in gram-negative rods using the RT BD MAX™ system and compared the in-house RT-PCR with the commercial assay, the Check-Direct CPE kit.

Methods
Culture methods
Bacterial isolates
116 multidrug-resistant gram-negative isolates were collected from urine, blood-culture, wound swabs, tracheal secretions and other clinical specimens. Patient material were plated on Mac Conkey agar (BD, Becton–Dickinson and company, Heidelberg) and incubated at 37 °C over night. Species identification of these bacterial isolates was confirmed using MALDI-TOF mass-spectrometer. Carbapenem-resistance was approved using phenotypically methods (antibiotic disk diffusion and Etests on Muller–Hinton agar with imipenem, meropenem and ertapenem (BD Heidelberg, 10 µg and BD Phoenix system). All isolates have been characterized by the National Reference Centre (NRZ) at the molecular level.

For the identification of carbapenemase-producers directly from positive blood-cultures, negative Bactec™ Plus Aerobic/F blood-culture bottles containing clinical blood samples were inoculated with carbapenemase-producing isolates and incubated in a shaking incubator at 37 °C. For this purpose, a bacterial cell suspension was prepared with NaCl until a density of 0.5 McFarland turbidity standard was achieved. The blood-culture was inoculated with 500 µL of the bacterial suspension.

As negative controls we analysed 15 *Pseudomonas aeruginosa* and 20 *A. baumannii* isolates which were resistant to carbapenems but negative for the carbapenemase genes.

Molecular methods
DNA extraction
Some colonies of an overnight bacterial culture were suspended in 1.5 mL of 0.9% NaCl and centrifuged at 13,000 rpm for 10 min. The supernatant was discarded, the pellet resuspended in 500 µL NaCl and incubated for 15 min at 95 °C. Thereafter the suspension was incubated for further 10 min at room temperature and centrifuged at 13,000 rpm for 10 min. The supernatant was transferred in a new tube and the DNA concentration was measured.

For the bacterial extraction from positive blood culture vials 1.5 mL of the blood-culture was centrifuged for 5 min at 900 rpm. 500 µL of the supernatant was transferred in a new tube, mixed with 500 µL SDS (2%) and centrifuged at 13,000 rpm for 2 min. The supernatant was discarded and the DNA was extracted from the bacterial pellet as described above.

BD MAX™ diagnostic system
The BD MAX™ diagnostic system is an open RT-PCR system which allows the application of user defined protocols (UDPs). The advantage of this technology is the combined automatization of sample lysis, extraction, amplification and detection. This diagnostic system is time saving and avoids human errors. The fluorescence detection of the BD MAX™ is based on LEDs and photodiode filtering components to monitor fluorescence up to five different channels.

Primer and probes design/sets for the detection of β-lactamase genes
The primers used in this study were designed after aligning variations of the target gene using MUSCLE (http://www.ebi.ac.uk/Tools/msa/muscle/). The used sequences were downloaded from the National Center for Biotechnology Information (NCBI).

The aligned sequence was then used to design primers with the NCBI primer designing tool (http://www.ncbi.nlm.nih.gov/tools/primer-blast) and ordered at Eurofins Genomics, Ebersberg. Initially, singleplex PCR

Comparison of in-house and commercial real time-PCR based carbapenemase gene...

205

using the mastercycler (Eppendorf, Hamburg) was done to proof the primer pairs. The probes for each designed primer were ordered at TIB MOLBIOL Syntheselabor. The primers and the corresponding probes are listed in the Table 1.

In-house RT PCR on BD MAX™ system

For amplification, we used the Absolute qPCR Mix, no ROX (2×) (Thermo Fisher Scientific) and suspended the mix with 0.5 μL of the OXA-23 primer, OXA-48 Light Mix Modular, 0.75 μL of KPC, NDM and VIM primers, 0.3 μL OXA-23 probe and with 0.45 μL KPC, NDM and VIM probes. The primers primer master stock concentration was 10 pmol/μL for VIM, KPC, OXA-23 and NDM, and the probe concentration was 0.5 pmol/μL. 0.5 μL of the extracted DNA with a concentration of 80 ng/μL was added and a final volume of 12.5 μL were pipet into the microfluidic PCR cartridge (BD, Heidelberg).

The PCR was run at 95 °C for 5 min for 45 PCR cycles (95 °C, 15 s; 59 °C, 30 s; 72 °C, 11.7 s) followed by melt curve analysis for OXA-23 and OXA-48 variants with SYBR green from 40 to 100 °C in 0.2 °C steps. For the amplification and the analysis of the results the BD MAX software 4.32 A was used.

Check Direct CPE on BD MAX™ system

Bacterial isolates were directly analysed from culture media. Therefore a bacterial cell suspension to an optical density of 0.5 McFarland was diluted 1:100 and approximately 500 μL of this suspension was transferred into the DNA sample buffer tube SB-1. The rack and instrument were prepared according to the manufacturers' guidelines as well as the amplification program and the interpretation of the results.

Kappa (κ) statistics

To rather analyse the concordance between the two RT-PCR methods (in-house and commercial) for the detection of the various carbapenemase genes we performed kappa statistical analysis by use of the VassarStats platform http://vassarstats.net/index.html.

Results

Detection of the carbapenemase genes from solid culture isolates by use of the in-house method

A total of 18 KPC (bla_{KPC-2} and bla_{KPC-3}), 19 NDM ($bla_{NDM-1/6, -2, -3, -5}$ and $_{-9}$) and 13 VIM ($bla_{VIM-1, -2, -4}$ and $_{-11}$) were detected by the in-house RT-PCR. Sixty seven (56.3%) of the 116 carbapenem-resistant gram-negative isolates harboured carbapenemase genes of oxacillinase-type carbapenemase (OTC)-variants ($bla_{OXA-23, -40, -48,}$ and $_{-58}$-like). Within this family we observed the highest diversity of subtypes. The prevalence rate of the gene variant $bla_{OXA-23-like}$ was 41.8% among the different carbapenemase genes, primarily in *A. baumannii* isolates. 57 (85.1%) of the OXA types were detected by multiplex RT-PCR by use of OXA-23/-48 primer pairs. The $bla_{OXA-23-like}$ variants were amplified with the OXA-23 primer pair and $bla_{OXA-48, -162, -204}$, and $bla_{OXA-232}$ with the OXA-48 primer pair. Weak signals were observed during the amplification of $bla_{OXA-181}$ (OXA-48-like) ($n = 4$ out of 5; 80%) with the OXA-48 primer pair. The remaining *A. baumannii* isolates and other gram-negative species carrying the genes bla_{OXA-40}-like and bla_{OXA-58}-like could not be detected by the in-house RT-PCR assay.

In comparison to the in-house RT-PCR assay the isolates were analysed by use of the commercial Check-Direct CPE kit on the BD MAX™ system as well. All isolates harbouring the bla_{KPC}, bla_{NDM} and bla_{VIM} genes were sufficiently detected by the commercial assay. One bla_{NDM} lost the resistance gene and has been excluded from the analysis. However, not all bla_{OXA} gene variants were detected by use of the Check-Direct CPE assay. Only two of the 28 bla_{OXA-23}-like and all the bla_{OXA-48}-like (including 16 OXA 48, one OXA-162, five OXA-181, one OXA-204, and two OXA-232) isolates were detected

Table 1 Primer and probe sequences for the in-house RT-PCR assay

Gene	Primer pairs	Product size, bp	Probe
bla_{KPC}	for-GCGATACCACGTTCCGTCTG rev-CGGTCGTGTTTCCCTTTAGC	183	6FAM-AGCGGCAGCAGTTTGTTGATTG–BBQ
bla_{NDM}	for-TTTGGCGATCTGGTTTTCCG rev-ATCAAACCGTTGGAAGCGAC	101	LC610-AGACATTCGGTGCGAGCTGGC–BBQ
$bla_{OXA-23-like}$	for-CGCGACGTATCGGTCTTGAT rev-CGCGACGTATCGGTCTTGAT	162	HEX-ACGTATTGGTTTCGGTAATGCTGA–BBQ
$bla_{OXA-48-like}$	for-GGCACGTATGAGCAAGATGC rev-GTTTGACAATACGCTGGCTGC	182	[a]
bla_{VIM}	for-CCGAGTGGTGAGTATCCGAC rev-GAATGCGTGGGAATCTCGTTC	337	Cy5-CGCTGTATCAATCAAAAGCAACTCATCA–BBQ

[a] The melting-curve analysis for the OXA gene variants was performed with the OXA-48 primer. For the multiplex RT-PCR analysis a Light Mix Modular from TIB MOLBIOL Syntheselabor GmbH Berlin was used for OXA-48

in the OXA-48-like channel of the BD MAX system. Moreover, the commercial system also detected incorrectly two of the 6 bla_{OXA-72} (OXA-40-like) isolates in the same channel. The two *A. baumannii* isolates harbouring bla_{OXA-23}-like and $bla_{NDM-1/-6}$ were only identified as NDM gene carrying isolates. Figure 1 illustrates the differences of the two assays in distinguishing the carbapenemase genes. The unweighted kappa (κ) for the KPC, NDM and VIM detection was 1—showing 100% concordance between the commercial and the in-house method—whereas for the OXA gene detection the unweighted κ was 0.4298 (95% CI 0.1251–0.7345). Noteworthy, both the in-house and the commercial RT-PCR assay did not detect any carbapenemase genes in our negative controls: 35 carbapenem non-susceptible *P. aeruginosa* and *A. baumannii* isolates. Therefore, the unweighted κ for the analysis of the non-carbapenmase isolates was 1.

Due to the high prevalence rate of bla_{OXA-23} and bla_{OXA-48} variants a stepwise diagnostic workflow by use of melting-curve analysis on BD MAX™ system was performed to rather differentiate these OXA subtypes. Figure 2 demonstrates the results of the in-house assay for OXA-23- and OXA-48-like with distinct melting points (T_m).

Detection of the carbapenmase genes from positive blood culture

Based on the in-house RT-PCR assay, 58 of 116 investigated carbapenemase-producing isolates were additionally analysed directly from spiked blood-culture vials and all the bla_{NDM} and bla_{VIM} isolates were sufficiently detected. One (7.1%) of the 14 bla_{KPC} carrying isolates and five (19.2%) of the 26 bla_{OXA} gene variants carrying isolates were not verified by the in-house assay. The amplification of one $bla_{OXA-232}$ (OXA-48-like) indicated weak signal and isolates carrying $bla_{OXA-181}$

(OXA-48-like) were not detected directly from positive blood-culture vials. The two *A. baumannii* isolates co-harbouring the genes $bla_{OXA-23-like}$ and $bla_{NDM-1/-6}$ were detected in both channels (Table 2).

Discussion

Multidrug resistance in gram-negative bacterial strains is increasing globally and turn out to be a very urgent challenge in health care facilities. Several phenotypic screening methods have been developed to detect or confirm carbapenemase production. These phenotypic methods are time consuming and might be difficult to interpret, e.g. occurrence of extended-spectrum betalactamases (ESBL) and porin loss or AmpC production. Therefore, the resistance gene detection by specific nucleic acid detection methods is the gold standard [3, 4, 6].

In this study we established and evaluated a multiplex RT-PCR assay in the PCR-only mode on the BD MAX™ system for the simultaneously detection of carbapenemase gene variants and the data were compared to those gained by commercial test kit. Another advantage is the combined sample lysis, extraction, amplification and detection using the fully automated BD MAX™ system. Hindiyeh et al. [7] detected bla_{KPC} genes and Naas et al. [8] bla_{NDM-1} using RT-PCR. However, these assays can only detect the presence of one carbapenemase gene. Hofko et al. [9] reported the detection of carbapenemase gene variants with a multiplex SYBR green RT-PCR assay on the BD MAX™ system using two different master mixes (master mix 1: IMP-1, IMP-2, GES, VIM-2, KPC and 16S rRNA; master mix 2: OXA-23-like, OXA-48-like, VIM-1 and NDM). Nevertheless, this assay detects the carbapenemase genes in one channel (wavelength 475/520). The melting-curve analysis was performed to rather differentiate the different genes. In our RT-PCR assay we identified four different carbapenemase genes

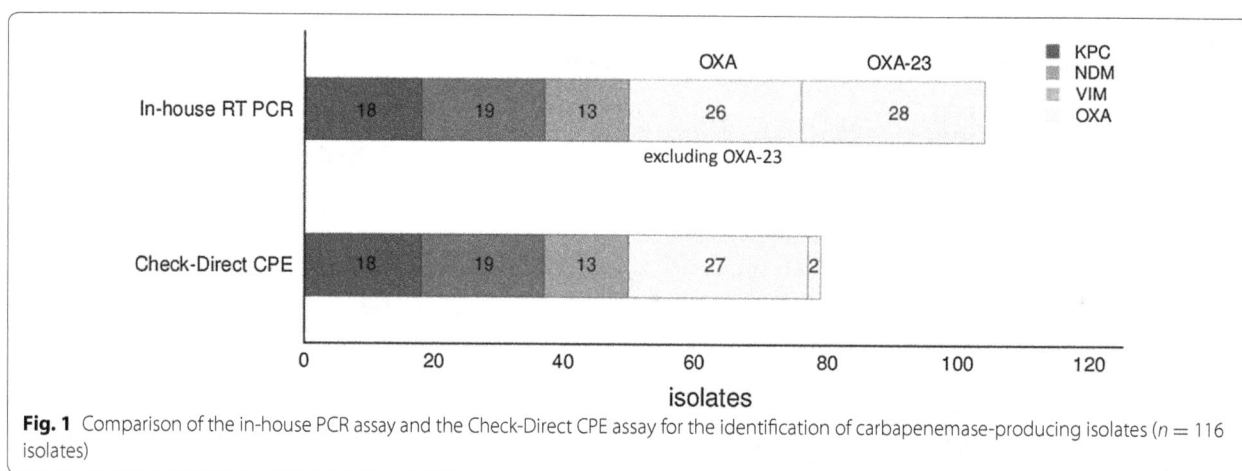

Fig. 1 Comparison of the in-house PCR assay and the Check-Direct CPE assay for the identification of carbapenemase-producing isolates ($n = 116$ isolates)

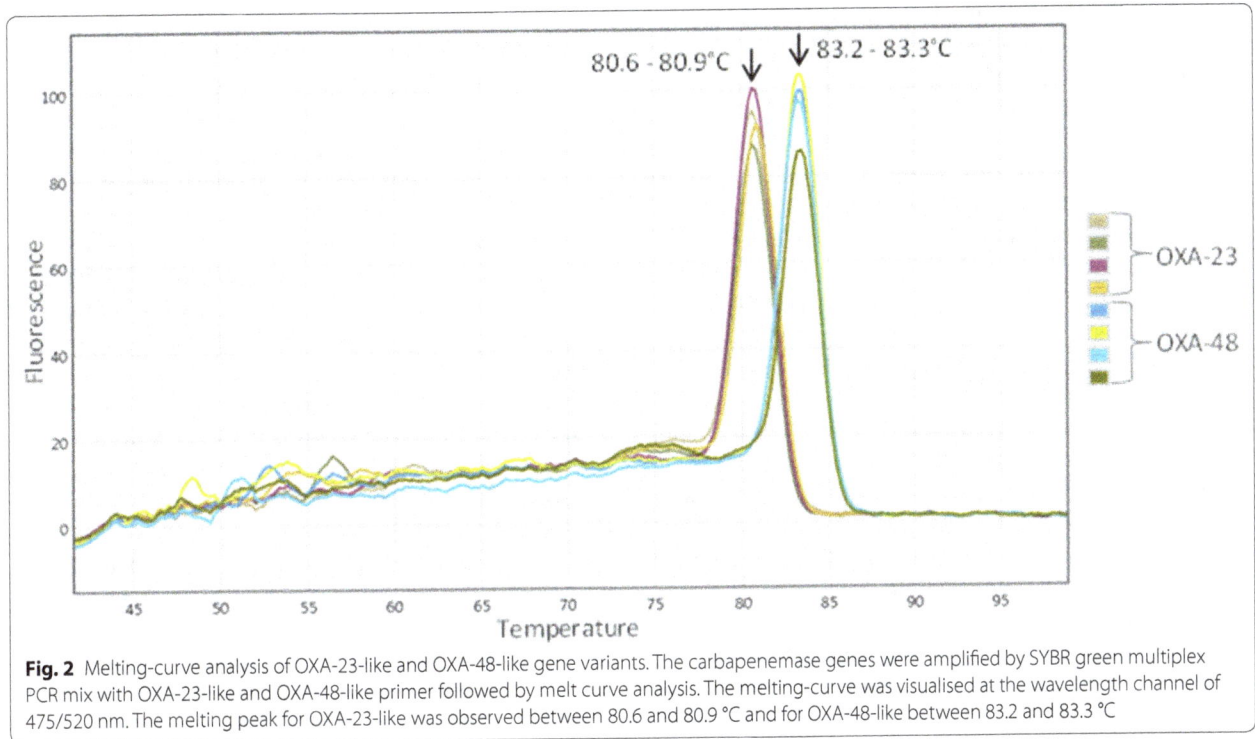

Fig. 2 Melting-curve analysis of OXA-23-like and OXA-48-like gene variants. The carbapenemase genes were amplified by SYBR green multiplex PCR mix with OXA-23-like and OXA-48-like primer followed by melt curve analysis. The melting-curve was visualised at the wavelength channel of 475/520 nm. The melting peak for OXA-23-like was observed between 80.6 and 80.9 °C and for OXA-48-like between 83.2 and 83.3 °C

Table 2 **Detection of carbapenemase genes directly from positive blood culture vials by use of the in-house multiplex RT-PCR ($n = 58$)**

Species	OXA23-/48-like ($n = 26$)	NDM ($n = 11$)	VIM ($n = 9$)	KPC ($n = 14$)
A. baumannii	18[a]	2[a]		
C. freundii	1		1	
E. asburiae		1		
E. cloacae			2	
E. coli	2	4		2
K. oxytoca			1	1
K. pneumoniae	5	4	1	11
P. aeruginosa			4	
Detected by in-house RT-PCR	21	11	9	13

[a] 2 isolates carrying $bla_{OXA-23-like}$ and $bla_{NDM-1/-6}$

(bla_{KPC}, bla_{NDM}, bla_{OXA} and bla_{VIM}) in four different channels using five different probes labelled with four fluorescent dyes for each primer pair. Based on the in-house PCR assay all investigated isolates carrying $bla_{KPC-2, -3}$ (18/18), $bla_{NDM-1/-6, -2, -3, -5, -9}$ (19/19) and $bla_{VIM-1, -2, -4, -11}$ (12/12) gene variants were correctly identified. In case of the two bacterial isolates carrying more than one carbapenem-resistance gene (bla_{OXA-23}-like and $bla_{NDM-1/-6}$) both variants were identified simultaneously.

The detection of oxacillinases seems to be more challenging. Today five main phylogenetic subgroups of the OXA-type carbapenemases (OTC) have been recognised

in A. baumannii: OXA-23-like, OXA-40-like, OXA-51-like, OXA-58-like and OXA-143-like. The master mix containing two different OXA primer pairs (OXA-23- and OXA-48-like) detected 53 of 67 (79.0%) bla_{OXA} genes. The in-house assay was specific in a manner that it did not detect bla_{OXA-40}- and bla_{OXA-58}-like variants. However, the detection of $bla_{OXA-181}$ (4 out of $n = 5$; OXA-48-like) in *Klebsiella pneumoniae* isolate was insufficient. Further primer pairs aligned to the undetected genes could be included to rather enable the detection of more OTC variants. This was also consistent with the commercial Check-Direct CPE kit which also missed some oxacillinases positive isolates. The kit identified all five investigated $bla_{OXA-181}$. Unfortunately, this kit was not specific by detecting two of the six bla_{OXA-40}-like isolates. The primers should not cover this enzyme sub-group. However, the identification of bla_{OXA-23}-like variant remains as one of the challenging issues that yet to be improved. Only two (7.1%) of the 28 *A. baumannii* isolates carrying this gene variant were identified with the Check-Direct CPE kit. Lau et al., Antonelli et al., and Nijhuis et al. [10–12] reported 100% sensitivity for the detection of carbapenemase-producing bacteria comprising of bla_{NDM}, bla_{KPC}, bla_{VIM} and bla_{OXA-48}-like performed by the Check-Direct CPE kit which is consistent with our results. The comparison of the simultaneous detection of bla_{OXA-23}-like gene variants and the other carbapenemase genes with previous studies was not possible due to the fact that no corresponding data exist yet. However, in comparison to the Rotor-Gene instrument Monteiro et al. [13] reported the detection of bla_{IMP}, bla_{OXA-48}-like, bla_{NDM-1}, bla_{GES}, bla_{VIM} and bla_{KPC} in 21 *Enterobacteriaceae*, 1 *A. baumannii* and 8 *P. aeruginosa* isolates ($n = 30$) using the Rotor-Gene 6000 instrument with 100% sensitivity. Compared to the BD MAX™ where the genes were differentiated in five separate channels by use of the Rotor gene instrument, the genes were distinguished via melting curve analysis. Ellington et al. [14] reported in 2016 100% sensitivity for the detection of bla_{KPC}, bla_{NDM}, bla_{OXA-48}-like and bla_{VIM} carbapenemase genes using a multiplex real-time PCR assay on the Rotor-Gene Q as well as on the ABI 7500 instrument. The ABI Prism 7500 Fast instrument was also used by another research group to simultaneously detect bla_{NDM} and bla_{KPC} genes [15]. Yang and Rui [16] reported the simultaneous detection of bla_{NDM}, bla_{OXA-23}-like, bla_{OXA-40}-like, and bla_{OXA-58}-like genes in *A. baumannii* and other *Acinetobacter* spp. by performing two multiplex RT-PCR assays on the ABI Prism 7500 FAST apparatus. However, their assays did not include the identification of different carbapenemase gene variants from other species, so that the comparison of the simultaneous detection of bla_{OXA-23}-like gene variants with bla_{KPC} and bla_{VIM} with our data was not possible.

Another insufficiency of the Check Direct CPE kit is that it was not able to detect bla_{OXA-40}-like and bla_{OXA-58} due to the fact that the assay was designed for the detection of OXA-48-like. In outbreak situations this may increasingly become a problem, especially in outbreaks with *A. baumannii* isolates, the detection for such emerging subtypes in clinical specimens is mandatory for preventive and control measures in hospital setting. Fournier [17] reviewed a large number of numerous outbreaks caused by *A. baumannii* occurred in France and in the United States. Many of the outbreak strains have

been found at intensive care units. Kohlenberg et al. [18] reported an outbreak of carbapenem-resistant *A. baumannii* carrying the carbapenemase gene OXA-23-like in a German university medical centre and Rolain et al. [19] reported this for Qatar during the period of 2011–2012.

In brief, the simultaneous identification of bla_{OXA}-like gene variants needs to be improved. However, our in-house assay displays a sensitivity rate of 100% for the detection of bla_{OXA-23}-like. With our in-house RT-PCR assay we were not able to differentiate the subtypes of the individual gene variants. Considering the high number of the analysed isolates positive for bla_{OXA-23}-like and bla_{OXA-48}-like variants a stepwise diagnostic workflow with melting-curve analysis was performed to rather differentiate the most prevalent OXA subtypes in this study. The peak between 80.6 and 80.9 °C was observed for OXA-23-like and between 83.2 and 83.3 °C for OXA-48-like. This assay is advantageous for the epidemiological surveillance for outbreaks with isolates carrying carbapenemase bla_{OXA} gene variants and might be extended for other carbapenemase gene variants. Roth et al. [6] reported the differentiation and identification of bla_{KPC-2} and bla_{KPC-3} genes with high-resolution melting analysis with 100% specificity and sensitivity for the detection of bla_{KPC}.

Regarding the importance of identification and antimicrobial susceptibility testing from positive blood-cultures due to septicaemia and septic shock [20] carbapenemase-producers were additionally identified directly from positive blood-culture isolates using the in-house assay. In brief, all investigated bla_{VIM} and bla_{NDM} isolates were identified by the in-house assay. In case of isolates carrying bla_{KPC} genes one (7.1%) out of 14 could not be detected. The bacterial pellet of this isolate was bloody after the second centrifugation step and not whitish as was observed for the other bacterial pellets, which might be the cause for the unsuccessful detection. For isolates containing bla_{OXA} gene variants the identification directly from positive blood vials could be observed for bla_{OXA-23}-like and bla_{OXA-48}-like (OXA-48 and -162). One $bla_{OXA-181}$ (bla_{OXA-48}-like) isolate could not be detected which is consistent with the PCR results from solid culture media. The amplification of one $bla_{OXA-232}$ showed weaker PCR product. It should be emphasized that we used negative blood-culture bottles spiked with bacterial isolates to investigate the performance of the in-house RT-PCR. Noteworthy, whereas the phenotypic assays, e.g. MHT, are eligible to detect the carbapenemase activity irrespective of the carbapenemase encoding gene sequence the RT-PCR based assay can only detect known carbapenemase encoding genes and the number of carbapenemase encoding genes and allelic variants thereof is expanding rapidly.

We would like to address a few limitations of our study, e.g. the low number and diversity of the gram-negative bacterial isolates producing VIM subtypes and OXA-48-like enzymes—in contrast to OXA-23-like—and thus representing only one or few isolates of particular subtype. Based on our findings, we plan to conduct a longitudinal surveillance study to further elucidate the epidemiology of carbapenem non-susceptible gram-negative bacteria in our region.

In conclusion, we have demonstrated that the in-house multiplex RT-PCR was a successful tool for the identification of carbapenemase gene variants directly from different solid culture isolates as well as from positive blood-culture vials. The assay is easy to perform, interpret and allows distinction between bla_{OXA-23} and bla_{OXA-48} variants, e.g. for outbreak analysis. Our in-house RT-PCR assay is an easy and rapid method for the detection of carbapenem resistance genes as compared to the routine microbiological diagnostic methods which need 2–3 days. Such same day analysis is crucial in hospital setting to rather implement the infection control and prevention measures, and moreover to administer the appropriate antimicrobial therapy in severe infections.

Authors' contributions
BG and MS proposed, designed, carried out the study, MS and BG analyzed the generated data and drafted the manuscript and performed the data analysis. MK provided with some of the strains from NRZ. MK and PAN participated in proofreading of the manuscript and in critical revision. All authors read and approved the final manuscript.

Author details
[1] Center for Clinical and Translational Research, Institute for Medical Laboratory Diagnostics, HELIOS University Clinic Wuppertal; Witten/Herdecke University, Heusnerstr. 40, 42283 Wuppertal, Germany. [2] Department of Medical Microbiology, Ruhr-University Bochum, Bochum, Germany. [3] Department of Infection Control, University Medical Center Göttingen, Göttingen, Germany.

Competing interests
The authors declare that they have no competing interests.

References
1. Saini A. Insights on the structural characteristics of NDM-1: the journey so far. Adv Biol Chem. 2012;02:323–34.
2. Cantón R, Akóva M, Carmeli Y, Giske CG, Glupczynski Y, Gniadkowski M, Livermore DM, Miriagou V, Naas T, Rossolini GM, Samuelsen Ø, Seifert H, Woodford N, Nordmann P. Rapid evolution and spread of carbapenemases among Enterobacteriaceae in Europe. Clin Microbiol Infect. 2012;18:413–31.
3. Nordmann P, Poirel L. Strategies for identification of carbapenemase-producing Enterobacteriaceae. J Antimicrob Chemother. 2013;68:487–9.
4. Birgy A, Bidet P, Genel N, Doit C, Decré D, Arlet G, Bingen E. Phenotypic screening of carbapenemases and associated β-lactamases in carbapenem-resistant Enterobacteriaceae. J Clin Microbiol. 2012;50:1295–302.
5. Ghebremedhin B, Halstenbach A, Smiljanic M, Kaase M, Ahmad-Nejad P. MALDI-TOF MS based carbapenemase detection from culture isolates and from positive blood culture vials. Ann Clin Microbiol Antimicrob. 2016;15:5.
6. Roth AL, Hanson ND. Rapid detection and statistical differentiation of KPC gene variants in gram-negative pathogens by use of high-resolution melting and ScreenClust analyses. J Clin Microbiol. 2013;51:61–5.
7. Hindiyeh M, Smollen G, Grossman Z, Ram D, Davidson Y, Mileguir F, Vax M, David DB, Tal I, Rahav G, Shamiss A, Mendelson E, Keller N. Rapid detection of bla_{KPC} carbapenemase genes by real-time PCR. J Clin Microbiol. 2008;46:2879–83.
8. Naas T, Ergani A, Carrer A, Nordmann P. Real-time PCR for detection of NDM-1 carbapenemase genes from spiked stool samples. Antimicrob Agents Chemother. 2011;55:4038–43.
9. Hofko M, Mischnik A, Kaase M, Zimmermann S, Dalpke AH. Detection of carbapenemases by real-time PCR and melt curve analysis on the BD Max system. J Clin Microbiol. 2014;52:1701–4.
10. Lau AF, Fahle GA, Kemp MA, Jassem AN, Dekker JP, Frank KM. Clinical performance of Check-Direct CPE, a multiplex PCR for direct detection of bla_{KPC}, bla_{NDM} and/or bla_{VIM} and bla_{OXA-48} from perirectal swabs. J Clin Microbiol. 2015;53:3729–37.
11. Nijhuis R, Samuelsen Ø, Savelkoul P, van Zwet A. Evaluation of a new real-time PCR assay (Check-Direct CPE) for rapid detection of KPC, OXA-48, VIM, and NDM carbapenemases using spiked rectal swabs. Diagn Microbiol Infect Dis. 2013;77:316–20.
12. Antonelli A, Arena F, Giani T, Colavecchio OL, Valeva SV, Paule S, Boleij P, Rossolini GM. Performance of the BD MAX™ instrument with Check-Direct CPE real-time PCR for the detection of carbapenemase genes from rectal swabs, in a setting with endemic dissemination of carbapenemase-producing Enterobacteriaceae. Diagn Microbiol Infect Dis. 2016;86(1):30–4.
13. Monteiro J, Widen RH, Pignatari ACC, Kubasek C, Silbert S. Rapid detection of carbapenemase genes by multiplex real-time PCR. J Antimicrob Chemother. 2012;67:906–9.
14. Ellington MJ, Findlay J, Hopkins KL, Meunier D, Alvarez-Buylla A, Horner C, McEwane A, Guivere M, McCraec LX, Woodforda N, Hawkey P. Multicentre evaluation of a real-time PCR assay to detect genes encoding clinically relevant carbapenemases in cultured bacteria. Int J Antimicrob Agents. 2016;47:151–4.
15. Zheng F, Sun J, Cheng C, Rui Y. The establishment of a duplex real-time PCR assay for rapid and simultaneous detection of bla_{NDM} and bla_{KPC} genes in bacteria. Ann Clin Microbiol Antimicrob. 2013;12:1.
16. Yang Q, Rui Y. Two multiplex real-time pcr assays to detect and differentiate Acinetobacter baumannii and Non-baumannii $bla_{OXA-58-Like}$ genes. PLoS ONE. 2016;11(7):e0158958.
17. Fournier PE. The epidemiology and control of Acinetobacter baumannii in health care facilities. Clin Infect Dis. 2006;42:692–9.
18. Kohlenberg A, Brümmer S, Higgins PG, Sohr D, Piening BC, De Grahl C, Halle E, Rüden H, Seifert H. Outbreak of carbapenem-resistant Acinetobacter baumannii carrying the carbapenemase OXA-23 in a German university medical centre. J Med Microbiol. 2009;58:1499–507.
19. Rolain J, Loucif L, Elmagboul E, Shaukat A, Ahmedullah H. Emergence of multidrug-resistant Acinetobacter baumannii producing OXA-23 Carbapenemase in Qatar. New Microbes New Infect. 2016;11:47–51.
20. Moore DF, Hamada SS, Marso E, Martin WJ. Rapid identification and antimicrobial susceptibility testing of gram-negative bacilli from blood cultures by the rapid identification and antimicrobial susceptibility testing of gram-negative bacilli from blood cultures by the automicrobic system. J Clin Microbiol. 1981;13:934–9.

Permissions

All chapters in this book were first published in ACMA, by BioMed Central; hereby published with permission under the Creative Commons Attribution License or equivalent. Every chapter published in this book has been scrutinized by our experts. Their significance has been extensively debated. The topics covered herein carry significant findings which will fuel the growth of the discipline. They may even be implemented as practical applications or may be referred to as a beginning point for another development.

The contributors of this book come from diverse backgrounds, making this book a truly international effort. This book will bring forth new frontiers with its revolutionizing research information and detailed analysis of the nascent developments around the world.

We would like to thank all the contributing authors for lending their expertise to make the book truly unique. They have played a crucial role in the development of this book. Without their invaluable contributions this book wouldn't have been possible. They have made vital efforts to compile up to date information on the varied aspects of this subject to make this book a valuable addition to the collection of many professionals and students.

This book was conceptualized with the vision of imparting up-to-date information and advanced data in this field. To ensure the same, a matchless editorial board was set up. Every individual on the board went through rigorous rounds of assessment to prove their worth. After which they invested a large part of their time researching and compiling the most relevant data for our readers.

The editorial board has been involved in producing this book since its inception. They have spent rigorous hours researching and exploring the diverse topics which have resulted in the successful publishing of this book. They have passed on their knowledge of decades through this book. To expedite this challenging task, the publisher supported the team at every step. A small team of assistant editors was also appointed to further simplify the editing procedure and attain best results for the readers.

Apart from the editorial board, the designing team has also invested a significant amount of their time in understanding the subject and creating the most relevant covers. They scrutinized every image to scout for the most suitable representation of the subject and create an appropriate cover for the book.

The publishing team has been an ardent support to the editorial, designing and production team. Their endless efforts to recruit the best for this project, has resulted in the accomplishment of this book. They are a veteran in the field of academics and their pool of knowledge is as vast as their experience in printing. Their expertise and guidance has proved useful at every step. Their uncompromising quality standards have made this book an exceptional effort. Their encouragement from time to time has been an inspiration for everyone.

The publisher and the editorial board hope that this book will prove to be a valuable piece of knowledge for researchers, students, practitioners and scholars across the globe.

List of Contributors

Xiao-hong Xu, Ying-ping Cao and Bin Li
Department of Clinical Laboratory, Fujian Medical University Union Hospital, 29# Xinquan Road, Fuzhou 350001, Fujian, China

Qing-wen He and Fang-jun Lan and Zhi-yun Wu
Department of Clinical Laboratory, Fujian Medical University Union Hospital, 29# Xinquan Road, Fuzhou 350001, Fujian, China
The Union Clinical Medical College of Fujian Medical University, Fuzhou 350004, Fujian, China

Zhi-chang Zhao
Department of Pharmacy, Fujian Medical University, Union Hospital, Fuzhou 350001, Fujian, China

Paul Cheddie
Department of Medical Technology, University of Guyana, Georgetown, Guyana

Francis Dziva
Faculty of Medical Sciences, The University of the West Indies, St. Augustine, Trinidad and Tobago

Patrick Eberechi Akpaka
Department of Para-Clinical Sciences, Faculty of Medical Sciences, The University of the West Indies, St. Augustine, Trinidad and Tobago

Jeongjin Kim and Ara Jo
Department of Medical Biomaterials Engineering, Kangwon National University, Chuncheon, Gangwon 24341, South Korea

Juhee Ahn
Department of Medical Biomaterials Engineering, Kangwon National University, Chuncheon, Gangwon 24341, South Korea
Institute of Bioscience and Biotechnology, Kangwon National University, Chuncheon, Gangwon 24341, South Korea

Ekachai Chukeatirote
School of Science, Mae Fah Luang University, Chiang Rai 57100, Thailand

Essam J. Alyamani, Rayan Y. Booq and Majed A. Majrashi
National Center for Biotechnology, King Abdulaziz City for Science and Technology, Riyadh 11442, Saudi Arabia

Anamil M. Khiyami
College of Medicine, Princess Nora Bint Abdul Rahman University, Riyadh 12484, Saudi Arabia

Fayez S. Bahwerth
Hera Hospital, Makkah, Saudi Arabia

Elena Rechkina
ID Genomics, Seattle, WA, USA

Idrissa Diawara, Khalid Katfy, Houria Belabbes, Khalid Zerouali and Naima Elmdaghri
Laboratoire de Microbiologie, Faculté de Médecine et de Pharmacie, Hassan II University of Casablanca, B.P 5696, Casablanca, Morocco
Service de Microbiologie, CHU Ibn Rochd, B.P 2698, Casablanca, Morocco

Kaotar Nayme
Laboratoire de Microbiologie, Faculté de Médecine et de Pharmacie, Hassan II University of Casablanca, B.P 5696, Casablanca, Morocco
Molecular Bacteriology Laboratory, Institut Pasteur du Maroc, Casablanca, Morocco

Abouddihaj Barguigua
Laboratoire Polyvalent en Recherche et Développement, département de Biologie-Géologie, Faculté polydisciplinaire, Université Sultan Moulay Slimane, Beni Mellal, Morocco

Mohammed Timinouni
Molecular Bacteriology Laboratory, Institut Pasteur du Maroc, Casablanca, Morocco

Aydir Cecília Marinho Monteiro and Eduardo Bagagli
Departamento de Microbiologia e Imunologia, Instituto de Biociências de Botucatu, UNESP–Univ. Estadual Paulista, Distrito de Rubião Junior, s/n, Botucatu, SP CEP: 18618-970, Brazil

Maria de Lourdes Ribeiro de Souza da Cunha
Departamento de Microbiologia e Imunologia, Instituto de Biociências de Botucatu, UNESP-Univ. Estadual Paulista, Distrito de Rubião Junior, s/n, Botucatu, SP CEP: 18618-970, Brazil
Departamento de Doenças Tropicais, Faculdade de Medicina de Botucatu, UNESP-Univ. Estadual Paulista, Distrito de Rubião Junior, s/n, Botucatu, SP CEP: 18618-970, Brazil

Carlos Magno Castelo Branco Fortaleza
Departamento de Doenças Tropicais, Faculdade de Medicina de Botucatu, UNESP-Univ. Estadual Paulista, Distrito de Rubião Junior, s/n, Botucatu, SP CEP: 18618-970, Brazil

Adriano Martison Ferreira
Laboratório de Análises Clínicas do Hospital das Clínicas de Botucatu, Faculdade de Medicina de Botucatu, UNESP-Univ. Estadual Paulista, Distrito de Rubião Junior, s/n, Botucatu, SP CEP: 18618-970, Brazil

Ricardo de Souza Cavalcante
Comissão de Controle de Infecção Relacionada à Assistência à Saúde, Hospital das Clínicas, Faculdade de Medicina de Botucatu, UNESP-Univ. Estadual Paulista, Distrito de Rubião Junior, s/n, Botucatu, SP CEP: 18618-970, Brazil

Alessandro Lia Mondelli
Departamento de Clínica Médica, Faculdade de Medicina de Botucatu, UNESP-Univ. Estadual Paulista, Distrito de Rubião Junior, s/n, Botucatu, SP CEP: 18618-970, Brazil

Kamelia Osman and Ahmed Orabi
Department of Microbiology, Faculty of Veterinary Medicine, Cairo University, Giza, Egypt

Avelino Alvarez-Ordóñez
Department of Food Hygiene and Technology and Institute of Food Science and Technology, University of León, León, Spain

Lorena Ruiz
Department of Nutrition, Bromatology and Food Technology, Universidad Complutense de Madrid, Madrid, Spain

Jihan Badr and Alaa Saad
Department of Poultry Diseases, Animal Health Research, Institute, Giza, Egypt

Fatma ElHofy
Department of Bacteriology, Immunology and Mycology, Faculty of Veterinary Medicine, Benha University, Moushtohor, Egypt

Khalid S. Al-Maary and Ihab M. I. Moussa
Department of Botany and Microbiology, College of Science, King Saud University, Riyadh, Kingdom of Saudi Arabia

Ashgan M. Hessain
Department of Health Science, College of Applied Studies and Community Service, King Saud University, Riyadh, Kingdom of Saudi Arabia

Mohamed Elhadidy
Department of Bacteriology, Mycology and Immunology, Faculty of Veterinary Medicine, Mansoura University, Mansoura 35516, Egypt
Foodborne Pathogens, Scientific Institute of Public Health, Juliette Wytsmanstraat 14, 1050 Brussels, Belgium

Mahmoud Elhariri and Rehab Elhelw
Department of Microbiology, Faculty of Veterinary Medicine, Cairo University, PO Box 12211, Giza, Egypt

Dalia Hamza
Department of Zoonoses, Faculty of Veterinary Medicine, Cairo University, PO Box 12211, Giza, Egypt

Sohad M. Dorgham
Department of Microbiology and Immunology, National Research Centre, Giza, Egypt

Belay Tessema and Feleke Moges
Department of Medical Microbiology, College of Medicine and Health Sciences, University of Gondar, Gondar, Ethiopia

Dereje Habte, Nebiyu Hiruy, Kassahun Melkieneh and Muluken Melese
Management Sciences for Health, Help Ethiopia Address the Low Performance of Tuberculosis (HEAL TB) Project, Addis Ababa, Ethiopia

Shewaye Yismaw
Department of Chemistry, College of Natural and Computational Sciences, University of Gondar, Gondar, Ethiopia

Yewulsew Kassie
USAID/Ethiopia, Addis Ababa, Ethiopia

Belaineh Girma
Monitoring and Evaluation TA, National Tuberculosis Program, Lilongwe, Malawi

Pedro G. Suarez
Management Sciences for Health, Health Programs Group, Arlington, VA, USA

Amal Awad
Department of Bacteriology, Mycology and Immunology, Faculty of Veterinary Medicine, Mansoura University, Mansoura 35516, Egypt

Mohamed Elhadidy
Department of Bacteriology, Mycology and Immunology, Faculty of Veterinary Medicine, Mansoura University, Mansoura 35516, Egypt
Foodborne Pathogens, Scientific Institute of Public Health, Juliette Wytsmanstraat 14, 1050 Brussels, Belgium

Nagah Arafat
Department of Poultry diseases, Faculty of Veterinary Medicine, Mansoura University, Mansoura 35516, Egypt

Noah Obeng-Nkrumah and Georgina Awuah-Mensah
Microbiology Department, School of Biomedical and Allied Health Sciences, University of Ghana, Accra, Ghana, West Africa

Appiah-Korang Labi and Naa Okaikor Addison
Department of Microbiology, Korle-Bu Teaching Hospital, Accra, Ghana, West Africa

Juliana Ewuramma Mbiriba Labi
Department of Internal Medicine, La General Hospital, Accra, Ghana, West Africa

Ping Shen, Lihua Guo, Ang Li, Jing Zhang, Chaoqun Ying, Jinru Ji, Hao Xu, Beiwen Zheng and Yonghong Xiao
Collaborative Innovation Center for Diagnosis and Treatment of Infectious Diseases, State Key Laboratory for Diagnosis and Treatment of Infectious Diseases, The First Affiliated Hospital, School of Medicine, Zhejiang University, Hangzhou 310003, China

Jianzhong Fan
Department of Clinical Laboratory, Hangzhou First People's Hospital, Hangzhou 310006, China

Jiahua Li
Department of Hospital Infection Control, Zhucheng People's Hospital, Zhucheng 252300, China

Kenneth A. Lawson and James Wilson
College of Pharmacy, University of Texas at Austin, Austin, TX, USA

Grace C. Lee, Natalie K. Boyd and Christopher R. Frei
College of Pharmacy, University of Texas at Austin, Austin, TX, USA
Pharmacotherapy Education and Research Center, School of Medicine, The University of Texas Health Science Center, 7703 Floyd Curl Dr, MC 6220, San Antonio, TX 78229-3900, USA

Ronald G. Hall
School of Pharmacy, Texas Tech University Health Sciences Center, Dallas, TX, USA
Dose Optimization and Outcomes Research (DOOR) Program, Dallas, TX, USA

Steven D. Dallas
Department of Clinical Laboratory Sciences, School of Health Professions, University of Texas Health Science Center, San Antonio, TX, USA

Chad Retzloff, Liem C. Du, Lucina B. Treviño and Sylvia B. Treviño
South Texas Ambulatory Research Network, The University of Texas Health Science Center, San Antonio, TX, USA

Randall J. Olsen
Department of Pathology and Genomic Medicine, Houston Methodist Hospital and Research Institute, Houston, TX, USA

Yufeng Wang
Department of Biology, The University of Texas San Antonio, San Antonio, TX, USA

Jens Andre Hammerl and Sascha Al Dahouk
Department of Biological Safety, Federal Institute for Risk Assessment, Diedersdorfer Weg 1, 12277 Berlin, Germany

Alexander Rohde
Department of Biological Safety, Federal Institute for Risk Assessment, Diedersdorfer Weg 1, 12277 Berlin, Germany
Department of Biology, Chemistry and Pharmacy, Free University Berlin, Takustr. 3, 14195 Berlin, Germany

Fithamlak Bisetegen Solomon, Fiseha Wada Wadilo, Amsalu Amache Arota and Yishak Leka Abraham
School of Medicine, College of Health Sciences, Wolaita Sodo University, PO Box: 138, Wolaita Sodo, Ethiopia

Kaiwen Pan
Key Laboratory of Mountain Ecological Restoration and Bioresource Utilization and Ecological Restoration Biodiversity Conservation Key Laboratory of Sichuan Province, Chengdu Institute of Biology, Chinese Academy of Sciences, Chengdu 610041, China

Akash Tariq
Key Laboratory of Mountain Ecological Restoration and Bioresource Utilization and Ecological Restoration Biodiversity Conservation Key Laboratory of Sichuan Province, Chengdu Institute of Biology, Chinese Academy of Sciences, Chengdu 610041, China
Department of Botany, Kohat University of Science and Technology, Kohat 26000, Pakistan

Muhammad Adnan and Sakina Mussarat
Department of Botany, Kohat University of Science and Technology, Kohat 26000, Pakistan

Rahila Amber
Department of Zoology, Kohat University of Science and Technology, Kohat 26000, Pakistan

Zabta Khan Shinwari
Department of Biotechnology, Quaid-i-Azam University Islamabad, Islamabad 44000, Pakistan

Elisa Demonchy and Karine Risso
Infectious Diseases Department, Hôpital Archet 1, Nice Academic Hospital, Infectiologie 151 Route de St Antoine de Ginestière, 06200 Nice, France

Johan Courjon and Pierre-Marie Roger
Infectious Diseases Department, Hôpital Archet 1, Nice Academic Hospital, Infectiologie 151 Route de St Antoine de Ginestière, 06200 Nice, France
Université Côte d'Azur, Nice, France

Raymond Ruimy
Université Côte d'Azur, Nice, France
Department of Bacteriology, Archet 2 Hospital, Nice Academic Hospital, Nice, France
INSERM U1065 (C3M), Bacterial Toxins in Host Pathogen Interactions, C3M, Archimed, Nice, France

Nicolas Degand
Department of Bacteriology, Archet 2 Hospital, Nice Academic Hospital, Nice, France

Tapan Kumar Dutta
Department of Veterinary Microbiology, Central Agricultural University, Selesih, Aizawl, Mizoram 796 014, India

Karuppasamy Chellapandi
Department of Veterinary Microbiology, Central Agricultural University, Selesih, Aizawl, Mizoram 796 014, India
Department of Microbiology, Assam University, Silchar, Assam, India

Indu Sharma
Department of Microbiology, Assam University, Silchar, Assam, India

Surajit De Mandal and Nachimuthu Senthil Kumar
Department of Biotechnology, Mizoram University, Aizawl, Mizoram, India

Lalsanglura Ralte
Department of MLT, Regional Institute of Paramedical and Nursing Sciences, Aizawl, Mizoram, India

Rupak Thapa, Pragya Shrestha and Suvash Awal
Department of Biotechnology, Veer Narmad South Gujarat University, Surat, Gujarat 395007, India

Chintan Bhagat and Pravin Dudhagara
Department of Biosciences (UGC-SAP-DRS-II), Veer Narmad South Gujarat University, Surat, Gujarat 395007, India

Daniel B. Chastain
University of Georgia College of Pharmacy, 1000 Jefferson Street, Albany, GA 31701, USA
Phoebe Putney Memorial Hospital, Albany, GA 31701, USA

W. Anthony Hawkins
University of Georgia College of Pharmacy, 1000 Jefferson Street, Albany, GA 31701, USA
Phoebe Putney Memorial Hospital, Albany, GA 31701, USA
Medical College of Georgia at Augusta University, Albany, GA 31701, USA

Carlos Franco-Paredes
Phoebe Putney Memorial Hospital, Albany, GA 31701, USA
Hospital Infantil de Mexico, Federico Gomez, Mexico City, Mexico

Ijang Ngando
Beaufort Memorial Hospital, Beaufort, SC 29902, USA

Christopher M. Bland
University of Georgia College of Pharmacy, Savannah, GA 31405, USA

Qhtan Asmaa and Yiping Li
College of Environment, Hohai University, Nanjing 210098, China

Salwa AL-Shamerii
Faculty of Medical Science, Taiz University, Taiz, Yemen

Mohammed Al-Tag
Department of Applied Microbiology, Taiz University, Taiz, Yemen

Adam AL-Shamerii
Faculty of Applied Science, Direction of Scientific Research, Taiz University, Taiz, Yemen

Bashir H. Osman
College of Engineering, Sinnar University, Sinnar, Sudan

Diego Vargas-Blanco, Aung Lynn, Jonah Rosch, Rony Noreldin, Anthony Salerni, Christopher Lambert and Reeta P. Rao
Life Science and Bioengineering Center, Worcester Polytechnic Institute, 60 Prescott Street, Worcester, MA 01609, USA

Zahra Meshkat, Hadi Farsiani and Kiarash Ghazvini
Antimicrobial Resistance Research Center, Bu Ali Research Institute, Mashhad, Iran
Department of Microbiology and Virology, Ghaem hospital, Mashhad University of Medical Sciences, Ahmadabad Boulevard, Mashhad, Khorasan Razavi, PO Box: 91766-99199 (155), Iran

Davoud Mansouri and Adel Najafi
Antimicrobial Resistance Research Center, Bu Ali Research Institute, Mashhad, Iran
Department of Microbiology and Virology, Ghaem hospital, Mashhad University of Medical Sciences, Ahmadabad Boulevard, Mashhad, Khorasan Razavi, PO Box: 91766-99199 (155), Iran
Student Research Committee, Faculty of Medicine, Mashhad University of Medical Sciences, Mashhad, Iran

Himen Salimizand
Department of Microbiology, Faculty of Medicine, Kurdistan University of Medical Sciences, Sanandaj, Iran

Yousef Amini
Department of Microbiology, Faculty of Medicine, Zahedan University of Medical Sciences, Zahedan, Iran

Mostafa Khakshoor
Microbiology Department, Islamic Azad University, Tehran, Iran

M. Smiljanic, P. Ahmad-Nejad and B. Ghebremedhin
Center for Clinical and Translational Research, Institute for Medical Laboratory Diagnostics, HELIOS University Clinic Wuppertal; Witten/Herdecke University, Heusnerstr. 40, 42283 Wuppertal, Germany

M. Kaase
Department of Medical Microbiology, Ruhr-University Bochum, Bochum, Germany
Department of Infection Control, University Medical Center Göttingen, Göttingen, Germany

Index